Pocket Emergency
MEDICINE

Fourth Edition

ERICA ASHLEY MORSE, MD
GRAHAM INGALSBE, MD
Denver Health Residency in Emergency Medicine

AMY FOLLMER HILDRETH, MD
Naval Medical Center San Diego

DAVID SILVESTRI, MD, MBA
National Clinician Scholars Program
Yale School of Medicine

Edited by
RICHARD D. ZANE, MD, FAAEM
The George B. Boedecker Professor and Chair
Department of Emergency Medicine
University of Colorado School of Medicine
Executive Director, Emergency Services
University of Colorado Health
Aurora, Colorado

JOSHUA M. KOSOWSKY, MD, FACEP
Assistant Professor
Harvard Medical School
Department of Emergency Medicine
Brigham and Women's Hospital
Boston, Massachusetts

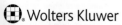 Wolters Kluwer

Philadelphia • Baltimore • New York • London
Buenos Aires • Hong Kong • Sydney • Tokyo

Senior Acquisitions Editor: Sharon Zinner
Development Editor: Ashley Fischer
Editorial Coordinator: Emily Buccieri
Strategic Marketing Manager: Rachel Mante Leung
Books Production Manager: David Orzechowski
Production Manager: Sadie Buckallew
Design Coordinator: Terry Mallon
Manufacturing Coordinator: Beth Welsh
Prepress Vendor: Aptara, Inc.

4th edition

Copyright © 2019 Wolters Kluwer.

© 2015 by WOLTERS KLUWER

9 8 7 6 5 4 3 2 1

Printed in China

Library of Congress Cataloging-in-Publication Data

Names: Morse, Erica Ashley, author. | Ingalsbe, Graham, author. | Hildreth, Amy Follmer, author. | Silvestri, David, author.
Title: Pocket emergency medicine / Erica Ashley Morse, Graham Ingalsbe, Amy Follmer Hildreth, David Silvestri ; edited by Richard D. Zane, Joshua M. Kosowsky.
Other titles: Pocket notebook.
Description: Fourth edition. | Philadelphia : Wolters Kluwer, [2019] | Series: Pocket notebook | Includes index. | Preceded by Pocket emergency medicine / John D. Anderson ... [et al.] ; edited by Richard D. Zane, Joshua M. Kosowsky. 3rd ed. Philadelphia : Lippincott Williams & Wilkins, c2015.
Identifiers: LCCN 2017046469 | ISBN 9781496372802
Subjects: | MESH: Emergencies | Emergency Medicine | Handbooks
Classification: LCC RC86.8 | NLM WB 39 | DDC 616.02/5–dc23
LC record available at https://lccn.loc.gov/2017046469

LWW.com

CONTRIBUTORS

Amy Follmer Hildreth, MD*
Emergency Medicine Physician
Naval Medical Center San Diego
San Diego, California

Graham Ingalsbe, MD
Chief Resident, 2016–2017
Department of Emergency Medicine
University of Colorado School of Medicine
Denver Health Residency in Emergency Medicine
Denver, Colorado

Erica Ashley Morse, MD
Resident Physician
Department of Emergency Medicine
University of Colorado School of Medicine
Denver Health Residency in Emergency Medicine
Denver, Colorado

David Silvestri, MD, MBA
National Clinician Scholars Program
Department of Emergency Medicine
Yale School of Medicine
New Haven, Connecticut

*The views expressed in this publication are those of the authors and do not reflect the official policy or position of the Department of the Navy, Department of Defense, or the United States Government.

ACKNOWLEDGMENTS

Practicing medicine is like having a front row seat at the play of life. If that is true, and I believe it is, emergency medicine is like being back stage. This book is for the dedicated men and women who are often back stage making life and death decisions without a net knowing that the expectation is that they get it right the first time, every time, without blinking.

Siobhan, Jake, Gaby, Finn, for whom I exist, thank you for tolerating my passion of academic medicine.

RICHARD D. ZANE, MD

To all those from whom I continue to gain wisdom—my teachers, my colleagues, my students, and perhaps foremost, my patients. And to Devorah, Harry, Jake, and Judah, whose support means the world to me.

JOSHUA M. KOSOWSKY, MD

PREFACE

The practice of emergency medicine, like all disciplines, is changing and evolving. More than ever, the care of our patients depends upon having accurate, actionable, and accessible information in real time. Now in its fourth edition, *Pocket Emergency Medicine* remains the essential, go-to reference for busy clinicians on the front lines of emergency care. Unlike traditional texts, *Pocket Emergency Medicine* is designed to be used at the bedside, organized around presenting conditions and mirroring the thought process of clinicians: from history and physical exam to differential diagnosis testing; from testing and therapeutics to disposition. Clinical pearls and updates in medical practice are highlighted throughout the text.

This book was written by four dedicated emergency medicine residents from the University of Colorado and Harvard University and edited by senior faculty; the text has been updated and referenced in exacting detail, while retaining the fundamental ease of use so cherished by busy providers. We hope our readers find this edition of *Pocket Emergency Medicine* to be a valuable tool in their daily practice.

RICHARD D. ZANE, MD
JOSHUA M. KOSOWSKY, MD

CONTENTS

SECTION IV: INFECTIOUS DISEASE

SECTION V: NEUROLOGY

SECTION VI: RENAL & GENITOURINARY

SECTION VII: OBGYN

SECTION VIII: DERMATOLOGY

SECTION XV: PSYCHIATRIC PATIENT

SECTION XVI: TOXICOLOGY

SECTION XVII: AIRWAY MANAGEMENT

SECTION XVIII: TRAUMA

SECTION XIX: APPENDIX

CHEST PAIN

Approach

- **Immediate:** All nontrivial CP get IV access, O₂, cardiac monitoring, ECG, CXR
  - Compare all ECGs to prior, repeat q15–20min if high suspicion for ACS; consider R-sided +/– posterior ECG if high suspicion (see *Electrocardiography* section)
- **History:** Obtain thorough pain HPI (position, quality, radiation, severity, timing, associated sx, alleviating & exacerbating factors), cardiac risk factors (eg, for CAD, aortic dz, PE, etc.), prior cardiac testing (timing & results of last stress test, catheterization, echo) & prior cardiac events/procedures (eg, myocardial infarction [MI], CABG, valve repair, etc.)
- **Empiric tx:** ASA 325 mg (if considering ACS & low suspicion for AoD), NTG for pain (unless R-sided ischemia, hypotension, PDE-inh)
- **Risk stratify** for dxs being considered: ACS (TIMI, GRACE, or PURSUIT), PE (Well's), AoD (Aortic Dissection Detection risk score)

Common or Life-Threatening Causes of Acute Chest Pain	
Pathophysiology	**Etiologies**
Cardiac	ACS (UA/NSTEMI, STEMI), Prinzmetal's/cocaine-induced angina, myocarditis, pericarditis, cardiac tamponade, constrictive pericarditis, CHF/acute pulmonary edema, post-MI cx
Vascular	PE, AoD, thoracic aortic aneurysm, pulmonary HTN
Pulmonary	PNA, PTX, pleural effusion/empyema, pleuritis, pulmonary infarct
GI	GERD, esophageal spasm, Mallory–Weiss tear, Boerhaave syndrome, PUD, biliary dz, pancreatitis
Musculoskeletal	MSK strain/contusion, costochondritis, OA/radiculopathy
Miscellaneous	Herpes zoster, anxiety, sickle cell chest crisis

ELECTROCARDIOGRAPHY

Approach

- Always check: correct pt, date, lead placement; calibration (mV, paper speed)
- Rate, rhythm, axis
- Waves (P, Q, R, T, U waves) & segments (PR, QRS, QT intervals, & ST segment)
- Conduction & bundle blocks
- Atrial enlargement, ventricular hypertrophy
- Ischemia/infarction
- Miscellaneous (stigmata of electrolyte abx, syncope, tox, PMs, PE, etc.)

Orientation: ECG Calibration and Standardization	
Voltage calibration	• Standard ECG voltage is usually set w/ a calibration box encompassing 2 large vertical squares (10 mm tall) & is equal to 1 mV (10 mm/mV): 1 small vertical box = 0.1 mV
Paper recording speed	• Standard ECG paper speed if usually set at 25 mm/s: • Large horizontal box (5 mm wide) = 200 ms (0.2 s) • Small horizontal box (1 mm wide) = 40 ms (0.04 s)

Determining Heart Rate (*nl* = 60–100 bpm)	
Quick approach	• Count the number of bold vertical lines b/w adjacent R waves: 0 = 300 bpm, 1 = 150 bpm, 2 = 100 bpm, 3 = 75 bpm, 4 = 60 bpm, 5 = 50 bpm.
Mathematical approach	• Multiply the number of QRS complexes on the ECG by 6 (at a standard paper speed of 25 mm/s), each ECG records 10 s of activity.

Determining Rhythm (see also section on *Dysrhythmia*)

• Determining the heart's rhythm is a complex process that requires synthesis of other features of ECG interpretation (esp rate, axis, intervals, & waves/segments)
• Key questions to help narrow the DDx of dysrhythmias include:
  1. Is the rate slow (eg, bradydysrhythmia) or fast (eg, tachydysrhythmia)?
  2. Is the QRS narrow (eg, SVT) or wide (eg, aberrancy, ventricular, electrolyte d/o)?
  3. Is the rhythm regular (eg, AFL, SVT, VT) or irregular (eg, AF, AFL w/ variable block, MAT, polymorphic VT)?
  4. Are P waves present? (If absent: AF vs. nodal/ventricular etiology)
  5. Is every P wave followed by a QRS & every QRS preceded by a P wave?
  6. For select tachydysrhythmias, is there response to vagal maneuvers or adenosine?

Determining Axis (nl QRS axis = −30° to +90°)		
Type	**Definition**	**Causes**
L axis deviation	QRS b/w −30° & −90° • Lead I: Positive • Lead II: Negative	LVH, LBBB, inferior MI, LAFB, ventricular pre-excitation w/ posteroseptal accessory pathway (WPW)
R axis deviation	QRS b/w +90° & +180° • Lead I: Negative • aVF: Positive	RVH, lateral MI, LPFB, ventricular pre-excitation w/ free wall accessory pathway (WPW), COPD, dextrocardia
Extreme axis deviation	QRS b/w +180° & −90° (−QRS lead I, −QRS aVF)	Ventricular tachycardia, Hyperkalemia, apical MI, RVH

ECG Waveforms and Segments	
Type	**Definition**
P wave	• Represents atrial depolarization (1st half represents predominant R atrial depolarization & 2nd half L atrial depolarization); best seen in leads II & V1 • Nl: Duration <0.12 s, Amplitude ≤0.2 mV (frontal) or ≤0.1 mV (transverse), axis upright in I, II, aVF, & V2–V4 & inverted in aVR • Can be absent (AF, MAT, AFL), aberrant shape (AT, SVT)
PR interval	• Represents time b/w onset of atrial depolarization (start of P) & onset of ventricular depolarization (start of QRS); isoelectric region represents conduction w/i AV node, bundle of His, bundle branches, & Purkinje fibers • Nl: duration normally 0.12–0.20 s (120–200 ms)
Q wave	• Defined as any initial negative deflection; represents onset of ventricular depolarization (specifically: L to R depolarization of septum) • Nl: Small Qw can be nl in all leads *EXCEPT* V1, V2, V3; Large Q waves can be nl variant in Lead III & aVR • Pathologic Q waves: Any Qw V1–V3, Qw >0.04 s (1 mm) & ≥0.2 mV (2 mm), or any Qw >25% of QRS complex
R wave	• Defined as any positive deflection w/i QRS; normally, Rw should become greater than Sw ~V3–V4 (called R-wave progression [RWP]) • Pathology suggested by poor RWP (LVH, LBBB, LAFB, ant-MI, WPW, COPD, infiltrative d/o, etc.), early RWP/dominant Rw in V1–V2 (RVH, RBBB, post-MI, WPW, HOCM, etc.), dominant Rw in aVR (TCA o/d)
QRS complex	• Represents ventricular depolarization (1st half: septum & RV; 2nd half: LV) • Nl duration 0.06–0.11 s (60–110 ms) measured in lead w/ widest QRS complex (see Causes of Abnl Interval Duration) • Pathology suggested by prolongation (see Causes of Prolonged QRS below) or low voltage (R + S <0.5 mV in limb leads or <0.1 mV precordial; suggests presence of fluid [pericardial/pleural effusion], air [COPD], or excess fat/tissue [obesity, infiltrative CMP, myxedema])
ST segment	• Represents plateau from end of ventricular depolarization (end of S) to start of repolarization (beginning of T); jxn of QRS & ST called J point • Normally isoelectric w/ TP segment • Pathology suggested by ST elevation (≥0.2 mV contiguous precordial leads, ≥0.1 mV limb leads, & ≥0.5 mV in R-sided & posterior leads) or depression (horizontal or downsloping depression ≥0.05 mV in 2 contiguous leads) (see Causes of ST Elevation)
T wave	• Represents ventricular repolarization • Normally smooth & round morphology, positive in all leads except aVR; may be biphasic in V1/V2; amplitude generally 2/3 that of the R wave • Pathology suggested by Tw inversions in I, II, aVL, V2–V6 (BBBs, LVH w/ strain pattern, Wellens' sign, myocardial ischemia, myopericarditis, cardiac contusion, MVP, SAH, hypokalemia, digoxin effect) or peaked-Tw morphology (hyperkalemia, early myocardial ischemia)
U wave	• Small wave following T wave; represents prolonged repolarization of mid-myocardial layer cells "M cells" • Nl amplitude <1.5 mm tall or ~10% on T-wave amplitude • Pathology suggested by prominent Uw (hypokalemia/hypocalcemia, sinus bradycardia, LVH, MVP, hyperthyroid, etc.)
QT interval	• Measured from start of QRS complex to end of T wave; represents duration of electrical activation & recovery of ventricle • Nl duration 390–450 ms in men; 390–460 ms in women (see Causes of Abnl Interval Duration)

Normal Intervals & Causes of Abnormal Interval Duration

Type	Normal	Shortened	Prolonged
PR	120–200 ms	↑ sympathetic tone, ectopic atrial PM, pre-excitation (WPW)	1° AVB, meds (digoxin, CCB, BB)
QRS	60–110 ms	↑ sympathetic tone, supraventricular tach, lytes (↓ K, ↓ Ca)	BBBs, ventricular conduction (including pacemakers), cardiomyopathies, lytes (↑ K) & channelopathies, meds (antiarrhythmics, TCAs), hypothermia
QTc	390–450 ms (M)* 390–460 ms (F)*	↑ sympathetic tone, digoxin toxicity, lytes (↑ K, ↑ Ca), congenital short QT syndrome	Myocardial injury: myocarditis, AMI, lytes (↓ K, ↓ Ca, ↓ Mg), hypothyroidism, hypothermia, mitral valve prolapse, increased ICP, meds (antiarrhythmics, psychotics, & histamines; quinolones, macrolides, methadone, etc.), long-QT syndromes

*Several formulas can be used to calculate QTc manually: [1] $QTc = QT/\sqrt{RR}$; [2] $QTc = QT/RR^{1/3}$; [3] $QTc = QT + 0.154 \times (1 - RR)$

Conduction Delays

Category	Definition
RBBB	1. QRS duration ≥120 ms (≥100–120 ms = "incomplete" RBBB) 2. Late intrinsicoid (R-wave peak time >0.05 s) M-shaped QRS (rsr′, rSr′, rSR′) in V1–V2 ("rabbit ears") 3. Early intrinsicoid, broad terminal slurred S wave in I, V5–V6 Causes: AMI, Right-heart strain (PE, pHTN), myopericarditis, CMP, endomyocardial fibrosis, Chagas dz, CHD (ASD, VSD, ToF)
LBBB	1. QRS duration ≥120 ms (≥100–120 ms = "incomplete" RBBB) 2. Wide, notched R wave & absent Q wave in V5–V6, I, aVL 3. Late intrinsicoid (R-wave peak time >0.06 s) in V5–V6 4. Wide S wave in V1 w/ rS or QS complex Causes: Anterior AMI, LVH, CMP, hyperkalemia, digoxin tox
LAFB	1. QRS duration ≤120 ms 2. LAD (usually ≥−60°) 3. QR pattern in I & aVL 4. rS pattern in II, III, & aVF 5. Late intrinsicoid (R-wave peak time >0.045 s) in aVL 6. Increased QRS voltage in limb leads Causes: Acute or remote MI, AS, OSA, CMP, endomyocardial fibrosis, Chagas dz, CHD
LPFB	1. QRS duration ≤120 ms 2. RAD (usually ≥+120°) w/o e/o RVH 3. rS pattern in I & aVL 4. QR pattern in II, III, & aVF 5. Late intrinsicoid (R-wave peak time >0.045 s) in aVF Causes: Acute cor pulmonale, CAD Lenègre's dz, CMP, endomyocardial fibrosis, Chagas dz, hyperkalemia
Bifascicular block	2 of RBB, LAFB, & LPFB; can be complete or incomplete
Trifascicular block	All 3 of RBBB, LAFB, & LPFB; can be complete or incomplete (ie, incomplete trifascicular block can present w/ fixed block of both fascicles w/ e/o delayed conduction in remaining fascicle as in a 1° or 2° AVB)
Intraventricular conduction delay	1. QRS duration >110 ms 2. Typical waveforms of RBBB & LBBB not present

Atrial Abnormality and Ventricular Hypertrophy	
Type	**Definition**
RAE (P pulmonale)	1. P ≥0.15 mV in V1/V2 2. P ≥0.25 mV in II or aVF 3. P-wave duration <0.12 s 4. P-wave axis (>75°–90°)
	Causes: TR, PS; pHTN (eg, ILD, COPD, CHF); ASD, VSD
LAE	1. Terminal negative P wave in V1 >0.04 s & >0.01 mV 2. Duration b/w peaks in P wave notches >0.04 s (in II) 3. P-wave duration >0.12 s
	Causes: MS/MR; AS; CHF; HTN; HOCM
RVH	1. Right atrial enlargement 2. Right-axis deviation 3. S wave in I + Q wave in III 4. R in V1 >0.7 mV or S in V5 or V6 >0.7 mV 5. QR complex V1 or raR' in V1 w/ R' >1 mV (w/ QRS duration <120 ms)
LVH	Sokolow–Lyon criteria: • S wave in V1 + R wave in V5 or V6 ≥3.50 mV (sens 22%, spec 100%) • R wave in aVL >0.9 (F) or >1.1 mV (M) (sens 11%, spec 100%) Cornell voltage criteria: • R wave aVL + S wave V3 >2 mV (women), >2.8 mV (men) (sens 42%, spec 96%)

Causes & Morphologies of ST Elevation (NEJM 2003;349:2128–2135)	
Differential	**Comments**
STEMI	Upward convex; coronary distribution; large T waves
Prinzmetal's angina	As above (STEMI), but transient due to coronary spasm etiology
Myo/pericarditis	Upward concave; diffuse (can be regional); +/– PR depression
Massive PE	Inferior & anteroseptal leads
LV aneurysm	Concave or convex; precordium common; ±pathologic Q waves; smaller T waves compared to STEMI
LBBB	Concave, usually discordant w/ QRS
LVH	Concave, other features of LVH present
Hyperkalemia	Seen w/ other features of hyperkalemia
Brugada	Usually incomplete RBBB, RAD, rSR' & downsloping STE V1, V2
nl (esp young men)	Concave, seen in healthy young men, most marked in V2
Early repolarization	Most marked at V4, notching at J point; tall upright T waves present
Cardioversion	Seen 1–2 min after DCCV; can be markedly elevated

ACUTE CORONARY SYNDROME

Overview
- Approach to patient w/ angina sx: See section on Chest Pain
- **Chronic Stable Angina:** Substernal chest discomfort (pain, tightness, pressure) of less than 10-min duration, provoked by exertion or stress & alleviated by rest or NTG; & nonprogressive (ie, stable) over long periods of time (see table; compare to unstable angina [UA])
  - Chronic angina should be a dx of exclusion in ED (after reviewing recent stress or cath results), as pts often present to EDs b/c sxs are worse in some capacity

Canadian Cardiovascular Society (CCS) Grading of Angina Pectoris (Circulation 1976;54:522)	
Grade	**Description**
Grade I	*Ordinary physical activity does not cause angina.* Angina w/ strenuous or rapid or prolonged exertion as work or recreation.
Grade II	*Slight limitation of ordinary activity:* walking or climbing stairs rapidly; walking uphill; walking or stair climbing after meals; in cold, wind, or under emotional stress; or only during the few hours after awakening; walking >2 blocks on level & climbing >1 flight of ordinary stairs at a nl pace & in nl conditions.
Grade III	*Marked limitation of ordinary physical activity.* Angina occurs on walking 1 or 2 blocks on the level & climbing 1 flight of stairs in nl conditions & at nl pace.
Grade IV	*Inability to carry on any physical activity w/o discomfort.* At rest.

- **Acute Coronary Syndrome:** Clinical spectrum of conditions ranging from UA through MI (NSTEMI & STEMI); due to vulnerable or high-risk plaque undergoing disruption of the fibrous cap causing thrombogenesis & ultimate imbalance b/w myocardial O_2 supply & demand (eg, tissue ischemia)
- **Myocardial Infarction** (see *Universal Definition*): death of myocardial cells due to myocardial tissue hypoxia, acutely causing release of intracellular cardiac biomarkers
  - Once diagnosed, important to consider subtype & etiology (see tables below)
    - MI DDx is broad: not always 2/2 acute plaque rupture (see table below)
  - Elevated troponin not always MI: consider nonischemic etiologies (see table below)

Universal Definition of Myocardial Infarction Classification System (*JACC* 2012;60(16):1581)

Summary of Criteria for Acute MI

Detection of a rise &/or fall of cardiac biomarker values (preferably cTn) w/ at least one value above the 99th percentile upper reference limit w/ *at least one* of the following:
- **Symptoms:** Sxs of ischemia
- **ECG:** New or presumed new significant ST-T changes, LBBB, Qw
- **Imaging:** e/o new loss of viable myocardium or new regional wall motion abx
- **Pathology:** Identification of an intracoronary thrombus by angiography or autopsy

Criteria for Prior MI

- **ECG:** Pathologic Q waves w/ or w/o sxs in the absence of nonischemic causes
- **Imaging:** e/o loss of viable myocardium in the absence of nonischemic causes
- **Pathology:** Pathologic findings of a prior MI

Universal Classification of MI

Type 1	Spontaneous MI related to atherosclerotic plaque rupture, ulceration, erosion, or dissection w/ resulting intraluminal thrombosis in 1 or more CAs
Type 2	MI secondary to an ischemic imbalance b/w myocardial O_2 supply &/or demand (ie, CA spasm, embolism, dysrhythmia, hypotension, etc.)
Type 3	MI resulting in death when biomarker values are unavailable
Type 4a	MI related to PCI
Type 4b	MI related to stent thrombosis
Type 5	MI related to CABG

Differential for MI and Injury

Causes		Examples
Ischemic injury	Atherosclerotic plaque rupture	Most common cause of 1° ACS
	Coronary artery dissection	1° (spontaneous, a/w pregnancy), or 2° (type A AoD w/ retrograde RCA dissection, post-PCI)
	Coronary artery spasm	Prinzmetal's variant, cocaine-induced
	Coronary artery embolism	Thrombus, endocarditis, myxoma
	Fixed atherosclerotic plaque w/ increased O_2 demand	↑ HR, ↑ BP, AoS (↑ O_2 demand) ↓ BP, anemia, hypoxia (↓ O_2 supply)
Nonischemic injury		Myocarditis, myocardial contusion, infiltrative dz, drug-induced myocardial injury

History

- Typical symptoms of angina: Substernal pressure, pain, or tightness; often radiating to neck, jaw, or arm(s); precipitated by exertion & relieved w/ rest or NTG
  - Associated sxs: dyspnea diaphoresis, N/V, palpitations, LH
  - Up to 23% of AMIs lack typical anginal sxs (*AJC* 1973;32:1)
- Concerning features: new, at rest, or crescendo (frequency, severity, duration, ↓ threshold)

Value of Specific Symptoms in Diagnosis of AMI (*JAMA* 2005;294:2623)

Pain Descriptor	LR (95% CI)	Pain Descriptor	LR (95% CI)
Increased Likelihood of AMI		**Decreased Likelihood of AMI**	
Radiation: R arm/shoulder	4.7 (1.9–12)	Described as pleuritic	0.2 (0.1–0.3)
Radiation: B/L arms/shoulders	4.1 (2.5–6.5)	Described as positional	0.3 (0.2–0.5)
Exertional	2.4 (1.5–3.8)	Described as sharp	0.3 (0.2–0.5)
Radiation to L arm	2.3 (1.7–3.1)	Reproducible w/ palpation	0.3 (0.2–0.4)
A/w diaphoresis	2 (1.9–2.2)	Inframammary location	0.8 (0.7–0.9)
A/w N/V	1.9 (1.7–2.3)	Nonexertional	0.8 (0.6–0.9)
Worse w/ previous angina or similar to previous MI	1.8 (1.6–2)		
Described as pressure	1.3 (1.2–1.5)		

Physical Exam

- Can be unremarkable unless c/b hypotension, heart block/arrhythmia, pulm edema
- Helpful for assessing for other causes of chest pain: bilateral UE BPs (AoD), lung exam (CHF, PTX, PNA), abdominal exam (biliary & pancreatic etiologies), chest wall ttp

Evaluation

- **ECG:** always check w/i 10 min, if sxs change, at 6–12 h; always compare w/ baseline; if pain persists or changes present, always repeat q15–20min; always consider posterior ECG (leads V7–V9) in pts w/ non-dx initial ECG to r/o L circumflex STEMI
  - Acute ischemia changes: ↑ or ↓ in ST or new TWI in anatomic distribution, new LBBB
  - Old ischemic changes: Qw or PRWP (indicates presence of CAD even if no known hx)
  - Sgarbossa criteria: Used to identify STEMI in the presence of old LBBB (see table)

Anatomic Distribution of ECG Findings Associated with AMI		
Anatomic Area	**ECG Leads**	**Coronary Artery**
Septal	V1–V2	Proximal LAD[1]
Anterior	V3–V4	LAD
Apical	V5–V6	Distal LAD, LCx, or RCA
Lateral	I, aVL, V5–V6	LCx
Anterolateral	aVR	L main CA
Inferior[2]	II, III, aVF	RCA (~85%), LCx (~15%)
RV	V1–V2 & V4R (most sens)	Proximal RCA
Posterior	ST depression V1–V2	RCA or LCx (obtain posterior leads)

[1]Wellen's syndrome: Biphasic T waves in V2–V3; specific for critical prox LAD lesion
[2]Always obtain R-sided leads in inferior STEMI to evaluate for RV infarc

Sgarbossa Criteria for Identifying AMI in Presence of Old LBBB				
Criteria & Points	**Sens (%)**	**Spec (%)**	**Pos LR**	**Neg LR**
5 pts: ≥1 mm STE concordant w/ QRS	73	92	9.5	0.3
3 pts: ≥1 mm STD in V1–V3	25	96	6.6	0.8
2 pts: ≥5 mm discordant w/ QRS	31	92	3.6	0.8

NOTE: Data above as originally reported by Sgarbossa et al. (*NEJM* 1996;334:481–487). Meta-analysis supports use of Sgarbossa criteria, though limits to Score ≥2 (Sens 18%, Spec 98%, Pos LR 7.9, Neg LR 0.8) (*Ann Emerg Med* 2008;52(4):329–336).

- **Cardiac biomarkers:** Troponin (I or T) preferred over CK-MB
  - Troponin: longer duration (↑ Sens) & higher specificity
  - CK-MB: only useful in addition to Tn if c/f new event w/i 1 wk from prior event in which +Tn (eg, return visit after recent PCI, MI, CABG, etc.)
    - Cardiac index: CI = (CK – MB/CK) × 100. CI <3 suggests skeletal source, CI 3–5 → indeterminate, CI >5 suggests cardiac source
  - Serial biomarker testing if signs/sx ACS: Perform serial troponin at 3–6 h after arrival, & at 6 h (+/– 12 h) if intermediate- or high-suspicion of ACS; if positive, continue measuring until levels peak & downtrend (*J Am Coll Cardiol* 2014;64(24):e139–228)
  - If initial Tn positive (eg, CKD), Δ Tn > +20% suggests new myocardial injury (if no AKI)
  - Non-MI causes of elevated biomarkers: myopericarditis; drug toxicity; acute neurologic diseases (eg, ICH); myocardial contusion; myocardial O₂ supply-demand mismatch 2/2 tachyarrhythmia, CHF, HTN, hypotension, PE, sepsis, burns, respiratory failure
- **Special note on novel high-sensitivity troponin I assays:** HS TnI assays can detect TnI levels far earlier, but may also detect nonnecrosis processes (eg, nl apoptosis), & thus can even be positive even in some healthy individuals
  - Single- & serial-HS-Tn protocols under investigation: Prelim studies suggest very high Sens at 0 h (99.6–100%) & 3 h (*Am Heart J* 2016;181:16–25; *Int J Cardiol* 2013;168(4):3896–3901); potentially helpful for ruling out AMI quickly
  - Due to lower Spec, Δ in serial HS-Tn may have greater clinical significance than elevation itself for ACS (*J Am Coll Cardiol* 2014;64(24):e139–e228), though absolute elevations may have prognostic value (*J Am Heart Assoc* 2014;3(1):e000403)

Characteristics of Cardiac Enzymes*					
Cardiac Enzyme	**Initial Elevation**	**Peak**	**Return to Baseline**	**Sens @ 8 h (%)**	**Sens @ 12 h (%)**
CK-MB	4–6 h	18 h	2–3 d	91	93–95
Troponin I	3–12 h	24 h	1–2 wk	90	95–100

*A single set of cardiac enzymes cannot r/o MI (& multiple sets cannot r/o ischemia w/o infarction)

- **Other labs:** Chem 7, CBC, coags, T/S (if intervention planned), tox (if cocaine suspected)
- **CXR:** Useful to r/o other causes of CP; check lungs, cardiac silhouette, mediastinum
- **Transthoracic echo:** If ECG is not interpretable (prior LBBB, paced) & suspicion for ACS is high, can obtain TTE to assess for regional wall motion abnormalities; +WMA in pt w/ ongoing CP may suggest benefit from earlier PCI (*J Am Coll Cardiol* 2014;64(24):e139–e228)
- **Risk-stratification testing:** See section on *Risk Stratification Testing*
- Coronary CTA, exercise stress testing, stress echocardiography, nuclear stress testing

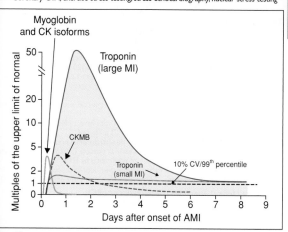

Figure 1.1

Treatment

Give ASA if considering ACS & no CIs (50–70% drop in D/MI for UA/NSTEMI (*NEJM* 1988;319(17):1105–1111); 23% drop in death in STEMI (*Lancet* 1988;2(8607):349–360)

Chronic stable angina: ASA (NNT = 50 in pts w/ known or suspected CAD), BP control, moderate- to high-intensity statin supported by mx RCTs (*NEJM* 2016;374:1167–1176; *Lancet* 2009;373(9678):1849–1860)

ACS: See *UA/NSTEMI & STEMI* for details

Disposition

Admit all STEMI, NSTEMI, & UA (see *UA/NSTEMI & STEMI* for details)

For patients w/ nondiagnostic hx, ECG, & biomarkers: Risk-stratify w/ HEART score
- **HEART** (score ≤ 3) > TIMI & GRACE in predicting major adverse cardiac events w/i 30 d (Sens 99%, NPV 98%) (*Int J Cardiol* 2016;221:759–764; *Int J Cardiol* 2017;227:65–661)

HEART Score for Chest Pain Patients in the ED (*Neth Heart J* 2008;16(6):191–196)			
History		**Troponin**	
Highly suspicious	2 pts	≥3× Nl limit	2 pts
Moderately suspicious	1 pt	>1 to <3× Nl limit	1 pt
Slightly/nonsuspicious	0 pts	≤ Nl limit	0 pts
ECG		**Risk Factors***	
Significant ST depressions	2 pts	≥3 risk factors**	2 pts
Nonspecific repolarization	1 pt	1 or 2 risk factors	1 pt
Nl	0 pts	No risk factors	0 pts
Age		*Risk factors include: Current DM, current or recent (<1 mo) smoker, HTN, HLD, FHx CAD, obesity	
≥65 y	2 pts		
>45 to <65 y	1 pt	**2 pts given for prior PCI, MI, CVA, PAD	
≤45 y	0 pts		
Total Score, Prognostic Value, and Disposition			
Score 0–3	2.5% MACE over next 6 wk	Discharge home w/ f/u	
Score 4–6	20.3% MACE over next 6 wk	Observation & risk-stratification testing	
Score 7–10	72.7% MACE over next 6 wk	Admit for early catheterization	

STEMI: Overview & Treatment

Definition
- Acute complete occlusion of coronary artery (usually proximal) due to unstable thrombus, causing transmural ischemia & myocardial necrosis; characterized by angina usually at rest usually >30 min, ECG e/o ST elevations (see below for criteria), & +troponin
- **ECG Criteria:** ≥0.2 mV precordial leads, ≥0.1 mV limb leads, & ≥0.5 mV in R-sided & posterior leads in at least 2 contiguous leads

Treatment Approach
- Initiate early medical therapies (ASA, heparin, nitrates prn, O_2 prn, analgesia)
  - Antithrombotic/adjunctive therapy should not delay transfer for pPCI
- Reperfusion: Immediate decision regarding availability of 1° PCI (see below)
  - pPCI or transfer to PCI-capable hospital preferred for all pts **except** if time b/w 1st medical contact (FMC) & pPCI is expected >120 min
  - Fibrinolysis may be preferred if delay to pPCI expected >120 min: after 120 min, no benefit of tfx to PCI-capable facility (*Circulation* 2011;124:2512–2521)
    - Goal time from FMC to lysis: <30 min
  - If FMC-to-pPCI time expected >120 min, consider: (*J Am Coll Cardiol* 2009;54(23):2205–2241)
    - Known CI to lysis (see below): pPCI preferred
    - Delay from sx onset (>3 h): pPCI preferred (lytics have ↓ efficacy w/ ↑ delays)
    - High-risk patient (shock, Killip class ≥3): pPCI preferred
    - Dx of STEMI in doubt (eg, AoD w/ RCA dissection): pPCI preferred
  - If planning PCI, call cardiology/PCI lab as early as possible (potentially even before the pt arrives in the ED—if reliable pre-notification by EMS)
  - If transferring for PCI, call for tfx early & ensure their door-to-balloon time is <90 min
- Monitor & treat complications (eg, CHB, cardiogenic shock, pulm edema, arrhythmias)

Adjunctive Medical Therapies (Fibrinolytics or pPCI)
- **Analgesia:** Morphine formerly used widely but may carry increased risk of adverse outcomes; use opioids only if absolutely needed (*Am Heart J* 2005;149(6):1043–1049)
- **O_2 supplementation:** No e/o benefit & may cause harm, possibly 2/2 free radical formation; use only in hypoxic pts w/ O_2 saturation <90% (*Cochrane* 2013;8:CD007160)
- **Nitrates:** No proven long-term mortality benefit, but may ameliorate sxs; typical dose 0.4 mg SL q5min × 3; CI w/ ↓ BP, RV infarct, PD-inh w/i 24–48 h (*Cochrane* 2009;4:CD006743)
- **Anti-plt tx:** Always give ASA (162–325 mg PO/PR), 23% ↓ in death c/w placebo (*Lancet* 1988;2:349); additional benefit from other anti-plt agents (see table); all patients should be administered additional anti-plt agents either in the ED or cath lab
- **Antithrombotic tx:** See table for recommended regimens
- **Beta-blockers:** Early IV BB ↓ VT/VF & reinfarction acutely & ↑ LVEF in long term, but also ↑ acute cardiogenic shock (esp if >70 y/o, SBP <120 mmHg, HR >110 bpm); give oral BB w/i 24 h of STEMI; consider IV BB acutely if no CI or ongoing ischemia (*Int J Cardiol* 2013;168(2):915–921; 2017;228:295–302. COMMIT/CCS-2; *Lancet* 2005;366:1622)
- Other: Often started as inpatients include oral BBs, statins, ACE inh/ARBs

Adjunctive Therapies for Fibrinolysis in STEMI (*Circulation* 2013;127(4):529–555)	
P2Y$_{12}$ receptor inh (loading dose)	**Clopidogrel:** 300 mg for pts ≤75 y/o, 75 mg for pts >75 y/o; ↑ artery patency, ↓ MACE if give w/ ASA; consider deferring decision to cardiology if potential need for CABG (CLARITY-TIMI 28, *NEJM* 2005;352:1179; COMMIT, *Lancet* 2005;366:1607)
Antithrombotic tx	**UFH:** IV bolus 60 U/kg (max 4,000 U) then gtt at 12 U/kg/h (max 1,000 U) maintain aPTT ~50–70 s × 48 h or until revasc
	Enoxaparin: If <75 y/o, 30 mg IV bolus, then 15 min later, 1 mg/kg SC q12h; if >75 y/o, no bolus, 0.75 mg/kg SC q12h; if CrCl <30 mL/min, 1 mg/kg q24h; continue 8 d or until revasc; no mortality diff c/w UFH, may ↑ recurrent MI & need for urgent revasc, but also ↑ bleeding (*NEJM* 2006;354:1477–1488)
	Fondaparinux: Initial 2.5 mg IV, then 2.5 mg SC the following day; continue × 8 d or until revasc; especially useful if hx of HIT; CI if CrCl <30; may ↓ mortality w/o ↑ bleeding c/w UFH (*JAMA* 2006;295(13):1519–1530)

Adjunctive Therapies for PCI in STEMI (Circulation 2013;127(4):529–555)		
P2Y12 receptor inh (loading dose)	Clopidogrel:	600 mg load; ↓ infarct size, cardiac fxn, stent thrombosis, & ↓ 30-d MACE c/w 300 mg load (J Am Coll Cardiol 2011;58(15):1592–1599. Lancet 2010;376(9748):1233–1243) but ↑ bleeding & ICU LOS if need for urgent CABG (Am Heart J 2011;161(2):404–410); discuss w/ cardiology if potential CABG w/i 5 d
	Prasugrel:	60 mg load; mild ↓ ischemic cx but ↑ bleeding c/w clopidogrel; best if young & no need for surgery w/i 1 y; avoid if hx of CVA/TIA (NEJM 2007;357:2001; TRITON-TIMI, Lancet 2009;373:732)
	Ticagrelor:	180 mg load; mild ↓ mortality, MI, stroke c/w clopidogrel, but ↑ nonprocedural bleeding (eg, ICH) (NEJM 2009;361:1045–1057)
Antithrombotic tx	UFH:	IV bolus 50–70 U/kg IV, then 12 U/kg/h (max 1,000 U), maintain aPTT ~50–70 s; may need higher doses
	Bivalirudin:	0.75 mg/kg IV bolus, then 1.75 mg/kg/h infusion w/ or w/o UFH; preferred over UFH w/ GP IIb/IIIa inh in pts at high risk of bleeding; useful if hx of HIT

NOTE: ACCF/AHA Guideline for Mgmt of STEMI recommends GIIb/IIIa inh (Class IIa recommendation) in selected patients, though often performed in cath lab. Options include: Abciximab 0.25 mg/kg bolus, then 125 mcg/kg/min (max 10 mcg/min); Tirofiban (high-bolus dose): 25 mcg/kg IV bolus, then 0.15 mcg/kg/min, ↓ by 50% in CKD; Eptifibatide (double bolus): 180 mcg/kg IV bolus, then 2 mcg/kg/min; a 2nd 180 mcg/kg bolus given 10 min after 1st bolus, ↓ by 50% in CKD, avoid in dialysis pts.

Fibrinolysis

Indications: STEMI AND sx onset <12 h prior AND time b/w 1st medical contact & pPCI >120 min; may consider up to 24 h after sx onset if persistent sx, ongoing STE, rising troponin, hemodynamic instability, & pPCI unavailable

Goal: Door-to-needle time should be ≤30 min

Benefits: ~20% ↓ mortality in anterior MI or new LBBB; 10% ↓ mortality in IMI

Risks: ICH (<1%), high-risk groups include elderly (~2% if >75 y), women, low weight

Fibrin-specific lytic (front-loaded tPA) 14% ↓ mortality c/w SK (1% abs Δ; GUSTO, NEJM 1993;329:673) although ↑ ICH (0.7% vs. 0.5%); 3rd-generation bolus lytics easier to administer, but no more safe or efficacious

Contraindications to Fibrinolysis in STEMI (Circulation 2013;127(4):529–555)	
Absolute CIs	**Relative CIs**
Intracranial neoplasm, aneurysm, AVM H/o intracranial hemorrhage H/o intracranial/spinal surgery w/i 2 mo H/o i-CVA/closed head trauma w/i 3 mo Active internal bleeding or bleeding d/o Suspected aortic dissection Severe HTN (unresponsive to IV tx) If considering using streptokinase: prior streptokinase use w/i 6 mo	Any known active intracranial path not listed w/i absolute contraindications H/o iCVA >3 mo prior Active PUD, pregnancy, or dementia Current use of anticoagulants H/o trauma or major surgery w/i 3 wk H/o recent internal bleeding w/i 2–4 wk H/o severe poorly controlled HTN, or SBP >180 or DBP >110 on presentation Traumatic or prolonged CPR (>10 min) Noncompressible vascular punctures

Fibrinolytic Agents for STEMI (Circulation 2013;127(4):529–555)		
Agent	**Dosing**	**Patency, 90 min**
Tenecteplase (TNK-tPA)	Single IV weight-based bolus: <60 kg (30 mg), 60–69 kg (35 mg), 70–79 kg (40 mg), 80–89 kg (45 mg), ≥90 kg (50 mg)	85%
Reteplase (rPA)	10 U + 10 U IV bolus given 30 min apart	84%
Alteplase (tPA)	Bolus 15 mg, infusion 0.75 mg/kg for 30 min (max 50 mg), then 0.5 mg/kg (max 35 mg) over 60 min; total dose not to exceed 100 mg	73–84%

Indications for Transfer for PCI After Fibrinolysis

- **Cardiogenic shock or severe acute HF:** Immediate tfx regardless of time from sx onset (can tfx even >48 h after MI); ↓ 6-mo mortality w/ immediate tfx; (NEJM 1999;341:625–634)
- **Failed reperfusion/re-occlusion:** Urgent tfx for rescue-PCI ↓ HF & recurrent MI, w/ trend toward ↓ mortality (Circulation 2013;127(4):529–555; NEJM 2005;353:2758)
- **Any pt:** As part of an invasive strategy in stable pts after successful fibrinolysis; ideally PCI performed >3 h & <24 h after fibrinolysis; greatest benefit in high-risk pts
- Routine angio ± PCI w/i 24 h of successful lysis: ↓ D/MI/Revasc (Lancet 2004;364:1045)

Primary PCI (NEJM 2007;356:47)

- **Indications:** STEMI sx onset <12 h prior, STEMI sx onset >12 h if CI to fibrinolytics or presence of severe acute HF, or cardiogenic shock; ongoing ischemia 12–24 h
- **Goal:** door-to-balloon <90 min by skilled operator at high-volume center
- **Benefits:** 27% ↓ death, 65% ↓ re-MI, 54% ↓ stroke, 95% ↓ ICH c/w lysis (Lancet 2003;361:13)
- PCI w/i 3 h of lytics in stable pts (w/o e/o failed re-perfusion) may cause harm (Lancet 2006;367:569; Lancet 2006;367:579; FINESSE, NEJM 2008;358:2205)

Disposition

- If no PCI available: transfer to PCI-capable center regardless of decision to use lytics
- If PCI available: admit to cath lab → CCU/cardiology

UNSTABLE ANGINA / NSTEMI: OVERVIEW & TREATMENT

Definition

- **Pathogenesis:** Nonocclusive coronary thrombus on pre-existing plaque, causing dynamic & progressive obstruction, inflammation, & ischemia
  - Coronary lesion can be located proximally or distally for UA, usually distal for NSTEM
- **Unstable Angina:** Any angina that is new-onset (if CCS III-IV severity), occurring a rest (if >20 min), or crescendo in nature (frequency, severity, duration, or more easily triggered), but *lacking* both ST elevations & positive troponin
- **NSTEMI:** Similar as UA, but characterized by positive troponin
- **ECG Criteria:** None; can have nl ECG, territorial STD, TWI, or NSSTW changes

Treatment Approach

- Initiate early medical therapies (ASA, heparin, nitrates prn, O_2 prn, analgesia)
- Determine risk using TIMI or GRACE risk scores to guide early vs. delayed timing o angiography (see section below) (Eur Heart J 2005;26(9):865–872)
- Monitor & treat complications (eg, CHB, cardiogenic shock, pulm edema, arrhythmias)

GRACE Risk Score for UA/NSTEMI (BMJ 2006;333(7578):1091)							
Age (y)							
≤30	0 pts	40–49	25 pts	60–69	58 pts	80–89	91 pts
30–39	8 pts	50–59	41 pts	70–79	75 pts	≥90	100 pts
Heart Rate (bpm)							
≤50	0 pts	70–89	9 pts	110–149	24 pts	≥200	46 pts
50–69	3 pts	90–109	15 pts	150–199	38 pts		
Systolic Blood Pressure (mmHg)							
≤80	58 pts	100–119	43 pts	140–159	24 pts	≥200	0 pts
80–99	53 pts	120–139	34 pts	160–199	10 pts		
Killip Class							
I (No heart failure)		0 pts	III (Crackles in whole lung field)				39 pts
II (Crackles in lower lung fields)		20 pts	IV (Cardiogenic shock)				59 pts
Serum Creatinine Level (mg/dL)							
0–0.38	1 pt	0.80–1.19	7 pts	1.59–1.90	13 pts	≥4	28 pts
0.39–0.79	4 pts	1.20–1.58	10 pts	2.0–3.99	21 pts		
Cardiac Arrest at admx		**ST-Segment Deviation**			**Troponin Elevation**		
Yes	0 pts	Yes		0 pts	Yes		0 pts
No	39 pts	No		28 pts	No		14 pts
Risk Classification and Prognosis							
Total score ≤100		Low risk			In-hospital death <1%		
Total score 101–170		Medium risk			In-hospital death 1–9%		
Total score ≥171		High risk			In-hospital death >9%		

TIMI Risk Score for UA/NSTEMI			*(JAMA 2000;284:835)*	
Age ≥65 y	1 pt	Severe angina (≥2 episodes w/i 24 h)		1 pt
≥3 RFs for CAD	1 pt	ST deviation ≥0.5 mm		1 pt
Known CAD (stenosis ≥50%)	1 pt	+cardiac marker (Tn, CK-MB)		1 pt
ASA use in past 7 d	1 pt			

Risk Classification and Risk of Death/MI/Urgent Revascularization w/i 14 d			
Total score	14d Risk: D/MI/Urg Revasc (%)	Total score	14d Risk: D/MI/Urg Revasc (%)
0–1 pt	5	4 pts	20
2 pts	8	5 pts	26
3 pts	13	6–7 pts	41

Adjunctive Medical Therapies

Analgesia: Morphine formerly used widely but may carry increased risk of adverse outcomes; use opioids only if absolutely needed *(Am Heart J 2005;149(6):1043–1049)*

O₂ supplementation: No e/o benefit & may cause harm, possibly 2/2 free radical formation; use only in hypoxic pts w/ O₂ saturation <90% *(Cochrane 2013;8:CD007160)*

Nitrates: No proven long-term mortality benefit, but may ameliorate sxs; typical dose 0.4 mg SL q5min × 3, continuous gtt if CP not improved w/SL (titrate until CP free; once CP free, titrate off); CI w/ ↓ BP, RV infarct, PD-inh w/i 24–48 h *(Cochrane 2009;4:CD006743)*

Anti-plt tx: Always give ASA (162–325 mg PO/PR), 23% ↓ in death c/w placebo *(Lancet 1988;2:349)*; additional benefit from other anti-plt agents (see table)

- **If allergic to ASA:** Clopidogrel 300–600 mg load (regardless of PCI approach)
- **If early invasive approach:** Once decision made to proceed to PCI made, give Clopidogrel (600 mg), Ticagrelor (180 mg), or GP IIb/IIIa inh (eptifibatide IV, tirofiban IV) in addition to ASA; discuss w/ cardiology, may have greatest value if expected delay to PCI; further agents (P2Y₁₂ inh, GPI) may have benefit when given peri-PCI in cath lab *(J Am Coll Cardiol 2013;61(23):e179–e347)*
- **If conservative approach:** If PCI uncertain or not planned, give Clopidogrel (300 mg or 600 mg) or Ticagrelor (180 mg) in addition to ASA; reasonable to consider addition of GP IIb/IIIa inh (eptifibatide IV, tirofiban IV) unless low risk score &/or high bleeding risk *(J Am Coll Cardiol 2013;61(23):e179–e347)*
- Inconclusive benefit from ED administration (vs. cath lab/inpatient unit) of DAPT in either early invasive or conservative approach, though generally earlier tx is better if UA/NSTEMI dx certain & low bleeding risk

Antithrombotic tx: See table for recommended regimens; continue until angiography (early invasive approach) or 48 h (conservative approach, if stress results indicate no need for angiography); hold anticoagulation on warfarin until INR <2.0; anticoagulants have short-term benefit (UFH ↓ mortality 33–56% at 2–12 wk), but long-term benefit unclear, as dz process resumes once anticoagulation discontinued

Beta-blockers: Early IV BB ↓VT/VF & reinfarction acutely & ↑ LVEF in long term, but also ↑ acute cardiogenic shock (esp if >70 y/o, SBP <120 mmHg, HR >110 bpm); give oral BB w/i 24 h of UA/NSTEMI; IV not routinely indicated *(Int J Cardiol 2013;168(2):915–921. Int J Cardiol 2017;228:295–302. COMMIT/CCS-2, Lancet 2005;366:1622)*

Other: Often started as inpatients include oral BBs, statins, ACE inh/ARBs

Antithrombotic Therapy in UA/NSTEMI	
Early invasive approach	**UFH:** IV bolus 60 U/kg (max 4,000 U) then gtt at 12 U/kg/h (max 1,000 U), maintain aPTT ~50–70 s x 48 h or until revasc
	Enoxaparin: If <75 y/o, 30 mg IV bolus, then 15 min later, 1 mg/kg SC q12h; if >75 y/o, no bolus, 0.75 mg/kg SC q12h; if CrCl <30 mL/min, 1 mg/kg q24h; mild ↓ in nonfatal MI c/w UFH
	Bivalirudin: 0.75 mg/kg IV bolus, then 1.75 mg/kg/h infusion w/ or w/o UFH; preferred over UFH w/ GP IIb/IIIa inh in pts at high risk of bleeding
Conservative approach	**UFH:** IV bolus 60 U/kg (max 4,000 U) then gtt at 12 U/kg/h (max 1,000 U), maintain aPTT ~50–70 s x 48 h or until revasc
	Enoxaparin: If <75 y/o, 30 mg IV bolus, then 15 min later, 1 mg/kg SC q12h; if >75 y/o, no bolus, 0.75 mg/kg SC q12h; if CrCl <30 mL/min, 1 mg/kg q24h
	Fondaparinux: Initial 2.5 mg IV, then 2.5 mg SC the following day; preferred if hx of HIT or ↑ bleeding risk

J Am Coll Cardiol 2013;61(23):e179–e347; 64(24):e139–e228

Early Invasive vs. Conservative Approach (*J Am Coll Cardiol* 2014;64(24):e139–e228)
- Ultimately, approach decided by interventional cardiology based on multiple factors: risk score, procedural risks, recent angiography results, clinical stability & sx, individual pt goals, etc.
- **Early invasive approach:** Routine angiography w/i 72 h, urgency based on presentation:
  - *Immediate-invasive (PCI <2 h):* Any HD instability, VT/VF, HF/MVR, refractory angina
  - *Routine-invasive (PCI w/i 12–48 h):* High-risk scores (TIMI ≥ 3, GRACE > 140), rising troponin, or new STD on ECG
  - *Delayed-invasive (PCI 25–72 h):* Medium-risk (TIMI ≥ 2, GRACE 109–140) or high-risk scores (w/o rising troponin or STD); +/− hx of PCI w/i 6 mo, prior CABG, CKD, ↓ EF
- **Conservative ("selective invasive") approach:** Best for initially stabilized pts w/o high-risk scores, ongoing symptoms, arrhythmias, heart failure; 2/2 marginal benefit but ↑ risks of early invasive approach (*Cochrane* 2016;26(5):CD004815)
  - Medical therapies (see above) for 48 h minimum, pre-discharge stress test
  - Angiography only if recurrent ischemia, arrhythmias, heart failure, positive stress test
- Early invasive approach: In meta-analysis, no ↓ all-cause mortality/nonfatal MI, may ↓ risk of MI, refractory angina, & rehosp at 6–12 mo c/w conservative approach; however, also ↑ bleeding risk & procedure-related MI (*Cochrane* 2016;26(5):CD004815)
- Higher-risk pts benefit most from earlier angiography (*J Am Coll Cardiol* 2013;61(23):e179–e347; TIMACS, *NEJM* 2009;360:2165–2175) as reflected in guidelines above

Disposition
- Admission to CCU/cardiology based on risk, clinical stability, arrhythmia risk
- If UA, low-risk score, −Tn, nondiagnostic ECG: consider admitting to a CP/observation unit for serial troponin testing & stress testing; admx if recurrent sx, Δ ECG, +Tn
Guidelines: J Am Coll Cardiol 2013;61(23):e179–e347; 2014;64(24):e139–e228.

Angiography Selection & Timing in UA/NSTEMI (*J Am Coll Cardiol* 2014;64(24):e139–e228)	
Immediate (<2 h) invasive	Hemodynamic instability Sustained VT or VF Signs or sx of HF or new or worsening mitral valve regurg Refractory angina
Selective (med tx, PCI prn) invasive	Low-risk score (eg, TIMI 0–1, GRACE <109) Low-risk Troponin-negative female pts Patient or clinician preference in absence of high-risk features
Early (<24 h) invasive	None of above, but high risk (TIMI ≥ 3, GRACE score > 140) Temporal change in Troponin New or presumably new STD on ECG
Delayed (25–72 h) invasive	None of above but DM Renal insufficiency (GFR <60 mL/min) Reduced LV systolic function (EF <0.40) Early postinfarction angina PCI w/i 6 mo Prior CABG Medium-risk score (TIMI 2, GRACE 109–140)

RISK STRATIFICATION TESTING

Approach
- **Definition:** Noninvasive eval for obstructive CAD in low-risk pts w/ acute CP/sx c/f ACS
  - Result usually qualitative ("positive" vs. "negative") for ischemia
- **Indications:** dx obstructive CAD, assess Δ clinical status in pt w/ known obstructive CAD, localize ischemia in pts w/ known symptomatic obstructive CAD
- **Contraindications:** severe acute illness, AMI w/i 48 h, high-risk UA, alternative critical dx (PE, AoD, myopericarditis, acute decompensated CHF, arrhythmias, severe AoS)
- Low-risk (HEART 0–3, TIMI 0–1, GRACE <109) pts may be safely discharged w/o stress testing if close f/u for outpatient stress testing can be arranged
  - ED stress testing in low-risk pts is low yield & high-cost (*Am J Cardiol* 2015;116(2):204–207)
  - 6-mo risk of MACE is low & may be unchanged regardless of whether pt receives stress in ED (*Int J Cardiol* 2017;227:656–661; *Crit Pathw Cardiol* 2016;15(4):145–151)

Exercise Treadmill Testing
- Patient runs on treadmill; monitoring includes ECG, symptoms, Δ hemodynamics (HR, BP)
  - "Diagnostic" test requires pt to achieve min of 85% of predicted HR (pHR = 220 − age)
- **Test characteristics:** 68% Sens, 77% Spec (*NEJM* 2011;364(24):1840–1845)

- **Benefits:** Lowest cost of risk stratification tests
- **Downsides:** requires nl resting ECG; ↓ Sens if low-risk pt; ↓ Sens & Spec in women; ↓ Sens if anti-ischemic drugs not d/c-ed (d/c BBs, digoxin, vasodilators, anti-HTN drugs ~2 d prior to testing if possible)
- Duke Treadmill Score: weighted index of treadmill time, ECG chgs, induced angina sx
  - DTS = Duration of exercise in min − (5 * max STD in mm) − (4 * angina index)
  - Angina index: No angina (AI = 0), nonlimiting angina (AI = 1), limiting angina (AI = 2)

Prognostic Value of Duke Treadmill Score in Exercise Stress Testing					
DTS Risk	1-y Mortality	No Stenosis ≥ 75%	1VD ≥ 75%	2VD ≥ 75%	3VD ≥ 75%
Male: Low	0.9%	52.6%	22.4%	13.6%	11.4%
Male: Mod	2.9%	17.8%	15.6%	27.9%	38.7%
Male: High	8.3%	1.8%	9.1%	17.5%	71.5%
Fem: Low	0.5%	80.9%	9.4%	6.2%	3.5%
Fem: Mod	1.1%	65.1%	14.2%	8.3%	12.4%
Fem: High	1.8%	10.8%	18.9%	24.3%	46.0%

Ann Int Med 1987;106:793–800. NEJM 1991;325;849–853. J Am Coll Cardiol 1998:32:1657–1664.

Pharmacologic Stress w/ Nuclear SPECT Imaging

- Ischemia induced by pharmacologic agents (dobutamine, adenosine, dipyridamole); radio-labeled tracers (eg, sestamibi) enter myocardial cells & reflect regional perfusion; ↓ tracer uptake during stress that resolves w/ time suggests viable area of tissue ischemia; fixed defect suggest existing infarct
  - Note: nuclear imaging can be performed after physical exercise as well
- **Test characteristics:** Adenosine SPECT Sens 90%, Spec 75%; dipyridamole SPECT Sens 89%, Spec 65%; dobutamine SPECT Sens 82%, Spec 75% (*Am Heart J* 2001;142(6):934–944)
- **Benefits:** Can use if abnl baseline ECG or unable to exercise; can localize ischemia
- **Downsides:** More expensive than exercise stress; ↓ Sens & Spec in women; ↓ Sens if anti-ischemic drugs not d/c-ed (d/c BBs, digoxin, vasodilators, anti-HTN drugs ~2 dys prior to testing if possible)

Pharmacologic/Exercise Stress w/ Echo Imaging

- Ischemia induced by pharmacologic agents (dobutamine, adenosine, dipyridamole) or exercise; echocardiography performed to assess for regional WMAs compared to rest
- **Test characteristics:** Adenosine Echo Sens 72%, Spec 91%; dipyridamole Echo Sens 70%, Spec 93%; dobutamine Echo Sens 80%, Spec 84% (*Am Heart J* 2001;142(6):934–944)
- **Benefits:** Can use if abnl baseline ECG or unable to exercise; can localize ischemia; can provide information re LVEF & valvular fxn
- **Downsides:** More expensive than exercise stress; ↓ Sens & Spec in women; ↓ Sens if anti-ischemic drugs not d/c-ed (d/c BBs, digoxin, vasodilators, anti-HTN drugs ~2 dys prior to testing if possible)

Coronary Computed Tomographic Angiography

- CT angiography of coronary arteries; images timed in conjunction w/ HR; assesses CAD burden & severity based on CA calcification; does not assess myocardial perfusion
- **Test characteristics:** Sens 85–99%, Spec 64–97%, NPV >95% (*Eur Heart J* 2016;37(30):2397–2405)
- **Benefits:** ↓ LOS & ↓ costs c/w conventional stress testing; especially useful for low-risk pts or intermediate-risk & nl serial ECGs/biomarkers, can evaluate global & regional LV fxn (*Circulation* 2006;114:1761; *JACC* 2008;48:1475; *NEJM* 2012;366(15):393; *NEJM* 2012;367(4):299)
- **Downsides:** Increased risk of downstream testing (2/2 ↓ Spec & detection of incidental findings), radiation exposure, requires relative bradycardia (often requires βB)
  - Radiation: 3× more radiation than ETT or stress echo, equivalent to nuclear stress; more important to avoid in young pts & women; newer protocols are being designed to minimize radiation exposure (*Eur Heart J* 2016;37(30):2397–2405)
- Combination of single negative conventional troponin & negative coronary CTA has equivalent risk of 28 d MACE c/w conventional stress (*Eur Heart J* 2016;37(30):2397–2405)

Disposition

- Inadequate quality study: discuss case w/ cardiology
- Adequate quality + Neg result + Low-risk: d/c w/ f/u
- Adequate quality + Neg result + Int-risk: discuss case w/ cardiology, likely d/c w/ f/u
- Adequate quality + Pos result: discuss w/ cardiology, admit
- For adequate study w/ high-risk test results, consider coronary angiography, ± admission depending on clinical presentation

Pearls
- False-positives: Positive risk-stratification testing in a pt who presented to ED w/ CP does not necessarily mean CP was 2/2 by CAD; esp if low pre-TP & other causes possible
- False-negatives: Negative risk-stratification testing in a pt who presented to ED w/ CP does not necessarily mean CP was not 2/2 by CAD; esp if high pre-TP

CARDIAC CATHETERIZATION

Overview
- **Indications:** ACS (see *STEMI & UA/NSTEMI* above for timing of PCI); high-risk stress test result OR indeterminate-risk stress test result & high PreTP for obstructive CAD; ongoing angina despite tx; r/o CAD in pts w/ CP suspected from nonatherosclerotic etiology (ie, spasm) or systolic dysfxn suspected of nonischemic etiology (ie, ni-CMP); after ROSC in pts w/ cardiac arrest (see below for criteria)
  - Postarrest PCI recommended if STEMI &/or absence of mx unfavorable features (unwitnessed arrest, no bystander CPR, initial non-VF rhythm, >30 min to ROSC, ongoing CPR, noncardiac / traumatic arrest, pH <7.2, lactate >7, age >85, ESRD); decision individualized for each case (*J Am Coll Cardiol* 2015;66(1):62–73)
- **Types of percutaneous coronary interventions:**
  - Balloon angioplasty: Effective but ↑ risk of CA dissection & restenosis 2/2 remodeling
  - Bare metal stent: ↓ restenosis, repeat revasc, & MACE c/w BA, but no Δ MI (most periprocedural), no Δ D (*Am Heart J* 2006;151(3):682–689); requires DAPT × 4 wk & lifelong ASA thereafter
  - Drug-eluting stent: ↓ restenosis & repeat revasc c/w BMS, but no Δ D/MI over 6 y (*NEJM* 2016;375;1242–1252); requires DAPT × 1 y & lifelong ASA thereafter

Post-PCI Complications
- **Bleeding (femoral access site):** Apply pressure, reverse/stop anticoag
- **Bleeding (retroperitoneum):** May c/o back pain, ±Hct drop, ↓ BP, ↑ HR; obtain abd/pelvic CT (I–); reverse/stop anticoag, consult IR/surgery
- **Vascular damage (pseudoaneurysm):** Pain, expanding mass, systolic bruit; obtain US; tx w/ manual compression, ± thrombin injection/surgery
- **Vascular damage (AV fistula):** May p/sx w 2/2 ↓ perfusion to LE (2/2 emboli, dissection, thrombus), continuous bruit, ↓ distal pulses; obtain US ± angiogram; consult card &/or surgery for repair (percutaneous or operative)
- **Renal failure:** Usually 2/2 contrast, occurs w/i 24 h, peaks 3–5 d
- **Stent thrombosis:** P/w acute CP & STE; consult cards/cath lab for urgent catheterization; may be more common in BMS than DES (*JACC Cardiovasc Interv* 2015;8(12):1552–1562); commonly 2/2 underexpanded stent, dissection, or d/c anti-plt Rx (*JAMA* 2005;293:2126)
- **Stent stenosis:** P/w subacute or chronic return of prior anginal sx months after PCI (but 10% p/w ACS); occurs 2° postprocedure remodeling, not atherosclerosis; despite advances, occurs still >10% cases (BA > BMS > DES) (*BMJ* 2015;351:h5392)

POST-MI COMPLICATIONS

Immediate Complications
- **LV systolic dysfunction/cardiogenic shock:** Common in L-sided (esp anterior) AMI; Dx w/ JVD, CXR or BSUS (B/L B-lines, ↓ EF); Tx w/ O₂ for hypoxia, ↑ preload (NTG SL → gtt), ↓ afterload (nitroprusside; IV ACE-I if CI; avoid hydral 2/2 reflex ↑ HR), inotropy PRN (norepi > dopamine 2/2 fewer arrhythmias [*NEJM* 2010;362(9):779–789]; ± dobutamine esp if SVR high), diuretics, minimize PEEP (if intubated), emergent reperfusion (lytics/pPCI), may need IABP in cath lab (*Lancet* 2000;356(9231):749–756).
- **RV systolic dysfunction/cardiogenic shock:** Common in RV AMI; Dx w/ R-sided leads, BSUS (few B-lines, ↑ RV:LV ratio, dilated IVC); Tx w/ O₂ for hypoxia, ↑ preload (IVF until e/o nonfluid responsive; ongoing IVF may aggravate), ↓ PVR (bronchodilators, inh NO or prostacyclins), inotropy PRN (milrinone > norepi), minimize PEEP/TV (if intubated), emergent reperfusion (lytics/pPCI) (*J Am Coll Cardiol* 2010;56(18):1435–1446)
- **Tachyarrhythmias (eg, VT/VF, AF):** Ischemia causes re-entry circuits in myocardium; place defibrillation pads on pt immediately on arrival; If unstable, tx w/ ACLS; If stable VT, tx w/ IV BB / membrane stabilization (amiodarone, metoprolol), check & replete lytes; emergent reperfusion (lytics/pPCI)
- **Bradyarrhythmias (eg, Heart block):** Heart block can be 2/2 strong vagal tone (1° AVNB) &/or ischemia to AV node (1°–3° AVNB); place pacer pads on pt immediately on arrival; Tx w/ IVF (for BP), atropine, TC/TV pacing if unstable; emergent reperfusion (lytics/pPCI)

Early Complications

- **Infarct expansion, re-infarction, postinfarction ischemia:** Usually w/i 4 d of MI; can present similarly to initial MI but diagnostics subtler; Δ ECG (2/2 nl evolution from prior MI vs. new ischemia), +Tn (may be ↓ from prior MI; ↑ suggests new ischemia), +CK-MB (suggests new ischemia); tx as w/ ACS; discuss w/ cardiology; depending on prior mgmt (pPCI vs. lytics; BA vs. BMS/DES), may need pPCI
- **Ventricular wall rupture:** Usually w/i 2–7 d after MI; RFs include ↑ age, female, anterior infarct, ↑ wall strain (↑ HR, ↑ afterload); occur at jxn of nl tissue & infarct
  - **Free wall rupture:** Rapid bleeding into pericardium causing s/sx of tamponade; Tx w/ IVF/blood; emergent pericardiocentesis & cardiac surgery; mortality >90%
  - **Pseudoaneurysm:** Bleeding contained w/i myocardial wall; may p/w arrhythmias, heart failure, systemic embolization, or be asx & dx'ed only on imaging; once identified, c/s cardiology & cardiac surgery
  - **Septal rupture:** May be asx or p/w sx of L → R shunt & ↓ L-sided CO (angina, shock, pulm edema); new pansystolic murmur; dx by echo; tx w/ urgent surgical closure
- **Papillary muscle rupture:** Usually w/i 7 d of MI; frequency i-MI & p-MI > a-MI; p/w sx of acute pulmonary edema, pansystolic murmur; BSUS differentiate from post-MI VSD; tx w/ ↓ preload & afterload (nitroprusside), diuretics, O_2, IABP, emergent surgical repair
- **Pericarditis:** Usually w/i 7 d of MI; most common w/ a-MI; p/w low-grade fever, chest pain, friction rub; ECG w/ diffuse STE w/o reciprocal chgs; BSUS ± pericardial effusion; tx w/ NSAIDs; NOTE: early pericarditis is distinct from Dressler's syndrome (below)

Delayed Complications

- **Left ventricular aneurysm:** Suspect if ECG w/ persistent STE post-MI; can p/w HF, embolic sx, arrhythmias; dx w/ echo; c/s cardiology (reperfusion), cardiac surgery
- **Left ventricular thrombus:** Most common in a-MI; RFs include ↓ EF, severe MVR, LV aneurysm (eg, slow, nonlaminar flow); tx w/ anticoagulation
- **Dressler's syndrome:** Usually 2–10 wk after MI; presumed autoimmune-mediated; p/w fever, chest pain, pleurisy; BSUS w/ pericardial & pleural effusions; self-limited w/ NSAIDs

PRINZMETAL'S (VARIANT) ANGINA

Overview

- **Definition:** Distinct syndrome of ischemic CP classically occurring at rest 2/2 focal coronary artery spasm, & a/w transient STE; exact etiology unknown
- Most vasospasm occurs in areas of pre-existing stenosis
- Can be a/w infarction, arrhythmia, & sudden cardiac death; consider in all pts w/ healthy SCD, particularly if arrest occurred in morning or cold settings

History

- Often young (35–50 y/o), F > M, tobacco use, EtOH use; PMH/FHx migraine, Raynaud's, pericarditis, MV prolapse; may have no known cardiac hx but CAD not uncommon
- Sxs include substernal pressure radiating to jaw & arm; can respond to NTG; often occur midnight to early AM (↑ vagal tone), or after hyperventilation or cold
- May be a/w marked diurnal variation in exercise tolerance (↓ tolerance in AM, ↑ in PM)

Evaluation

- EKG reveals transient territorial STE & reciprocal ST Δs; may induce a variety of conduction disturbances or arrhythmias
- Stress testing may induce no ST Δs, STDs, or STEs, or STEs may be seen during recovery phase of stress testing
- Dx definitively w/ angiography & provocative intracoronary ACH &/or ergot derivative (>90% Sens, >90% Spec; even better if combined); noninvasive approach w/ hyperventilation & exercise (65% Sens, >90% Spec) (*J Am Coll Cardiol* 2013;63(2):103–109)

Treatment

- High-dose CCB (nifedipine, verapamil, diltiazem), nitrates (SL prn); d/c smoking

Disposition

- Admit, given risk of MI & arrhythmia during acute episodes

COCAINE-INDUCED ANGINA

Overview
- Definition: Anginal sx occurring after cocaine use, 2/2 ↑ myocardial O_2 demand (↑ HR, ↑ afterload, ↑ contractility & end-systolic wall stress) & ↓ O_2 supply (vasoconstriction); generally not 2/2 acute thrombosis, though cocaine a/w premature CAD/ACS
- Overall incidence of cocaine-associated MI is 0.7–6% of those presenting w/ CP after cocaine (Acad Emerg Med 2000;36:469; COCHPA, Acad Emerg Med 1994;1:330)
- Can be c/b arrhythmia & heart failure (~90% occur w/i 12 h of presentation)

History
- CP that may be a/w dyspnea, anxiety, palpitations, diaphoresis, dizziness, or nausea
- Sxs typically occur w/i 3 h of ingestion, but cocaine metabolites may persist up to 24 h to cause delayed or recurrent vasoconstriction
- RF for cocaine-induced MI: Male gender, current smoker, non-white

Evaluation
- Similar to ACS (see above)
- Maintain high index of suspicion for aortic dissection as well
- Urine toxicology: Usually detects cocaine metabolite benzoylecgonine (urine $t_{1/2}$ of 6–8 h) up to 24–48 h (range 16–66 h); however, chronic cocaine users may have detectable levels for weeks after last use

Treatment
- Given risk of MI, tx similarly to ACS (see ACS, "Adjunctive Medical Therapies")
  - ASA, analgesia PRN, O_2 PRN, NTG PRN, antithrombotic tx all as per ACS guidelines
  - Avoid BB given risk of unopposed α-adrenergic effect (↑ CA vasospasm, ↑ BP)
- IV Benzodiazepines (↓ central stimulatory effects of cocaine)
- IV Anti-HTN (NTG, sodium nitroprusside, phentolamine; avoid BB)
- If STEMI: pPCI preferred over lytics 2/2 ↑ ICH risk after cocaine
- VT/VF immediately after cocaine is 2/2 local anesthetic (Na channel) effect & may respond to sodium bicarbonate tx in addition to standard therapies

Disposition
- Admit: If +Tn, ongoing CP, persistent unstable VS
- EDOU: If sx & VS controlled, -Tn, nonischemic ECG; no difference in 30-d outcomes if pts w/ & w/o stress-testing, consider if CAD RFs & poor f/u (Circulation 2008;117:1897–1907)
- Provide drug-abuse counseling to all pts prior to d/c

DVT AND PULMONARY EMBOLISM

DEEP VEIN THROMBOSIS

Overview
- Definition: In situ thrombosis of LE/UE deep veins, often provoked by stasis/turbulence, hypercoagulability, endothelial injury (Virchow's triad)
- RFs: Hypercoagulable state (cancer, pregnancy, OCPs, APLAS); recent surgery or trauma; prolonged immobilization; venous outlet obstruction; excess extremity use (eg, sports, occupation; for UE DVT); increased age; obesity; FHx of DVT/PE
- Lower-extremity DVT: Comprise 90% of DVTs; but as many as ~50% may be isolated distal DVT of the calf (only require tx if severe sx or propagating; see below)
- Upper-extremity DVT: Comprise the minority (10%) of DVTs; c/w LE DVT, ↓ risk of PE (6% vs. 15–32%), ↓ risk of recurrence (2–5% vs. 10%); can be 1° (20%) or 2° (80%) (NEJM 2011;364(9):861–869; Circulation 2012;126:768–773)
  - Primary: thoracic outlet compression of SC vein (eg, ribs, clavicle), microtrauma to SC vein from repeat UE movements (often young, athletes or occupation), idiopathic
  - Secondary: catheter-associated, cancer-associated (hypercoag, compression surgery (immobilization, endothelial trauma), systemic hypercoag state (preg, etc.)
- Management based on location (proximal vs. distal), depth (deep vs. superficial)

History & Physical Exam
- HX: May have unilateral discomfort, swelling, paresthesia, weakness, erythema, warmth
  - Always ask about RFs; obtain ROS to assess for s/sx of concurrent PE
- EX: Physical exam notoriously insensitive for DVT (JAMA 1998;279:1094–1099)

Evaluation

- Use Well's score to determine pre-TP of DVT (see table)

Well's Criteria for DVT (JAMA 1998;279:1094–1099; NEJM 2003;349(13):1227–1235)			
Active cancer (tx ongoing or w/i 6 mo or palliative)			1 pt
Paralysis, paresis, or recent immobilization of LE			1 pt
Recently bedridden >3 d or major surgery w/i 4 wk			1 pt
Localized tenderness along deep venous system			1 pt
Entire leg swelling			1 pt
Calf swelling by >3 cm c/w asx (10 cm below tibial tuberosity)			1 pt
Pitting edema (greater in symptomatic leg)			1 pt
Collateral superficial veins (nonvaricose)			1 pt
Previously documented DVT			1 pt
Alternative dx as likely or greater than that of DVT			–2 pts
Points	**Pre-Test Prob**	**D-dimer Sensitivity (%)**	**Prevalence of DVT (%)**	**NPV of D-dimer (%)**
–2 to 0 pts	Low	86	5	99
1 to 2 pts	Moderate	85	17	95
≥3 pts	High	90	53	81

RFs not incorporated into score but a/w inc risk of DVT include FHx of DVT (>2 1st-degree relatives), hospitalization w/i 6 mo; erythema.

- UE DVT: Compression US (Sens 97%, Spec 96%); if negative US but high pre-TP, obtain serial US or D-dimer (Sens 100%, Spec 14%) (NEJM 2011;364(9):861–869)
- LE DVT (initial eval): lab & imaging directed based on pre-TP (see Algorithms below)
  - D-dimer: Assays include enzyme-linked immunofluorescence assays (Sens 96%, Spec 46%), microplate ELISA (Sens 94%, Spec 53%), immunoturbidimetric (Sens 93%, 53%), whole-blood assay (Sens 83%, Spec 71%), & quantitative latex agglutination assays (Sens 95%, 53%) (Chest 2012;141(2Suppl):e351S–418S)
  - Lower-extremity ultrasound (two types: Proximal compression, Whole-leg)
    - WL-US: Superior to PC-US alone in detection of DVT (mostly distal)
      - Increased chance of dx isolated distal DVT of unclear significance (see Tx)
    - PC-US: should be used w/ D-dimer to increase sensitivity (see Algorithm)
      - If PC-US neg & D-dimer pos, repeat PC-US in 1 wk
    - 3-mo rate of PE after negative WL-US: 0.3% (low pre-TP), 0.8% (mod pre-TP), 2.5% (high pre-TP) (Chest 2012;141(2Suppl):e351S–418S)
      - No difference c/w combined PC-US + D-dimer (& prn repeat PC-US): No difference in 3-mo risk of PE (0.6%) (Chest 2012;141(2Suppl):e351S–418S)
  - CT venography: Highest sensitivity but risk of radiation & contrast; use selectively if mod or high pre-TP, positive PC-US & unable to obtain WL-US or repeat PC-US in 1 wk (Chest 2012;141(2Suppl):e351S–418S)
- LE DVT (recurrent): Risk of false-positives (2/2 scarring, postthrombotic syndrome) high
  - Recommended approach: Combined D-dimer (usually nl w/i 3 mo of starting tx for DVT) & PC-US; if PC-US neg or undiagnostic, repeat in 1 wk (if unable: CTV, MRV)

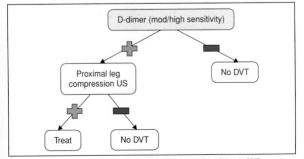

Figure 1.2 Diagnosis and Treatment of DVT, Low Pre-Test Probability. (Chest 2012;141(2)(suppl):e351S)

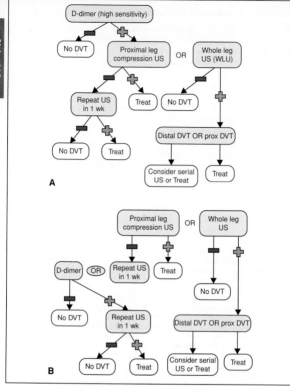

Figure 1.3 Diagnosis and Treatment of DVT, Mod Pre-Test Probability. (**A**) Starting with D-dimer assessment, and (**B**) Starting with ultrasonography (Chest 2012;141(2)(suppl):e351S)

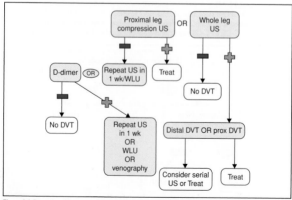

Figure 1.4 Diagnosis and Treatment of DVT, High Pre-Test Probability (Chest 2012;141(2)(suppl):e351S)

Treatment

- UE DVT: Anticoagulation × 3–6 mo, though comparative data lacking on specific regimens
  - Cather-associated DVT: Catheter removal only indicated if catheter malfxn or infxn, no further need for catheter, or strong CIs to systemic A/C (NEJM 2011;364(9):861–869)
  - Isolated basilic/cephalic vein thrombosis: very low risk of PE, no A/C required
- LE DVT: Anticoagulation × 3–6 mo unless strong CIs (Chest 2012;141(2) (Suppl):e419S–e494S)
  - Anticoagulation regimen should be selected based on comorbidities, ability to take PO medications, patient preference (monitoring, etc.), risks of bleeding:
    - SC LMWH (1 mg/kg BID; renally dose): slight ↓ risk of death, recurrence, major bleeding c/w UFH; preferred w/ malignancy; relative CIs include CKD & obesity
    - SC Fondaparinux (5 mg QD [<50 kg], 7.5 mg QD [50–100 kg], 10 mg QD [>100 kg]; renally dose): Similar risk of death, recurrence, major bleeding c/w LMWH; preferred w/ hx of HIT
    - IV UFH (80 U/kg bolus, 18 U/kg/h gtt): As above, may be preferred over LMWH if CKD/ESRD; risk of HIT higher than LMWH
    - PO Warfarin (INR 2.0–3.0): Bridge w/ LMWH/Fondaparinux until INR therapeutic
    - PO Rivaroxaban (15 mg BID x 3 wk, 20 mg QD thereafter)
    - PO Apixaban (10 mg BID x 7 d, 5 mg BID thereafter)
  - Duration of treatment generally depends if provoked (3 mo) or nonprovoked (6 mo if no bleeding risk, 3 mo if bleeding risk)
  - If strong contraindications to A/C: SVC filter until bleeding risk resolves
  - Isolated distal DVT: Tx as above if severe sx or e/o extension on repeat U/S (1–2 wk)

Complications

- **Phlegmasia alba dolens:** Emergent complication; P/w swollen white leg 2/2 extensive DVT obstructing collaterals (but not involving them), largely impeding arterial inflow; Tx w/ IV Heparin (in case need for surgery), +/– catheter-directed thrombolytic tx
- **Phlegmasia cerulea dolens:** Emergent complication; P/w severely swollen cyanotic leg 2/2 extensive DVT including thrombosis of collaterals & capillary beds, fully impeding arterial flow, causing massive fluid sequestration in affected limb (2/2 hydrostatic pressure), circulatory shock, death (20–40% cases); Tx w/ IV Heparin (in case need for surgery), catheter-directed thrombolytic tx, aspiration thrombectomy, or open surgical thrombectomy

PULMONARY EMBOLISM

Overview

- Definition: embolization of systemic venous thrombus into pulmonary arterial system
  - Diff from amniotic fluid embolism (RF: peripartum) & fat embolism (RF: long bone fx)
- RFs: See section on DVT above; Major identifiable RFs include recent surgery (OR 21.0), trauma (OR 12.7), immobility (hosp or nursing home) (OR 8.0), cancer (OR 4.1–6.5), paraplegia (OR 3.0), estrogen tx (OR 3.0) (JAMA 2003;290(21):2849–2858)

Approach

- IV access (if PE), ECG, O₂ prn, Monitor, CXR to r/o alternative dx
- If HD stable: diagnostic tests depending on pre-TP
- If unstable, consider empiric antithrombotic tx ± lysis if potential benefit > bleeding risk

History & Physical Exam (Chest 1991;100:598; Am J Card 1991;68:1723)

- HX: Dyspnea (73%), pleuritic CP (66%), cough (37%), syncope, ↓ BP, PEA
- Assess PreTP: May use PERC (to decide whether any testing is necessary) or Wells criteria (to decide whether D-dimer is sufficient w/u)
- EX: Unexplained ↑ HR, ↑ RR, ↓ SpO₂, fever, JVD

PERC Criteria for Pts w/ Low Risk of PE	
Age ≥ 50	Recent trauma or surgery or hosp w/i 4 wk
HR ≥ 100	Hemoptysis
O₂ Sat on room air <95%	Exogenous estrogen
Prior hx of DVT/PE	Unilateral leg swelling

Using the PERC Criteria: If any of above criteria present, PE cannot be r/o PE w/o additional dx tests. If all criteria negative, PE unlikely (Sens 97.4%, Spec 21.9%). (Thromb Haemost 2008;6:772)

Wells Criteria for PE

Criteria	Original	Modified	Simplified
Clinical signs & sx of DVT (OR 5.8)	3 pts	2 pts	1 pt
Tachycardia >100 bpm (OR 3.0)	1.5 pts	1 pt	1 pt
Immobilization or surgery w/i 4 wk (OR 2.5)	1.5 pts	1 pt	1 pt
Previous DVT/PE (OR 2.5)	1.5 pts	1 pt	1 pt
Hemoptysis (OR 2.4)	1 pt	1 pt	1 pt
Malignancy (OR 2.30	1 pt	1 pt	1 pt
PE more likely than alternative dx (OR 4.6)	3 pts	2 pts	1 pt
Cut-off for "PE unlikely" (sum of points)	≤4 pts	≤2 pts	≤1 pt

Rates of PE Based on Score

Original		Modified		Simplified	
≤4 pts	12.6%*	≤2 pts	11.5%*	≤1 pt	11.0%*
>4 pts	38.5%**	>2 pts	37.3%**	>1 pt	35.8%**

Rates of PE Based on "PE Unlikely" Score & Negative D-dimer

Original	0.5%	Modified	0.3%	Simplified	0.5%

*Order D-dimer to r/o out PE.

**Order imaging (CTA, V/Q) to r/o PE. *Thromb Haemost 2000;83(3):416–420; Thromb Haemost 2008;99(1):229–234*

Revised & Simplified Geneva Score for PE

Criteria	Revised	Simplified
Age >65	1 pt	1 pt
Previous DVT/PE	3 pts	1 pt
Surgery (under GA) or fx (LE) w/i 1 mo	2 pts	1 pt
Active malignancy or cure <1 y	2 pts	1 pt
Unilateral LE pain	3 pts	1 pt
Hemoptysis	2 pts	1 pt
HR 75–94	3 pts	1 pt
HR ≥ 95	5 pts	1 pt
Pain w/ LE deep vein palpation & unilateral edema	4 pts	1 pt
Cut-off for "PE unlikely" (sum of points)	**NA**	**≤2 pts**

Rates of PE Using Simplified Geneva Score

	≤1 pt (%)	2–4 pts (%)	5–7 pts (%)	0–2 pts (%)	3–7 pts (%)
Rate of PE	8	29	64	13	42
Rate of PE if D-dimer neg	1	3	12	1–3***	5–14******

*Order D-dimer in "PE Unlikely" to r/o PE.

**Range of rates includes both high- & low-sensitivity D-dimer.

***Order imaging (eg, CTA, V/Q) in "PE Likely" to r/o PE. *Arch Intern Med 2008;168(19):2131–2136.*

Evaluation

- ECG (Sinus tach, S1Q3T3 not sens/spec, diffuse TWI), CBC, PT/PTT, Cr
- CXR: R/o other dx; "classic" PE findings (Hampton's hump, Westermark's sign) not Sens/Spec
- Patients w/ low clinical gestalt for PE & negative PERC score may not need D-dimer
  - Combined low gestalt & PERC negative: Sens 97.4%, Spec 21.9%
- If unable to r/o by PERC criteria, compute Well's score (or modified Geneva)
- If "PE unlikely" by Well's score, obtain D-dimer (ELISA: Sens 95–98%, Spec 40–55%, NPV >99% for pts w/ low pre-TP) *JAMA 2006;295:172)*
  - Know your hospital's D-dimer test characteristics; wide variation among assays
  - False-positive D-dimer: Pregnancy, trauma, infection, malignancy, inflammatory conditions, surgery, ↑ age, SCD, AF, ACS, CVA, acute UGIB, DIC
- If "PE likely" by Well's score or D-dimer positive, obtain additional testing:
  - Bedside Ultrasound: Echo for RV dilatation (RV:LV >1) or dysfxn (hypokinesis, paradoxical septal wall motion, McConnell's sign) can suggest dx but not r/o (Sens 50%, Spec 98%, PPV 88%, NPV 88%) *(Ann Emerg Med 2014:63(1):16–24)*; combined thoracic & LE ultrasound can reduce need for CTA by dx'ing DVT or suggesting alternative dx *(Chest 2014;145(4):818–823)*
  - CT angiography (CTA Sens 83%, CTA/CTV Sens 90%, Spec 95%): *(NEJM 2006;354:2317)*
    - May miss small/subsegmental PEs (of uncertain clinical significance if asx w/ no further clot burden on LENIs); If negative for PE but suspicion is high, consider additional test (D-dimer, US, pulmonary angiogram); requires dye load (relative CI if CrCl <50 *NEJM 2006;354:379)*

- V/Q scan (if CI to CTA): Requires nl baseline CXR; tx if results are high-probability; 2/3 of all cases may result in low/intermediate probability
- MR angiography (MRA Sens 78%, Spec 99%; MRA/MRV Sens 92%, Spec 96%): Use in pts w/ CI to CTA; high proportion of studies limited qual (Ann Intern Med 2010;152(7):434–443)
- Pulmonary angiogram: Gold standard, though rarely used
- Risk stratify: ↑ HR, ↓ BP, ↓ SpO₂, CTA RV/LV dimension >0.9, ↑ Tn or BNP, echo e/o RV dysfxn, D-dimer >4,000 all predict bad outcomes

Treatment

- Supportive: O₂, IV fluids for ↓ BP (preload dep)
- Anticoagulation regimen should be selected based on comorbidities, ability to take PO medications, patient preference (monitoring, etc.), risks of bleeding:
  - SC LMWH (1 mg/kg BID; renally dose): slight ↓ risk of death, recurrence, major bleeding c/w UFH; preferred w/ malignancy; relative CIs include CKD & obesity
  - SC Fondaparinux (5 mg QD [<50kg], 7.5 mg QD [50–100 kg], 10 mg QD [>100 kg]; renally dose): Similar risk of death, recurrence, major bleeding c/w LMWH; preferred w/ hx of HIT
  - IV UFH (80 U/kg bolus, 18 U/kg/h gtt): As above, may be preferred over LMWH if CKD/ESRD; risk of HIT higher than LMWH
  - PO Warfarin (INR 2.0–3.0): Bridge w/ LMWH/Fondaparinux until INR therapeutic
  - PO Rivaroxaban (15 mg BID × 3 wk, 20 mg QD thereafter)
  - PO Apixaban (10 mg BID × 7 d, 5 mg BID thereafter)
- IV thrombolysis (tPA: 100 mg over 2 h): Indicated if massive PE / HD instability (SBP <90 mmHg), HD unstable & might suspicion of PE, or submassive PE w/ high risk of hypotension (e/o significant pHTN or RV dysfxn)
  - Submassive PE: tPA + UFH ↓ mortality & deterioration c/w UFH alone (NEJM 2002;347:1143–1150)
  - Consider lytics in unexplained PEA arrest if possibly 2/2 massive PE
- Catheter or surgical thrombectomy (PE): For pts w/ HD instability & massive PE if (1) CI to lysis, (2) failed lysis w/ tPA, or (3) experienced center & +RV dysfxn. Consult cardiac surgery; improved outcomes c/w UFH alone (Circulation 2014;129:479–486)
- IVC filter: When a/c fails or CI; no long-term mortality benefit (NEJM 1998;338:409).

Disposition

- HD stable, few comorbidities, no e/o RV strain: Observation Unit for A/C, LENIs, echo
- HD stable, comorbidities, e/o RV strain: Admit, tele floor
- HD unstable, mx comorbidities, e/o RV strain: Admit, ICU

DECOMPENSATED HEART FAILURE

Overview

- Heart failure: Any chronic state in which the heart's ability to pump blood w/ nl efficiency to meet the body's metabolic demands is impaired; either 2/2 ↓ systolic fxn (reduced EF: HFrEF) or ↓ diastolic relaxation (preserved EF: HFpEF); can be primarily L-sided, R-sided, or biventricular; although a chronic illness, characterized by intermittent decompensation 2/2 volume disequilibrium
- Manifestations of decompensated L-sided HF: pulmonary edema (↑ PCWP 2/2 hydrostatic forces), pleural effusions (↑ PCWP 2/2 hydrostatic forces), atrial arrhythmias (↑ atrial size), systemic hypoperfusion (HFrEF: ↓ LV end-diastolic volume → ↓ contractility [once over Frank–Starling curve] → ↓ EF; HFpEF: ↓ LV end-diastolic volume 2/2 impaired relaxation → ↓ EF)
- Manifestations of decompensated R-sided HF: pleural effusions (↑ systemic venous pressure → ↑ thoracic duct / lymphatic pressure → ↓ absorption of nl pleural fluid), peripheral edema (↑ systemic venous pressure), liver dysfxn (congestion)
- Acute decompensations can occur 2/2 many causes (see table)

Common Precipitants of Acute Decompensated Heart Failure	
Medication change or nonadherence*	Hypertensive crisis (↑ afterload)
Dietary indiscretion (↑ Na)	Overdoses (βB, CCB) or toxins (EtOH)
Myocardial infarct/ischemia	Myopericarditis, endocarditis
Tachyarrhythmia (eg, AF)	Sepsis
COPD/PE (↑ RH pressures)	Valvular heart dz (see table at end of section)
Renal failure (↑ volume)	Structural heart dz (see table at end of section)

*Especially diuretics, anti-HTN, or rate-controlling agents; however, review any med changes, as may have pharmacokinetic properties that affect cardiac meds

Approach
- Initiate immediately: IV access, O_2 PRN, ECG, Monitor, CXR
- If e/o severe respiratory distress, early CPAP/BiPAP, NTG gtt (unless ↓ BP)
- Early use of bedside U/S (thoracic & echo) can reduce time to dx

History & Physical Exam
- HX: SOB/DOE, CP, cough (clear → pink sputum), orthopnea/PND, LE/abd swelling
  - Always ask: timing (acuity), severity (fxnal capacity), behavioral chgs (sleeping upright), chg in home O_2, frequency of wt monitoring & any change from dry wt
  - Always assess for possible precipitants (see table above)
- EX: ↑ BP, ↑ HR, ↑ RR, cardiac dysrhythmia; +S3 (HFrEF) +S4 (HFpEF); Rales or ↓ BS, wheeze (L-sided); Leg edema, JVD, ↑ liver size, +hepatojugular reflex (R-sided)

Acute Decompensated HF: Value of Specific Hx Components			_(JAMA 2005;294:1944)_
Increase Likelihood of ADHF		**Decrease Likelihood of ADHF**	
Historical Factor	**Likelihood Ratio (95% CI)**	**Historical Factor**	**Likelihood Ratio (95% CI)**
H/o heart failure	5.8 (4.1–8)	No h/o HF	0.45 (0.38–0.53)
H/o MI	3.1 (2–4.9)	No DOE	0.48 (0.35–0.67)
PND	2.6 (1.5–4.5)		
Orthopnea	2.2 (1.2–3.9)		
Historical Features w/ Minimal Diagnostic Utility			
H/o CAD, HLD, DM, HTN, COPD, smoking. Sxs of edema, cough, fatigue, & weight gain.			

Acute Decompensated HF: Value of Specific PEx Components			_(JAMA 2005;294:1944)_
Increase Likelihood of ADHF		**Decrease Likelihood of ADHF**	
Exam Factor	**Likelihood Ratio (95% CI)**	**Exam Factor**	**Likelihood Ratio (95% CI)**
S_3 on auscultation	11 (4.9–25)	No rales	0.51 (0.37–0.7)
JVD	5.1 (3.2–7.9)		
Rales	2.8 (1.9–4.1)		
Any murmur	2.6 (1.7–4.1)		
LE edema	2.3 (1.5–3.7)		
Exam Features w/ Minimal Diagnostic Utility			
Abdominojugular reflex, SBP <100 mmHg or >150 mmHg, wheezing, ascites			

Evaluation
- Acute decompensated HF is primarily a clinical dx, aided by lab & imaging evaluations
- ECG: L-atrial enlargement, LVH, tachyarrhythmia, ischemia, e/o old infarction(s)
- Labs: CBC, lytes, Cr, troponin, LFTs, VBG, BNP/NT-proBNP (see below)
- Bedside thoracic U/S (Sens 94%, Spec 92%): >3 B-lines/field in 2+ fields bilaterally (Acad Emerg Med 2014;21(8):843–852); operator-dependent (some studies w/ Sens as low as 60%), but w/ skilled operator may be superior to CXR in dx of L-sided HF (Chest 2015;148(1):202–210); BSUS also used to eval for other dx:
  - Pleural effusions (2/2 CHF or other dx)
  - Focal B-lines (eg, 2/2 PNA, infarct > asymmetric pulm edema)
  - Reduced EF & pericardial effusion
  - IVC inspiratory collapsibility: <50% collapsibility w/ inspiration suggests volume overload; cannot be used if pt on PPV (Am J Emerg Med 2015;33(5):653–657)
- CXR (Sens 70%, Spec 82%): Pulm edema, pl effusion, ↑ heart size (Chest 2015;148(1):202–210)
- BNP (>100 ng/L), NT-proBNP (>300 ng/L): Imp to compare w/ dry weight BNP if hx of CHF; levels correlate w/ dz severity (NHYA) of underlying CHF (NEJM 2002;347:161–167)
  - False-negatives: Obesity (Int J Cardiol 2014;176(3):611–617)
  - False-positives: Large PE, cor pulmonale, ESRD, AMI
  - NT-proBNP may also be elevated w/ ↑ age; higher cut-offs suggested (>900 ng/mL if over 50 y)

Pooled Sensitivity & Specificity of BNP/NT-proBNP for Acute Decompensated HF					
BNP Level	**Sens (%)**	**Spec (%)**	**NT-proBNP Level**	**Sens (%)**	**Spec (%)**
≤100 ng/L	95	63	≤300 ng/L	99	43
100–500 ng/L	85	86	300–1800 pg/ml	90	76
≥500 ng/L	35	78	≥1800 ng/L	67	72

Based on pooled meta-analysis of 42 studies. _BMJ 2015;350:h910._

Treatment

- **Diuresis (↓ volume):** Patients w/ refractory edema have impaired PO absorption & may need IV diuresis; give 2× home dose in IV form (see conversions below); give home nonloop diuretics (eg, metolazone) for sequential nephron blockade (NEJM 2010;362(3):228–238)
  - Conversions: Furosemide:Torsemide:Bumetanide 40:10:1; Furosemide (PO:IV) 2:1; Torsemide (PO:IV) 1:1; Bumetanide (PO:IV) 1:1
  - If allergy to furosemide/torsemide/bumetanide, can use ethacrynic acid
- **Nitrates (↓ preload):** Nitrates (0.4 mg SL or 10–300 mcg/min IV): Caution in pts w/ AS → ↓ BP 2° preload dep; nitroprusside if NTG ineffective; nesiritide if ↑ Cr/ mortality compared to noninotropic tx (JAMA 2005;293:1900)
- **Positive Pressure Ventilation:** CPAP/BiPAP for ↓ SaO₂ (if no CIs); ↓ mortality, ↓ need for intubation (JAMA 2005;294:3124; Lancet 2006;367:1155); Intubate profound AMS, resp failure
- **Inotropes:** Cardiogenic shock (see section on Shock)
- **Other:** Positioning (sit up > supine), Foley may be necessary to assess ins/outs, IABP/LVAD (severe cardiogenic shock)

Disposition

- Mild exacerbation, benign etiology (ie, dietary indiscretion), & close f/u: Discharge after discussion w/ cardiologist; may ↑ diuretic for a few days
- Selected HF pts can be managed by a rapid tx protocol in the Observation Unit w/ fewer bed days & similar readmission rates to admitted pts (Acad Emerg Med 2013;20(6):554)
- Most pts require admission/∆s to tx regimen before d/c home: Cardiology/Tele
- All pts on PPV or severe resp distress: ICU

Structural Causes of Heart Failure	
Dilated CMP	**Pathophys:** Ventricular dilatation → ↓ contractility → ↑ EDV → ↓ EF **Causes:** Idiopathic, familial, ischemia, valvular, infxn (Chagas), EtOH, cocaine, autoimmune **Presentation:** L or R HF sx; embolic events; arrhythmia **Evaluation:** ECG (PRWP, Qw, BBB, AF), CXR (↑ heart size), Echo (LV dilatation, ↓ EF, LV ± RV HK) **Treatment:** See standard HF tx below **Pearl:** Always consider in chronic EtOH users w/ SOB
Hypertrophic CMP	**Pathophys:** LV outflow tract obstruction, worse if ↓ EDV → ↓ EF **Causes:** 50% are familial; asymmetric septal hypertrophy (eg, 2/2 HTN) may result in HOCM physiology (not true HOCM) **Presentation:** SOB/angina; arrhythmias; sudden death **Evaluation:** Systolic crescendo/decrescendo murmur; ECG (LVH, septal Qw), CXR (↑ heart size), Echo (↑ septal thickness) **Treatment:** βB, CCB (verapamil) **Pearl:** Avoid diuretics/preload reduction (inc PPV), digoxin, exercise
Restrictive CMP	**Pathophys:** ↓ compliance → ↓ EDV → ↓ EF **Causes:** Amyloidosis, sarcoidosis, hemochromatosis, XRT, cancer **Presentation:** R > L HF; embolic events; poor response to diuretics **Evaluation:** ↑ JVP, S3, S4, ECG (low voltage), CXR (pulm edema w/o ↑ heart size), Echo (symmetric wall thickening, LAE/RAE) **Treatment:** Treat underlying cause, gentle diuresis
Constrictive pericarditis	**Pathophys:** ↓ compliance → ↓ EDV → ↓ EF **Causes:** Postviral, XRT, TB, Postcardiac surgery, idiopathic **Presentation:** R > L HF **Evaluation:** ↑ JVP, pericardial knock; Echo (septal bounce) **Treatment:** Diuresis, pericardiotomy

Valvular Heart Disease	
Aortic Stenosis	**Causes:** Calcification (age >70 y), bicuspid valve, rheumatic heart dz **Presentation:** Angina, syncope, CHF **Exam:** Midsystolic, crescendo–decrescendo @ RUSB **Eval:** Echo (transvalvular velocity, EF, AVA) **Acute tx:** ↓ Afterload; minimize ↓ preload & negative inotropy; if severe acute HF decompensation 2/2 critical AS, c/s cardiac surg for consideration of urgent AVR **Pearl:** Indications for AVR (if sx) include: V_{max} ≥4 m/s; V_{max} <4 m/s + EF<50% + AVA ≤1.0 cm²; or V_{max} <4 m/s + AVA ≤0.6 cm² (NEJM 2014;372:744–756)

Aortic Regurg	**Causes:** Rheumatic heart dz, bicuspid valve, endocarditis, HTN **Presentation:** Acute or chronic CHF **Exam:** Diastolic decrescendo murmur, wide pulse pressure **Eval:** Echo: Severity of AI → width of regurgitant jet **Acute tx:** ↓ Afterload (nifedipine, ACEi); vasodilators ± dobutamine; if severe & unstable, c/s cardiac surg for consideration of urgent AVR **Pearl:** Limited data on mortality benefit of AVR; indications for AVR mostly based on sx severity (NYHA III/IV) *(NEJM 2004;351:1539–1546)*
Mitral Stenosis	**Causes:** Rheumatic heart dz **Presentation:** Pulmonary edema, AF, Emboli **Exam:** Diastolic murmur, opening snap **Eval:** ECG (LAE), Echo (valve area, pressure gradients) **Acute tx:** Careful diuresis, βBs; however percutaneous balloon valvuloplasty (PBV) & MVR have best outcomes **Pearl:** Most have sx if MVA <1 cm²; MVR/PBV based on sx (NYHA III/IV sx [+/– NYHA II]); PBV favorable c/w MVR, but 10–40% may have delayed re-stenosis & require repeat *(Lancet 2009;374:1271–1283)*
Mitral Regurg	**Causes:** MVP, endocarditis, rheumatic heart dz, ruptured chordae, papillary muscle dysfxn **Presentation:** Pulmonary edema **Exam:** Blowing holosystolic murmur **Eval:** ECG (LAE), Echo (width of regurgitant jet) **Acute tx:** Vasodilators (ACEi), βB; however, MVR is only intervention w/ proven outcome benefit *(Lancet 2009;373:1382–1394)*

AORTIC DISSECTION

Overview
- **Definition:** Any extent of tearing of the aortic *tunica intima* that enables blood to enter into & traverse the aortic wall b/w *tunica intima* & *tunica media* layers
  - Intramural "false lumen" can obstruct nl flow in true aortic lumen, including critical vascular branches (esp carotid, celiac, sup/inf mesenteric, renal, & spinal arteries)
  - Can also manifest w/ penetrating ulcer, pseudoaneurysm, & traumatic rupture
- Classification of dissection impacts management & prognosis (see table)

Prognosis for Aortic Dissection *(IRAD, JAMA 2000;283:897)*					
Stanford Type	% of Cases	Anatomical Distribution	Organs at Risk	Prognosis w/ Medical Tx	Prognosis w/ Surgical Tx
Type A	62%	Ascending aorta +/– descending	Brain Coronary Art Spinal cord Abd/kidneys Legs	58%	26%
Type B	38%	Descending aorta w/o ascending	Spinal cord Abd/kidneys Legs	10.7%	31%

Approach
- Immediate IV, ECG, pCXR, Analgesia, BP control (if HTN)
- Consult cardiothoracic surgery early, esp for type A dissection if clinically suspected
- Attention to extent of dissection, size of T/F lumens, involvement of branches, presence of periaortic/mediastinal hematoma or pleural effusion

Risk Factors for Aortic Dissection *(Circulation 2010;121:e266)*	
Mechanism	Associated Disorders
↑ Aortic wall stress	Hypertension, cocaine/stimulant use, extreme valsalva (eg, power lifting), blunt trauma/deceleration injury, aortic coarctation, pheochromocytoma
Vulnerability of Ao wall	Genetic disorders (Ehlers–Danlos, Marfan, Turner, Loeys–Dietz, Noonan syndromes, congenital bicuspid valve, familial dissection), inflammatory vasculitides (SLE, GCA, Behçet's), infectious vasculitides (syphilis, TB)
Iatrogenic wall injury	Cardiac/valve surgery, IABP use, aortic cannulation, cath
Other	Male, >50 y/o, pregnancy, PCKD, chronic steroids, immunosupp

History & Physical Exam

- Individual elements of hx in isolation notoriously insensitive &/or nonspecific (see table)
- HX: Abrupt onset & often worst-ever CP (ascending), interscapular back pain (descending), or neck pain; often maximal at onset, ripping/tearing in quality, & can migrate; can be a/w syncope, neurologic deficits
  - Note that up to 10% of pts may not p/w pain
  - As for RFs & consider in all blunt trauma pts w/ CP or back pain
- EX: Check for murmur, B/L UE BP asymmetry >20 mmHg (↓ Sens, but ominous finding), pulse deficit (27% of pts), neurologic deficits including Horner syndrome, abd pain +/- guaiac exam (+ result can suggest bowel ischemia), flank pain

	Aortic Dissection: Frequency of History, Exam, & CXR Findings			
	Component	Overall (%)	Type A (%)	Type B (%)
History	Severe/worst-ever pain	90	90	90
History	Abrupt onset of pain	90	91	89
History	Chest or back pain	85	85	86
History	Pain presenting w/i 6 h of sx	—	79	—
History	Abdominal pain	30	22	43
Exam	Hypertension at presentation	49	36	69
Exam	Hypotension, shock, or tamponade	18	27	3
Exam	Any focal neuro deficit	12	17	5
Exam	Any pulse deficit	27	31	21
Exam	Aortic regurgitation	32	44	12
CXR	CXR w/ widened mediastinum	60	63	56
CXR	CXR w/ abnl aortic contour	48	47	49
CXR	CXR nl	16	11	21

IRAD, Circulation 2004;110(suppl1):237–242. Lancet 2008;372:55–66.

Aortic Dissection: Sensitivity of Components of History			
	Sens (95% CI)		Sens (95% CI)
Hx of HTN	64% (54–72)	Hx of Marfan syndrome	5% (4–7)
Any pain	90% (85–94)	Back pain	32% (19–47)
Chest pain	67% (56–77)	Abdominal pain	23% (16–31)
Anterior chest pain	57% (48–66)	Syncope	9% (8–12)
Posterior chest pain	32% (24–40)		
Severe pain	90% (88–92)	Ripping/Tearing pain	39% (14–69)
Sudden-onset pain	84% (80–89)	Migrating pain	31% (12–55)

IRAD, JAMA 2002;287(17):2262.

Evaluation

- ECG: Assess for inf-STEMI (Type A dissection can involve RCA; ~4–8% of thoracic dissections will present w/ signs of STEMI), LVH (e/o chronic HTN)
  - In pts w/ inferior STEMI, consider Type A dissection always
- Labs: Type & Cross, CBC, Lytes, Cr (↑ w/ renal ischemia), Troponin, Lactate (↑ w/ any ischemia, ↑↑ suggests abd viscera ischemia), PT/PTT
- CXR: may be nl in 20%; characteristic findings include wide mediastinum, abnl aortic knob, L apical cap, trachea shift → R, depressed L bronchus, L pl effusion
- Combined use of D-dimer & Aortic Detection (ADD) Risk Score: Early data support combined use of ADD & D-dimer; ADD <1 & neg D-dimer can r/o AoD (Sens 100%, NPV 100%); ADD 1 & neg D-dimer also very high Sens (98.7%) & NPV (99.2%), & likely improved further if CXR nl (60% of pts w/ AoD have wide mediastinum) (see table)
  - D-dimer not appropriate in pts w/ ADD 2–3, given ↓ Sens & ↓↓ Spec
- Bedside cardiac US: Limited data suggest high diagnostic utility (Sens 88%, Spec 94%), esp in conjunction w/ ADD 0 (Sens 96%, Spec 98%); positive study includes any of following findings: intimal flap, intramural hematoma, ascending Ao dilatation, AV insuff, pericardial effusion; operator-dependent (*Intern Emerg Med 2014;9(6):665–670*)
  - May be most useful in low-risk pts w/ chronically elevated D-dimer (eg, cancer, age)
- Definitive diagnostic modalities: TEE (Sens 98%, Spec 95%), CTA (Sens 100%, Spec 98%), MRI (Sens 98%, Spec 98%) (*Arch Intern Med 2006;166:1350–1356*)

Aortic Dissection Detection (ADD) Risk Score

High Risk Conditions	High Risk Pain Features	High Risk Exam Features
• Marfan syndrome • FHx aortic dz • Known AoV dz • Recent aortic manipulation • Known thoracic AA	• Chest, back, or abd pain described as: • Abrupt in onset • Severe in intensity • Ripping or tearing	• Evidence of perfusion deficit (pulse deficit, SBP differential) • Focal neuro deficit in conjunction w/ pain) • Hypotension/shock

Test Characteristics of ADD & Combined Approach Using ADD + D-Dimer

No. ADD High Risk Categories Present	ADD Alone* Sens (%)	ADD Combined w/ D-Dimer** Sens (%)	Spec (%)	NPV (%)	PPV (%)
0 (Low risk)	95.7*	100	30.4	100	8.3
1 (Int risk)	63.5	98.7	35.7	99.2	25.6
2–3 (High risk)	40.8	97.5	37.1	95.8	50.3

*Note that half (48.6%) of low-risk pts with AoD in derivation data had widened mediastinum on CXR. *Circulation* 2011;123:2213–18.

**Int J Cardiol 2014;175:78–82.

Diagnostic Characteristics of Advanced Imaging for AD (Arch Intern Med 2006;166:1350)

Imaging Study	Sensitivity	Specificity	+LR	−LR
TEE	98% (95–99%)	95% (92–97%)	14.1 (6–33)	0.04 (0.02–0.08)
CTA	100% (96–100%)	98% (87–99%)	14 (4.2–46)	0.02 (0.01–0.11)
MRI	98% (95–99%)	98% (95–100%)	24 (11–57)	0.05 (0.03–0.10)

Treatment (Lancet 2008;372:55–66)
- In general, surgical tx preferred for Type A, medical tx for Type B
- Tx revolves around close BP & HR control; Goal HR 60–80, SBP 100–120
  - First-line: IV BB gtt preferred to bolus (esmolol, labetalol)
  - Second-line (CI to BB, need for further control): IV CCB gtt (eg, nicardipine, diltiazem)
  - If refractory HTN/tachy: Vasodilator (nitroprusside)
  - A-line for close monitoring (pref RUE or farthest from false lumen)
- Analgesia: Short-acting narcotics preferred in case of hemodynamic changes
- Urgent surgical consultation should be obtained (cardiac surgery for Type A, vascular surgery for Type B) for all pts diagnosed w/ thoracic aortic dissection regardless of the location as soon as the Dx is made or suspected
  - Type A: Evaluate for emergent surgical repair (1–2% mortality/h in 1st 24 h)
  - Type B: Manage medically w/ consideration for endovascular repair (esp if e/o mal-perfusion, enlarging aneurysm, inability to control BP/sx)

Disposition
- All patients w/ acute aortic dissection are admitted to ICU (+/− via OR)

THORACIC AORTIC ANEURYSM

Overview
- Nl aortic diameter ↑ w/ age, sex (M > F), body surface area, imaging modality
- **Thoracic Aortic Aneurysm:** Permanent localized of aortic wall dilatation involving all 3 layers (tunica intima, tunica media, tunica externa) & reaching 1.5 × nl aortic diameter; dilatation b/w >1 & <1.5 × nl dilatation referred to as ectatic.
- **Thoracic Aortic Pseudoaneurysm:** See TAA, but involves <3 aortic wall layers
- Can occur at the aortic root (annular aortic ectasia) &/or ascending aorta (50%), descending aorta (40%), aortic arch (10%), or thoracoabdominal aorta (10%)
  - Up to ~25% of pts w/ TAA may also have an AAA
- Most TAAs are caused by degenerative dz resulting in dilation of the aorta
- RFs: See section on Aortic Dissection (see above)
- Complications vary based on diameter; average rate of expansion 0.10–0.42 cm/y

Yearly Complication Rates as a Function of Aortic Size (Ann Thorac Surg 2002;74:S1877)

Aortic Size	>3.5 cm (%)	>4 cm (%)	>5 cm (%)	>6 cm (%)
Rupture	0	0.3	1.7	3.6
Dissection	2.2	1.5	2.5	3.7
Death	5.9	4.6	4.8	10.8
Any of above	7.2	5.3	6.5	14.1

History, Physical Exam, & Evaluation

- HX: Often discovered incidentally on imaging; sx can vary widely:
  - Compressive sx: Hoarseness (compression of recurrent laryngeal nerve), stridor (compression of trachea/bronchi), dyspnea (lung compression), dysphagia (esophageal compression), plethora/edema (SVC compression)
  - Heart failure sx: May occur 2/2 aortic regurgitation
  - Embolization of atherosclerotic debris w/ end-organ sxs may occur
  - May lead to dissection (see Aortic Dissection section) or rupture
- EX: May have nl exam; see Aortic Dissection section exam above
- Imaging: CTA (Good Sens, quick, noninvasive); MRI (best for Ao Root); TTE (limited for eval of Ao Root or descending TA); TEE (Better than TTE for Ao Root & descending TA)

Treatment

- Risk factor modification: Lipid profile optimization, smoking cessation, BP control (BB, ACEi), avoid intense exercise or valsalva
- Urgent open vs. endovascular repair as indicated (see table)

Indications for Urgent Cardiac Surgical Consultation *(Circulation 2010;121:e266)*
• Asymptomatic pts w/ degenerative TAAs, chronic aortic dissection, intramural hematoma, penetrating atherosclerotic ulcer, mycotic aneurysm, or pseudoaneurysm for whom the ascending aorta or aortic sinus diameter is ≥5.5 cm
• Pts w/ Marfan syndrome or other genetically mediated disorders (see above) for whom the ascending aorta or aortic sinus diameter is 4–5 cm
• Pts who have a growth rate of more than 0.5 cm/y in an aorta that is <5.5 cm
• Pts w/ sxs suggestive of expansion of TAA

Disposition

- Admit: Patients meeting indications for urgent repair, symptomatic patients
- Discharge (w/ vascular/cardiac surgery f/u): Pts w/ large but asx (ie, incidental) TAA
- Discharge (w/ PCP f/u for surgery referral): Pts w/ small & asx (ie, incidental) TAA
- All discharged pts: DC w/ RF modification (eg, improved BP control) & serial monitoring

ACUTE PERICARDITIS

Definition *(NEJM 2014;371(25):2410–2416)*

- Acute inflammatory dz of the pericardium due to a variety of causes:
  - Idiopathic (80% in developed nations)—Presumed post-viral
  - Infectious (TB, fungal, less likely staph/strep)
  - Post-MI (Dressler's)
  - Systemic dz (cancer, connective tissue d/o, myxedema, uremia)
  - Trauma or treatment (postsurgical, XRT, posttraumatic)
- Dx requires the absence of more likely cause of CP (eg, ACS, etc.) & ≥2 of the following:
  1. Characteristic CP (see below)
  2. Pericardial friction rub (high pitched, scratch sound heard best at left sternal border)
  3. Suggestive ECG findings (see below)
  4. New or worsening pericardial effusion
- Can be relapsing in 10–30%: Incessant (d/c of tx or attempts to wean cause relapse in <6 wk) or intermittent (symptom-free intervals >6 wk, but recurs)
- Can be a/w pericardial effusion w/ or w/o tamponade, or can be constrictive

History & Physical Exam

- HX: Characteristic CP—Sudden onset, retrosternal, pleuritic, positional (better w/ leaning forward or upright); pain can radiate to neck, arms, shoulders similar to ACS
  - Ask about recent viral illness
  - May have low-grade fever, SOB, dysphagia
- EX: Friction rub (high pitched, scratch sound heard best at LLSB apex), ↑ HR, ↑ RR, nl BP

Evaluation

- ECG: findings occur in 4 stages (see table), generally characterized by diffuse STE & PR depressions, though subtle PR depressions may be only sign
  - Assess for electrical alternans (suggests pericardial tamponade, see next section)

Stages of ECG Changes in Pericarditis		
Stage 1	Acute	ST ↑ I, V5, V6; reciprocal STD aVR & V1 PR ↓ II, aVF, V4–V6; PR ↑ Avr
Stage 2	Early resolution	Normalization of ST & PR segments
Stage 3	Late resolution	TWI I, V5, V6 which can be widespread
Stage 4	Complete resolution	Normalization of ECG

- Labs: CBC, BUN/Cr (r/o uremia), LFTs, ESR/CRP (↑ CRP in 75%), cardiac enzymes (as much as 1/3 cases a/w myocarditis) *(NEJM 2014;371(25):2410–2416)*
  - Further testing unnecessary unless WBC >13 k, T >38.5 F, or comorbidities or hx suggests specific underlying cause; PRN TSH, serologies (infxn, inflam)
- CXR: r/o other dx; can see cardiomegaly if >250 cc pericardial effusion
- Bedside echo: Assess for (1) pericardial effusion, (2) tamponade physiology (late diastolic collapse of RA, persistence of RA collapse >1/3 cardiac cycle, early diastolic collapse of RV, collapse of LA, dilated IVC w/ <50% respiratory collapse)
- Although not routinely indicated, CT & MRI can help make dx (pericardial thickening)

Treatment
- Pharmacologic tx is mainstay:
  - NSAIDs: Ibuprofen (600–800 mg q6h–q8h), Indomethacin (25–50 mg q8h), aspirin (2–4 g qd in divided doses) x 1–2 wk; Give w/ PPI for gastric protection
    - ASA preferred among NSAIDs in early post-MI period
  - Colchicine (0.5 mg QD if ≤70 kg; 0.5 mg BID if >70 kg): Used in conjunction w/ NSAIDs; c/w placebo, ↓ risk of recurrence & persistent sx at 72 h by 50% *(NEJM 2013;369:1522–1528)*
    - Use cautiously in CKD, hepatobiliary dz, bleeding dyscrasias, GI motility d/o
    - In conjunction w/ NSAIDs, usually improves sx w/i 1–3 d
  - Steroids (prednisone 1 mg/kg/d w/ slow taper after 2–4 wk): First-line for autoimmune or uremic etiologies, or those who fail NSAID or colchicine therapy; may ↑ risk of recurrence (COPE, *Circulation* 2005;112:2012).
  - Optimal duration of tx unclear: 3 mo course recommended *(NEJM 2013;369:1522–1528)*
- Tx underlying condition PRN (abx, dialysis, chemo, etc.)
- Pericardiocentesis indicated for purulent (postsurgical, TB, etc.) or neoplastic pericarditis
- Cardiology consult: If tamponade/echo is being considered
- CT surgery consult: Recent cardiac surgery or if pericardial window needed

Disposition
- 85% of pts can be discharged home
- Admit anyone w/ HD abnlty, myocarditis, uremia, large effusion

CARDIAC TAMPONADE

Overview
- Definition: A life-threatening state in which intrapericardial pressure (2/2 fluid, blood, pus) > RVEDP → ↓ LV preload → ↓ LVEDP → equilibration of L & R heart pressures → ↓ CO
- Tamponade more related to rate of fluid accumulation than volume of fluid
- Can be caused by blood (Type A AoD, post-MI free wall rupture, postsurgical, trauma), or fluid (myxedema, uremia, malignancy, SLE, XRT)

History & Physical Exam
- HX: If atraumatic, can p/w progressive SOB/DOE, orthopnea, PND, CP, LH, AMS, weakness; Traumatic usually w/ gross penetrating wound or blunt aortic injury
- EX: ↑ HR, ↑ RR, **Beck's triad** (↓ BP, distended neck veins, muffled heart sounds), narrow pulse pressure, pulsus paradoxus (see below)

Performing Pulsus Paradoxus Test: Assessing the Reversed Bernheim Effect

- Using a sphygmomanometer, inflate the cuff to 20 mmHg above systolic pressure, then deflate until the 1st Korotkoff sound is heard, which you should only hear during expiration. Record this number. Next, deflate the cuff until Korotkoff sounds are heard equally during both inspiration & expiration. Subtract this number from the 1st.
- If the difference b/w these 2 numbers is >10 mmHg, the pt has a pulsus paradoxus of a magnitude equal to that difference
- DDx: Cardiac tamponade, severe asthma/COPD, PE, constrictive pericarditis

Evaluation
- ECG: Low voltage, electrical alternans, ±signs of pericarditis
- CXR: Globular heart, but may be nl if rapid accumulation (eg, trauma)
- Bedside Echo: Can confirm dx; effusion (can be variable size) w/ septal shift, late diastolic collapse of RA, persistence of RA collapse >1/3 cardiac cycle, early diastolic collapse of RV, collapse of LA, dilated IVC w/ <50% respiratory collapse
- Pericardial fluid: If atraumatic, consider sending fluid culture & Gram stain, BUN, Cr, ANA, RF, malignancy screen/cytology

Treatment

- IVF Bolus: Preload dependent state; ↑ preload to RV causes ↑ RVEDP > intrapericardial pressure → ↑ LV preload → ↑ CO
  - Preload is purely temporizing to pericardiocentesis; ultimately, w/ excess preload pts will develop pulm edema & hypoxia; any need for PPV must be avoided at all costs given profound effect on ↓ preload
- Pericardiocentesis: cardiac tamponade w/ HD compromise requires urgent drainage (bedside if unstable; preferred in OR if time)

Disposition

- Admit all patients w/ cardiac tamponade. If drained effectively & stable, can be admx to tele floor (ie, cardiology). If admitted while awaiting drainage, ICU.

MYOCARDITIS

Overview

- Definition: Acute lymphocytic inflammatory dz of the myocardium of varying severity ranging from subclinical dz to fulminant systolic failure & death
- Frequently a/w viral infections (coxsackie, enterovirus, adenovirus), Chagas dz, toxins/meds (cocaine, lithium, doxorubicin), SLE, scleroderma

History & Physical Exam

- HX: Dyspnea (72%), CP (32%), arrhythmias (18%); May have systemic sxs including fever, arthralgia, malaise; Can present similar to HFrEF
- EX: Ranges from subtle signs of systolic dysfxn (crackles, LE edema) to fulminant respiratory failure (JVD, tachypnea, dec BS, LE edema), arrhythmia, or cardiac arrest

Evaluation

- ECG: Sinus tach, STE/STD/NSSTW Δs, VT/VF, heart block, Δs of pericarditis (see above)
- CXR: ↑ cardiac size
- Labs: Cardiac enzymes (Troponin > CKMB; 34% Sens, 89% Spec; ↑ Sens w/↑ extent of dz), BNP, CBC w/diff (can see eosinophilia), ↑ ESR/CRP (NEJM 2009;360:1526–1538)
- Cardiac MRI: Useful for establishing definitive dx &/or planning bx

Treatment

- Largely supportive; treat CHF, cardiogenic shock, or arrhythmias

SYNCOPE

Overview

- Definition (syncope): Loss of consciousness & postural tone arising from an abrupt drop in cerebral perfusion w/ spontaneous recovery.
- Definition (pre-syncope, near-syncope): As above, but sxs resolve before complete LOC or loss of tone; may experience AMS & weakness before return to nl
- Objective in ED is to distinguish from other causes of sudden LOC, & differentiate benign etiologies from those requiring further eval or tx (see table)

Common or Concerning Causes of Syncope	
Primary Cardiac Etiologies	
Tachydysrhythmia	**Mechanism:** ↑ HR (eg, VT, AF, AT, SVT, WPW), ↓ LVEDV, ↓ CO; **HX:** May be unheralded or prodrome of LH, CP, palp, diaphoresis, nausea, SOB; **DX:** ECG, Tele, o/p cardiac monitor; **TX:** rhythm-specific; **DISPO:** Admx
Bradydysrhythmia	**Mechanism:** ↓ HR (eg, SSS, BB, CCB, Heart block esp 3°), ↓ CO; **HX:** May be unheralded or prodrome of LH, CP, weakness, diaphoresis, nausea, SOB; **DX:** ECG, Tele, o/p cardiac monitor; **TX:** rhythm-specific; **DISPO:** Admx, may need PPM
Valvular Heart dz (usually AoS)	**Mechanism:** ↓ Preload w/ fixed severe AS, ↓ CO; **HX:** May be unheralded, often a/w position (standing), dehydration, dysrhythmia (↓ CO), can have chronic DOE/known AoS; **DX:** Murmur, echo; **TX:** Optimize preload, AVR; **DISPO:** Admx (see Valvular Ht Dz table)
HFrEF (eg, post-MI)	**Mechanism:** ↓ EF (esp if ↑ neg inotropic med); **HX:** Weakness, DOE, PND/orthopnea, recent MI or hx HF, med Δs; **DX:** Echo; **TX:** HF optimization (↓ afterload, ↓ preload if not hypovolemic, +/– ↑ inotropy); **DISPO:** Admx for med optimization. (see CHF section)

HOCM	**Mechanism:** ↑ HR, ↑ EDV, ↓↓ SV 2/2 outflow obstruction (can also ↑ risk of VT/VF); **HX:** Often a/w exercise (↑ HR), missed meds (↑ HR), or dehydration (↓ preload); **DX:** Echo; **TX:** BB, CCB, ↑ Preload; **DISPO:** Admx, may need AICD (see Cardiomyopathy table)
Tamponade	**Mechanism:** ↑ intrapericardial pressures > RV filling pressure, ↓ L-sided filling pressures, ↓ CO; **HX:** Progressive weakness, SOB, DOE, orthopnea, PND, +/− CP; **DX:** Echo; **TX:** ↑ preload, pericardiocentesis; **DISPO:** Admx (see Tamponade section)
Primary Vascular Etiologies	
Pulm Embolism	**Mechanism:** ↑ PA obstruction, ↓ L-sided preload, ↓ CO; **HX:** May be unheralded, or sudden SOB, CP, sense of doom; **DX:** Risk stratify, then: D-dimer or CTA or V/Q; **TX:** Lysis vs. anticoagulation; **DISPO:** Admx (if cause of syncope) (see PE section)
Pulm HTN	**Mechanism:** ↓ LV preload 2/2 any ↑ PVR; **HX:** Often a/w exertion, PMH of IPH, CTD, MS/MR, COPD; **ECG:** RAE, RBBB, RVH; CXR (enlarged pulm vasc, RA, RV); BNP, echo (↑ RSVP, PR/TR); cardiology c/s ± right-heart cath; **TX:** O2 (↓ hypoxic vasoconstriction), diuresis, ↑ inotropy (digoxin, dobutamine), +/− inh NO if decomp, prostacyclins, PDE5 inh, discuss w/ cardiology; **DISPO:** Admx
AoD (Type A>B)	**Mechanism:** False lumen ↓ carotid inflow, OR tamponade present; **HX:** Sudden CP, back pain; **DX:** Echo, CTA; **TX:** Emergent cardiac surgery (Type A); **DISPO:** Admx (see Aortic Dissection section)
TAA/AAA	**Mechanism:** Sudden expansion, contained leak, or rupture of AA; **HX:** Sudden but not always severe CP, back pain, flank pain, abd pain; **DX:** Abd U/S, CTA; **TX:** Optimize BP/HR, Emergent vasc surgery c/s; **DISPO:** Admx (see TAA section)
Subclavian (SCA) steal syndrome	**Mechanism:** Sudden ↓ SBP or ↑ SCA (eg, UE movement) overlying chronic prox SCA stenosis → retrograde vert artery flow ipsilaterally, ↓ postcirculation perfusion; **HX:** Can be a/w movements of affected UE, dehydration, med Δs, sometimes also w/ vertigo; **DX:** B/L SBP Δ >45 mmHg, Asymmetric pulses, CXR (1st rib), Duplex U/S, CTA, MRA; **TX:** Open or endovascular surgery; **DISPO:** Vascular c/s, Admx
Carotid stenosis	**Mechanism:** ↓ SBP (any cause) w/ chronic o/w asx carotid stenosis can ↓ cerebrovascular perfusion (if impaired autoreg), ↓ CPP & syncope; **HX:** May be unheralded, often a/w position (standing), dehydration, dysrhythmia (↓ CO); **DX:** Duplex U/S; **TX:** Optimize BP, HR, +/− o/p CEA; **DISPO:** Admx
Vertebrobasilar insufficiency	**Mechanism:** ↓ SBP (any cause) w/ chronic VB stenosis (eg, CAD) can ↓ cerebrovascular perfusion (if impaired autoreg), ↓ CPP & syncope; **HX:** May be unheralded, often a/w position (standing), dehydration, dysrhythmia (↓ CO), a/w dizziness/vertigo, dysarthria, ataxia, vision chg; **DX:** CTA, MRA, Neuro c/s; **TX:** Med mgmt of atherosclerosis, rarely surgery; **ADMX:** Admx
Non-Cardiovascular Etiologies	
Vasovagal	**Mechanism:** ↑ vagal tone a/w emotional or physiologic stressor; **HX:** Common emotional precipitants inc sight of blood, sudden emotional shock; physiologic stressors inc fatigue, long standing, warmth, n/v, coughing, swallowing, micturition, defecation; **DX:** Clinical dx, ↓ HR (sinus brady) & BP during event; **TX:** None needed; **DISPO:** Home
Carotid sinus hypersensitivity	**Mechanism:** ↑ vagal tone after mechanical pressure on carotid sinus; **HX:** often after shaving, head turning; **TX:** None indicated; **DX:** Clinical; **DISPO:** Home
Orthostatic hypotension	**Mechanism:** ↓ vascular compliance → ↓ SBP w/ position chgs; **HX:** Often elderly (stiff vessels), can be a/w GI bleed, ectopic preg; **DX:** CBC, imaging if c/f underlying condition, orthostatic VS ↓ Sens (sx w/ standing may be more helpful & Sens vs VS); **TX:** IVF, +/− blood if e/o ongoing losses; **DISPO:** Varies depending on if underlying condition identified; if none found & pt stable gait, can dc home w/ FU

Autonomic dysfxn	**Mechanism:** Impaired fxn of autonomic nervous system; **HX:** May be a/w dysfxn of other autonomic fxns (GI, bladder, sweating), may have hx of DM, EtOH, HIV, SLE, Neuro dz; check med Δs; often hx of similar episodes in the past; **DX:** Tilt table testing, c/s neurology **TX:** Tx underlying condition, salt tabs, +/– midodrine (discuss w/ cardiology & neurology); **DISPO:** Admx; can d/c w/ close o/p f/u if low-risk pt & low-frequency events
Medications	Common medications (new or ↑ dose) a/w syncope: vasodilators (α-blockers, nitrates, ACEI/ARB, CCB, hydralazine, phenothiazines, antidepressants), diuretics, negative chronotropes (BB, CCB), antiarrhythmics (class IA, IC, III), psychoactive meds (antipsych, TCAs, barbs, benzos), substances (EtOH)
Syncope mimics	Seizure,* TIA/stroke,* ICH,* migraine*

*Can mimic syncope, but not considered true syncopal events. (modified from: *NEJM* 2002;347:878; *JACC* 2006;47:473)

History & Physical Exam

- HPI: Always ask about preceding activity (inc. posture), precipitants, prodromal sxs (weakness, LH, diaphoresis, visual chgs), duration (<5 s suggests cardiac; >5 s suggests vasovagal), assoc sx (CP, palp, focal neuro deficits, HA, abd pain, nausea)
  - Differentiate from seizure: C/w seizure, syncope typically more abrupt, shorter duration, quicker return to nl (seconds–minutes), no tongue biting or incontinence, lack of rigidity; note syncope commonly can occur w/ slow & irregular myoclonic jerking mistaken as seizure/convulsive activity.
- ROS, PMH (cardiac dz, meds, & FHx (sudden cardiac death) are very important
  - High-risk hx: Older age, structural heart dz, h/o CAD
  - Lower-risk hx: Young, healthy, nonexertional, no hx or e/o cardiac dz, no FHx SCD
- EX: Guided by hx; evaluate neuro exam (inc stability w/ standing/gait), murmurs, carotid bruits, abd exam +/– guaiac

Evaluation

- ECG in all pts: Evaluate for stigmata of malignant dysrhythmia (HOCM, ARVD, Brugada syndrome, prolonged QTc, pre-excitation syndrome, coronary artery abnormalities)

Characteristic ECG Findings in Patients with Selected Cardiac Causes of Syncope	
Cardiac Dz	**ECG Findings**
Brugada syndrome (*Circulation* 2005;111:659)	• *Type I:* Coved ST-segment elevation ≥2 mm followed by a negative T wave in >1 R precordial lead (V1–V3) • *Type II:* STE w/ saddle-back appearance w/ a high takeoff STE ≥2 mm, a trough displaying STE ≥1 mm, & then either a + or biphasic T wave • *Type III:* Either saddleback or coved appearance w/ STE <1 mm • *Other:* Prolonged QT, P wave, PR interval, QRS
HOCM (*Am J Emerg Med* 2007;25:72)	• Characteristic findings of LVH (see ECG section) • Deep narrow Q waves in inferior (II, III, aVF) & lateral (I aVL, V5,V6) leads in pts w/ septal hypertrophy • Deep inverted T waves in mid & lateral precordial leads in pts w/ isolated apical hypertrophy
Arrhythmogenic R ventricular dysplasia (*Am J Med* 2004;117:685)	• Epsilon waves (small amplitude deflections at transition of QRS & ST segment) in R precordial leads • Prolonged QRS complex to >110 ms in V1–V3 w/o RBBB • Inverted T waves in nV1–V3 in absence of RBBB • Reduced R-wave amplitude
Long QT syndrome (*Circulation* 1995;92:2929; *Circulation* 2000;102:2849)	• Prolongation of QT interval, usually >500 ms • LQT1 has a broad T wave, LQT2 has small &/or notched T wave, LQT3 has unusually long onset T wave
Pre-excitation syndrome (WPW) (*Am Heart J* 1930;6:685)	• Short PR interval • Slurred upstroke of QRS complex (delta wave) • Increased QRS duration

- Labs & imaging: All guided by history/exam & specific dx's being considered; consider CBC, electrolytes (+/– Hcg) in most pts; however, obvious vasovagal syncope in a young o/w healthy male may not require any labs at all
- Consider cardiac markers, UA, stool guaiac, head CT in elderly
- Any pt w/ ICD who has syncope should have their ICD interrogated by an appropriate specialist given the high likelihood of malignant dysrhythmia in such pts, which was likely the initial indication for ICD placement prophylactically.

Disposition (Ann Emerg Med 1997;29:4)
- Home if low-risk cardiac features: (1) Age <45, (2) nl ECG, (3) nl exam. Consider outpatient f/u.
- Admit if high-risk cardiac features: (1) Age (unknown age threshold, but continuous variable), (2) h/o cardiac dz (esp e/o heart failure or structural heart dz), (3) one or more Criteria of San Francisco Syncope rule
- Other if diagnosed or suspected life-threatening diseases (eg, MI, aortic dissection, GI bleed), acute neurologic abnlty (eg, stroke, sz), ± for congenital heart dz, FHx sudden death, exertional syncope in pt w/o obvious cause

Decision Rules in Evaluation of Syncope
- Note at present no single clinical decision rule should outweigh clinical judgment

San Francisco Syncope Rule	
Clinical Features ("CHESS")	
CHF (past or present)	SBP <90 mmHg initially
Hct <30%	SOB
ECG abnl (new change or nonsinus)	

Using SFSR to Guide Disposition Decisions
- If any of above features, admit patient.
- Predicts risk of serious outcome (mortality, MI, arrhythmia, PE, CVA, SAH, significant hemorrhage, return to ED) w/i 7 d; Sens 86% (CI 83–89%), spec 49% (CI 48–41%) (Ann Emerg Med 2010;56(4):362)
- If none of above features present, consider d/c. Note that at publication of this book, pooled studies on SFSR have revealed a considerable population of pts w/ serious outcomes that did not have any of the five SFSR clinical features; however, all of these patients were admitted for other reasons. Combination of clinical gestalt & SFSR may have higher Sens & NPV than SFSR alone.
- Note: most robust syncope rule in terms of external validation

Ann Emerg Med 2004;4:224; 2006;47:448; 2007;49:420; 2008;427:e1; CMAJ 2011;183(15):E1116

OESIL Score (Osservatorio Epidemiologico sulla Sincope nel Lazio)	
Clinical Features	**Points**
Age >65 y	1
Syncope w/o prodrome	1
H/o Cardiovascular dz: Clinical or lab dx of any form of structural heart dz (ischemic, valvular, 1° myocardial dz, CHF, PAD, TIA/CVA)	1
Abnl ECG: Abnl rhythm (AF/AFL, SVT, MAT, frequent or repetitive PATs/PVCs, sustained or nonsustained VT, paced rhythms), AV or interventricular conduction d/o (CHB, Mobitz I or II AVB, BBB, IVCD), LVH, RVH, left-axis deviation, definitive or possible e/o prior MI	1

Prognostication Based on OESIL Score		
Points	**All-Cause Mortality w/i 12 mo of ED Visit (%)**	**Notes:**
0	0	• Sens 95% (CI 88–98%), spec 31% (CI 29–34%) (Ann Emerg Med 2010;56(4):362)
1	0.8	• Best at long-term outcomes, poor w/ short term
2	19.6	• Not rigorously externally validated compared to other syncope scores; derived & validated in Italian community ED settings.
3	34.7	
4	57.1	

Eur Heart J. 2003;24(9):811–819.

Boston Syncope Criteria for Predicting Adverse Event or Critical Interventions	
Clinical Features	
Ischemic symptoms	CP of possible cardiac origin, Ischemic ECG chgs (STE or >0.1 mV STD), Other ECG chgs (VT/VF, SVT, rapid AF, or new STTW changes), SOB
Signs of conduction dz	Multiple syncopal episodes w/i last 6 mo, rapid HR by hx, syncope during exercise, QT >500 ms, 2° or 3° AVB or intraventricular block
H/o underlying cardiac dz	H/o CAD (inc deep Q waves, hCMP, dCMP), CHF or LV dysfxn, VT/VF, PPM/AICD

Family Hx (1st degree)	Sudden death, HOCM, Brugada, or long QT synd
Persistent (>15 min) abnl VS w/o need for intervention	RR >24, O₂ <90% RA, HR <50 or 100 bpm, SBP <90 mmHg
Volume depletion	GIB by hx or hemocult, Hct <30%, Dehydration not corrected in ED by treating EP discretion
1° CNS event	(eg, SAH, CVA/TIA)

- Predicts critical intervention (PM/ICD placement, PCI, surgery, blood transfusion, CPR, alteration in antidsrhythmic therapy, endoscopy w/ intervention, or correction of carotid artery stenosis) or an adverse outcome (death, PE, CVA, severe infection/sepsis, ventricular/atrial dysrhythmia, ICH, hemorrhage, AMI, cardiac arrest, or other life-threatening sequelae) w/i 30 d
- Authors recommend admission for any + finding
- Diagnostic utility of any + finding: Sens 97% (CI 93–100%), spec 62% (CI 56–69%)
- Has not been externally validated

J Emerg Med 2007;33:233

HYPERTENSION AND HYPERTENSIVE EMERGENCIES

Approach
- Must differentiate chronic elevations in BP from an acute elevation
- Must differentiate transient elevations (ie, from anxiety or pain) from other causes
- Search for life-threatening causes of elevations in BP, including e/o end-organ damage (see HTN emergency)

Differential for Hypertension	
Pathophysiology	Differential
Other	Anxiety, pain, medications (cocaine, steroids, NSAIDs), rebound HTN (clonidine, βBs), EtOH withdrawal, preeclampsia–eclampsia, ICH, CVA
Cardiovascular	Essential HTN, ADHF, aortic dissection, coarctation of aorta, polycythemia vera
Renal	CRF, renal artery stenosis, glomerulonephritis, fibromuscular dysplasia
Endocrine	Cushing, pheochromocytoma

Definition (JAMA 2003;289:2560)
- HTN: SBP ≥140 or DBP ≥90
- HTN urgency: SBP ≥180 or DBP ≥110 w/ no acute organ damage; this term is also referred to as "hypertensive crisis" & has largely fallen out of favor
- HTN emergency: Elevated BP w/ acute organ damage (cardiac, CNS, renal)

History
- H/o CAD, CHF, TIA, stroke, peripheral a. dz, renal insufficiency, meds (sympathomimetics, cocaine, amphetamines), med noncompliance

Evaluation
- Check BP in both arms, check cuff/cuff size
- In ED pts w/ asymptomatic markedly elevated BP, routine screening for acute target organ injury (ie, serum Cr, US, ECG) is not required
- In select pt populations (ie, those w/ poor f/u), screening for an elevated Cr level may identify kidney injury that affects disposition

Treatment
- Goal BP <140/90 mmHg; if DM or renal dz goal is <130/80 mmHg
- Tx HTN results in 50% ↓ CHF, 40% ↓ stroke, 20–25% ↓ MI (Lancet 2000;356:1955)
- In pts w/ asymptomatic markedly elevated BP (ie, ≥180/≥110), routine ED medical intervention is not required
- In selected pt populations (ie, those w/ poor f/u), EPs may treat markedly elevated BP in the ED &/or initiate therapy for long-term control
  - For initiation of long-term therapy, it may be reasonable to start a thiazide-type diuretic for most pts, but may consider ACEI, ARB, BB, CCB, or combination (Hypertension 2003;42:1206)
  - In this situation, consider HCTZ 12.5–50 mg QD or Chlorthalidone 12.5–25 mg QD. Chlorthalidone may be superior to HCTZ (MRFIT, Circulation 1990;82(5):1616; SHEP, JAMA 1991;265;265(24):3255; ALLHAT, JAMA 2002;288(23):2981)

Antihypertensive Medications for Specific Causes		
Dz	**Drug Choice**	**Dose**
Cardiac ischemia	Metoprolol NTG	2.5–10 mg IV 10–200 mcg/min IV
CHF	NTG	10–200 mcg/min IV
ICH, HTN encephalopathy	Nitroprusside Labetalol	0.3–10 mcg/kg/min IV 10 mg IV, up to 300 mg
Aortic dissection	Esmolol + nitroprusside, or labetalol alone	Esmolol: Bolus 0.25–0.5 mg/kg over 1–2 min, then 10–200 mcg/kg/min gtt; see above for nitroprusside & labetalol
Renal artery stenosis	ACEI or ARBs	Captopril 25 mg PO BID, Losartan 50 mg PO QD
Pheochromocytoma	Phenoxybenzamine Phentolamine	10 mg PO BID 5 mg IV during HTN crisis
Preeclampsia–eclampsia	Magnesium Hydralazine	1–4 g IV over 2–4 min 10 mg IV

Disposition
- Asymptomatic pts may be d/c home w/ PCP f/u

Pearls
- HTN in the ED is often a/w anxiety/pain. Always re√ BP once pt is calm & pain free
- Tx of pts w/ *asymptomatic* HTN in the ED is *not* necessary if outpatient f/u is available
- In neonates, suspect renovascular dz, coarctation of the aorta, or kidney malformation

Hypertensive Emergency
Approach
- Look for e/o acute end-organ damage
- Neurologic: Encephalopathy, hemorrhagic or ischemic stroke, papilledema
- Cardiac: ACS, CHF, aortic dissection
- Renal: ARF
- Other: Preeclampsia–eclampsia

History
- Look for precipitants: Progression of essential HTN, medication noncompliance, rebound HTN (clonidine), worsening renal dz, pheochromocytoma, Cushing drug use (cocaine, amphetamines, MAOIs + tyramine), cerebral injury
- CP, dyspnea, HA, blurry vision, confusion, oliguria, hematuria

Findings
- Assess MS, e/o papilledema, visual acuity

Evaluation
- BUN/Cr, lytes, CBC, UA, ECG (e/o LVH), CXR, cardiac enzymes (if ischemia suspected), head CT (if ICH suspected)

Treatment
- ↓ MAP by 25% w/i 1–2 h using IV meds, then f/u w/ PO version
- Avoid tx HTN during acute stroke unless pt is getting lysed, has extreme HTN (>220/110), aortic dissection, active ischemia, or CHF (Stroke 2003;34:1056)
- Treat by underlying cause as noted above

Disposition
- True hypertensive emergencies require ICU admission for BP monitoring
Guideline: Wolf SJ, Lo B, Shi RD, et al. Clinical policy: Critical issues in the eval and management of adult patients in the emergency department w/ asymptomatic elevated blood pressure. Ann Emerg Med 2013;62:59–68.

HYPOTENSION AND SHOCK

Approach
- ABCs: Always address airway/breathing prior to circulation
- Differentiate hypotension from shock

Definition
- Hypotension: BP below pt's baseline, often defined as SBP <90 mmHg
- Shock: Insufficient perfusion pressures for organs' metabolic needs

Differential for Hypotension			
Pathophysiology		**Differential**	
Shock	↓ intravascular volume	Hypovolemic shock	
	↓ CO	Cardiogenic shock	
		Obstructive shock	PE
			Cardiac tamponade
			Tension PTX
	Peripheral vasodilation (ie, distributive)	Septic shock, anaphylactic shock, neurogenic shock	
Hypotension*	Adrenal insufficiency, medications (eg, nitrates, narcotics, antihypertensives), orthostatic hypotension, neurocardiogenic syncope, pregnancy, hypoglycemia, pseudohypotension (ie, inaccurate measurement, faulty BP cuff)		

*Some causes of hypotension can lead to shock.

History
• AMS, CP, SOB

Findings
• ↓ BP, ↑ HR, hypoxia, ↑ RR, UOP <1 mL/kg/h

Evaluation
• CBC, Chem 7, PT/PTT, cardiac markers, LFTs, blood gas, lactate, T/S, stool guaiac, ECG e/o ischemia
• POC ultrasonography: RUSH (Rapid Ultrasound in Shock, *Emerg Med Clin N Am* 2010;28:29) protocol incorporates a 3-part bedside physiologic assessment simplified as:
  • **the pump** (POC cardiac US to assess for pericardial effusion, global LV contractility, relative size of LV to RV)
  • **the tank** (POC IVC US to assess respiratory dynamics of IVC & volume status, as well as lung, pl & abdominal US to assess for pathology that could alter vascular volume; ie, PTX, pl effusion, free intra-abdominal fluid)
  • **the pipes** (POC thoracic & abdominal aortic US to assess for AD/AAA & LE compression US to assess for DVT)

RUSH Protocol: US Findings of Classic Shock States				
RUSH Evaluation	**Hypovolemic Shock**	**Cardiogenic Shock**	**Obstructive Shock**	**Distributive Shock**
Pump	Hypercontractile heart Small chambers	Hypocontractile heart Dilated heart	Hypercontractile heart Pericardial eff Cardiac tampon RV strain Cardiac thromb	Hypercontractile heart (early) Hypocontractile heart (late)
Tank	Flat IVC Flat IJ Peritoneal fluid Pl fluid	Distended IVC Distended IJ Lung rockets Pl fluid Peritoneal fluid	Distended IVC Distended IJ No lung sliding (PTX)	nl or small IVC Peritoneal fluid Pl fluid
Pipes	AAA AD	nl	DVT	nl

(Emerg Med Clin N Am 2010;28:29)

Treatment
• Priority should be to obtain adequate IV access. If peripheral large-bore IVs cannot be placed in timely manner, consider IO (humeral/tibial/sternal) or stat central venous access w/ large internal diameter catheters (ie, cordis).
• Priority should be to restore hemodynamics before time-consuming diagnostic w/u:
  • 1–2 L of isotonic crystalloid infusion as rapid as possible (ie, on pressure bag if indicated)
  • Consider stat uncrossmatched blood in life-threatening hemorrhage; consider using rapid infuser device; consider permissive hypotension in hemorrhagic shock
  • Consider peripheral vasoactive agents if persistently hypotensive after IVF bolus as bridge to obtaining central venous access

Vasoactive Agents and Dosing (*Emerg Med Clin N Am* 2008:26:759)				
Vasoactive Agent	Primary Receptor Activity	Relative Effects	Typical IV Dosing	Adverse Effects
Phenylephrine	α1 +++	↑ SVR ↓ HR	20–200 mcg/min	Reflex bradycardia
Norepinephrine	α1 ++++ α2 +++ β1 +++ β2 0(+)	↑ HR ↑ SV ↑ SVR	1–40 mcg/min	Tachydysrhythmia
Epinephrine	α1 ++++ α2 +++(+) 1 +++ β2 0(+)	↑↑↑ HR ↑↑↑ SV ↑↑↑ SVR Brchdilate	1–20 mcg/min	Tachydysrhythmia Splanchnic ischemia Acute MI
Dopamine	α2+, β1+, β2+, D++ α1/2+, β1++, β2+, D++ α1+(++), α2+, β1++, β2+, D++	Natriuresis ↑↑ HR ↑↑ SV ↑ SVR	Dose dependent: 1–5 mcg/kg/min 5–10 mcg/kg/m 10–20 mcg/kg/m	Tachydysrhythmia
Vasopressin	V1 receptor	↑ SVR ↓ HR	0.01–0.03 U/min	Limb ischemia Acute MI Bradycardia
Dobutamine	α1 0(+) α2 0(+) β1 ++++ β2 +++	↑↑ HR ↑↑↑ SV ↓ SVR	2–20 mcg/kg/min	Tachydysrhythmia HypoTN Acute MI
Milrinone	PDE inhibition	↑ HR ↑↑↑ SV ↓ SVR	0.25–0.75 mcg/kg/min	Tachydysrhythmia HypoTN Acute MI

• Use MS, UOP, & MAP as early e/o adequate end-organ perfusion

Pearls
• Not all hypotension is clinically significant. Use clinical context, pt's baseline BP, & check the BP cuff.
• Pulses provide a marker of baseline SBP, but may overestimate the absolute value (*BMJ* 2000;321:673)

Cited Correlations of Pulse and SBP (*Note: poorly evidence based*)	
Pulse Present	Minimum SBP (mmHg)
Radial artery	80
Femoral artery	70
Carotid	60

HYPOVOLEMIC SHOCK

Approach
• Dehydration is a Dx of exclusion; consider other etiologies (hemorrhage, ectopic pregnancy, etc.)

Definition
• Intravascular volume depletion → ↓ perfusion, most commonly 2° blood loss

Differential for Hypovolemic Shock	
Pathophysiology	Differential
Hemorrhage	Trauma (internal, external), GI bleed, ruptured AAA
Other	Dehydration, ectopic pregnancy, placenta previa, placental abruption

History
- Trauma, melena, hematochezia, hematemesis, ↓ PO intake

Findings
- E/o trauma, guaiac + stool, pelvic exam

Evaluation
- As above +UA/HCG, FAST (blood in abdomen or chest); consider CT chest/abd/pelvis, pelvic US, type/screen

Treatment
- **Identify/treat cause,** IV fluid bolus; consider PRBCs; **consult** immediately for life-threatening disorders requiring definitive tx (surgery, GI, OB/Gyn)

Disposition
- Admit vs. OR

CARDIOGENIC SHOCK

Approach
- Consider intubation early, look for & **treat underlying cause**

Definition
- ↓ CO + nl intravascular volume → ↓ systolic contractility + ↑ diastolic filling

Differential
ACS, myocarditis, dysrhythmia, valvular failure, severe CMP, cardiac contusion, pulmonary HTN

Findings
- ↑ HR, ↓ BP, ↑ RR, hypoxia, pulmonary rales, S3, S4

Evaluation
- CBC, Chem 7, Ca, Mg, PO_4, ECG, CXR, stat echo (systolic/diastolic dysfxn, papillary muscle rupture, ventricular wall rupture, VSD, pericardial effusion, R heart strain)

Treatment
- Treat underlying dz, IV fluids (if ↓ intravascular volume)
- Dopamine: ↑ myocardial contractility & BP, but ↑ O_2 demand
- Dobutamine: ↑ HR & inotropy, less O_2 demand, but causes vasodilation (best if not tachycardic or severely hypotensive)
- Central venous catheter: Consider for CVP monitoring, administration of pressors
- Cardiology consult
- Revascularization: Early revasc → ↓ mortality (NEJM 1999;341:625; JAMA 2001;285:190)
- Other: Thrombolytics, IABP, ventricular assist device

Disposition
- Admit to ICU

SEPTIC SHOCK

Approach (NEJM 2006;355:1699)
- Identify & treat early → best outcomes when treated w/i 6 h
- Look for source of infection

Definition
- Sepsis = SIRS (severe inflammatory response syndrome) + source infection
- SIRS: ≥2 of the following: Temp ≥38°C or ≤36°C, HR ≥ 90, RR ≥ 20, WBC (≥12,000, ≤4,000, or >10% bands)
- Severe sepsis: Sepsis + sepsis-induced hypoperfusion (hypotension persisting after initial fluid challenge or blood lactate >4 mmol/L) or organ dysfxn (see organ dysfxn variables below)
- Septic shock: Severe sepsis + ↓ BP despite adequate fluid resuscitation

Common Causes of Sepsis	
Pathophysiology	Differential
Respiratory	PNA, empyema
Abdominal	Peritonitis, abscess, cholangitis
Skin	Cellulitis, fasciitis
Renal	Pyelonephritis
CNS	Meningitis, brain abscess

Evaluation

- CBC w/ diff, Chem 10, LFTs, lactate, blood (×2)/urine/sputum culture, PT/PTT, cardiac markers, VBG, CXR; consider CT brain/LP, CT chest &/or abdomen, RUQ US based on pt
- Consider 1,3 beta-D-glucan assay & galactomannan assay if available & invasive candidiasis is in the DDx as cause of infection

Diagnostic Criteria for Sepsis
Inflammatory variables: Leukocytosis (WBC >12,000 μL^{-1}) Leukopenia (WBC <4,000 μL^{-1}) nl WBC w/ >10% immature cells (band forms) Plasma CRP >2 SD above nl Plasma procalcitonin >2 SD above nl
Organ dysfxn variables: Arterial hypoxemia (PaO_2/FiO_2 <300) Acute oliguria (UOP <0.5 mL/kg/h for at least 2 h despite fluid resuscitation) Cr increase >0.5 mg/dL Coagulation abx (INR >1.5 or aPTT >60 s) Ileus TTP (plt count <100,000 μL^{-1}) Hyperbilirubinemia (plasma Tbili >4 mg/dL)
Tissue perfusion variables: Hyperlactemia (>1 mmol/L) Decreased cap refill/mottling

Treatment

- EGDT (NEJM 2001;345:1368); ↓ mortality/hospital stay in 1 study, though no prospective validation study
- Protocolized quantitative resuscitation of pts w/ sepsis-induced hypoperfusion. *Goals during the 1st 6 h:*
  - **CVP 8–12 mmHg** → crystalloid (NS or LR) is the initial fluid of choice; *initial fluid challenge 30 cc/kg;* consider albumin when pts require substantial IVFs
    - Central venous access should be obtained as soon as practical
  - **MAP ≥65 mmHg** → use of vasopressors, whereby:
    - Norepinephrine is 1st choice
    - Epinephrine (added to or substituting NE) when additional agent needed
    - Vasopressin 0.03 U/min can be added to NE to raise MAP or decrease NE dose
    - Dopamine as alternative to NE only in highly selected pts (low-risk arrhythmia)
    - Phenylephrine not recommended except special circumstances
    - Arterial catheter should be placed as soon as practical
  - **UOP ≥0.5 mL/kg/h**
    - Foley catheter should be placed as soon as practical for I/O monitoring
  - **ScvO2 or mixed venous O2 saturation 70% or 65%, respectively**
    - Trial of dobutamine up to 20 mcg/kg/min should be given or added to vasoactive agent in the presence of myocardial dysfxn (elevated filling pressure/low CO) or ongoing signs of hypoperfusion, despite CVP & MAP goals ($ScvO_2$ <70%)
- Abx: Broad spectrum, given prior to drawing cultures (cover gram+, gram–, anaerobes; consider double coverage for pseudomonas)
- Start abx w/i 1 h of recognition, regardless of whether source is known
- Source control
- **Hydrocortisone:** Consider hydrocortisone use in pts w/ severe sepsis refractory to IV fluids & pressors; corticotropin test + routine steroid use → no benefit & possibly harm (NEJM 2008;358:111)
- **Blood products:** PRBCs to target Hgb 7–9 g/dL; Plts if <10,000 μL^{-1} w/o bleed, <20,000 μL^{-1} w/ risk of bleeding, <50,000 μL^{-1} for active bleeding, surgery, procedure
- **Oxygenation/ventilation:** Supplemental O_2; consider need for intubation early; if intubated use VTs of 6 cc/kg predicted BW (NEJM 2000;342:1301) use of sedation/paralytics → ↓ O_2 consumption
- **Glucose control:** q1–2h measurements; initiate protocolized blood glucose management when 2 consecutive measurements >180 mg/dL to a target <180 mg/dL
- **Renal replacement therapy:** Use continuous therapies (ie, CVVH) to facilitate managing fluid balance in HD unstable pts
- **Activated protein C:** Use is controversial; ↓ mortality in severe sepsis based on 1 phase 3 trial (NEJM 2001;344:699; Crit Care Med 2003;31:12), but ↑ bleeding, ↑ cost, & no benefit in less sick (APACHE II <25) populations (NEJM 2005;353:1332); recently taken off market

Disposition
- Admit

Guideline: Dellinger RP, Levy MM, Rhodes A, et al. Surviving sepsis campaign: International guidelines for management of severe sepsis and septic shock: 2012. *Crit Care Med.* 2013;41(2):580–637.

NEUROGENIC SHOCK

Approach
- Cervical spine injury → risk of apnea, may require intubation; evaluate according to ATLS

Definition
- Transection of the spinal cord → disruption of sympathetic pathways → loss of vascular sympathetic tone → vasodilation (typically cervical or high thoracic lesions)

History
- Trauma w/ severe injury to the spinal cord

Findings
- ↓ HR, ↓ BP, anesthesia, paralysis below an spec dermatome; saddle anesthesia, ↓ rectal tone, areflexia, Horner syndrome, absent bulbocavernosus reflex, priapism (unopposed PNS stimulation)

Evaluation
- CT spine (esp cervical, thoracic); consider CT head, chest, abd/pelvis if h/o trauma

Treatment
- C-spine immobilization: Aspen or Philadelphia collar for prolonged immobilization
- Strict log-roll precautions
- IV fluids: Prior to starting pressors
- Vasopressors: Dopamine, norepinephrine, phenylephrine
- Consult neurosurgery immediately

Disposition
- Admit

Pearl
- Any trauma pt w/ hypotension should be suspected of having hemorrhagic shock until proven o/w, thus neurogenic shock should be treated if suspected but should not be the 1° DDx in the hypotensive trauma pt.

DYSRHYTHMIA

Approach
- Follow ACLS protocols for anyone unstable or symptomatic (CP, SOB, AMS, abnl VS)

Differential		
Type		**Differential**
Bradycardia		Sinus bradycardia, SA node block/escape rhythm, sick node dysfxn, AV blocks (2nd- & 3rd-degree AV block)
Tachycardia	Regular — Narrow-complex	Sinus tachycardia, SVT (AVNRT, AVRT), AT, AFL
	Regular — Wide-complex	Ventricular tachycardia, SVT w/ aberrancy, SVT w/ pre-excitation (eg, WPW), tachycardia w/ PM
	Irregular — Narrow-complex	AF, AFL w/ variable AV block, multifocal atrial tachycardia
	Irregular — Wide-complex	AF w/ aberrancy, polymorphic VT

BRADYCARDIA

Approach
- Follow ACLS protocols for anyone unstable or severely symptomatic (CP, SOB, AMS)
- Anticipate need for external/transvenous pacing & cardiology consult early

- Always obtain ECG & rhythm strip
- Medication hx is crucial
- In children, be highly suspicious of toxic ingestion
- In neonates, consider congenital cardiac dz

Definition
- HR <60 in an adult, <80 in a child <15 y/o, <100 in an infant <1 y/o. Caused by depressed function of the SA node or conduction system block/delay.

Sinus Bradycardia (NEJM 2000;342:703)
History
- Fatigue, syncope/presyncope, DOE, medication hx (esp βBs)

Differential
- Physiologic (athletic young adults), medications (nodal agents), hypothyroidism, ↑ vagal tone (including inferior MI), hypothermia, ↑ ICP

Evaluation
- ECG (HR <60 in adults, nl PR intervals, P wave preceding each QRS), rhythm strip

Treatment
- Asymptomatic bradycardia does not require tx. Tx only if symptomatic or life-threatening cause is suspected w/ atropine &/or pacing.

Disposition
- Admit anyone who is symptomatic

SA Node Block/Escape Rhythm
History
- Same as for sinus bradycardia

Differential
- Same as for sinus bradycardia. Also a/w ↑ K, ↑ vagal tone.

Evaluation
- ECG (absent atrial depolarization & missing P waves), rhythm strip, lytes, consider TSH, cardiac markers

Treatment
- Asymptomatic bradycardia does not require tx. Tx only if symptomatic or life-threatening cause is suspected.

Disposition
- Admit anyone who is symptomatic

Sinus Node Dysfunction (Sick Sinus Syndrome/Tachy–Brady Syndrome)
Definition
- Sinus node dysfxn includes a series of ECG abnormalities characterized by failure to generate appropriate cardiac potentials from the sinus node
- In sick sinus syndrome, there are frequent long sinus pauses that may degenerate to absent atrial depolarization for a period of time before the resumption of regular cardiac conduction (sinus arrest)
- In tachy–brady syndrome, episodes of sinus bradycardia or sinus arrest are interspersed w/ episodes of supraventricular tachycardia (often AF)

History
- Syncope, presyncope, fatigue, weakness, DOE, palpitations
- Typically observed in 70–80 y/o, suggesting age-related degeneration

Differential
- Consider other life-threatening arrhythmias

Evaluation
- ECG (frequent sinus pauses, bradycardia/tachycardia rhythms); consider electrolytes, cardiac markers, CBC; Holter or event monitoring

Treatment
- Acute tx only for symptomatic or life-threatening arrhythmia; ultimately may require combination of rate control for tachycardia & PPM for bradycardia

Disposition
- Admit anyone who is symptomatic for permanent PM placement
- If minimal or no sxs are present, d/c home w/ close f/u

AV NODE BLOCK

Definition
- These occur when conduction from the atria to the AV node & into the His bundle is disrupted
- These blocks can anatomically be located above, w/i, or below the His bundle
- Classified as 1st-degree, 2nd-degree Mobitz I (Wenckebach), 2nd-degree Mobitz II, & 3rd-degree blocks based on characteristic ECG patterns:

Differential		
Classification	ECG Findings	Differential
1° AV block	• Prolonged PR interval >0.2 s, nl QRS	↑ vagal tone, MI, age-related degeneration, drugs (BB, CCB, digoxin), infection, endocarditis
2° AV block Mobitz type I	• Progressive ↑ PR interval w/ RR interval shortening until QRS dropped • Appears as grouped beats • Block at level of AV node	↑ vagal tone, *inferior* MI, age-related degeneration, drugs (BB, CCB, digoxin), infection, endocarditis, RF
2° AV block Mobitz type II	• Stable PR & RR interval w/ occasional dropped QRS • Can be regular (2:1) or irregular • Block at level of His-Purkinje	Age-related degeneration, *anteroseptal* MI
3° AV block	• Complete AV dissociation • P waves are not conducted & never produce a QRS • Escape rhythm is a regular narrow junctional or wide ventricular response	MI (IMI w/ AV node ischemia or anteroseptal MI w/ H-P ischemia), age-related degeneration, drugs (BB, CCB, digoxin), infection, endocarditis, myocarditis, RF, congenital

Approach
- Differentiate 1st, 2nd Mobitz I (Wenckebach), 2nd Mobitz II, & 3rd-degree blocks
- 2° Mobitz II & 3° blocks are never nl → look for underlying cardiac dz
- In children, be highly suspicious of toxic ingestion
- In neonates, consider congenital cardiac dz
- Determine (1) rate, (2) wide or narrow QRS, (3) rhythm regular or irregular, (4) P waves present or absent, (5) every P wave followed by QRS & every QRS preceded by P

History
- 1°: Asymptomatic, incidental finding on ECG
- 2° Mobitz I (Wenckebach): Often asymptomatic; irregular heartbeat, fatigue
- 2° Mobitz II: May be asymptomatic; presyncope/syncope, fatigue, DOE
- 3°: Usually symptomatic; presyncope/syncope, fatigue, weakness, DOE

Findings
- See above

Evaluation
- ECG & rhythm strip
- 2° Mobitz II & 3°: Labs in anticipation of PPM placement

Treatment
- 1° & 2° Mobitz I: No tx generally necessary
- 2° Mobitz II & 3°:
  - Continuous tele monitoring
  - Symptomatic pts require transcutaneous &/or transvenous pacing; if HD unstable, consider a beta-adrenergic agent (dopamine, epinephrine, or isoproterenol) as bridge to pacing. Dopamine has been demonstrated to have equivalent survival outcomes & adverse events to transcutaneous pacing (*PrePACE*, Resuscitation 2008;76(3):341)
  - Treat active cardiac ischemia
  - Consult cardiology

Disposition
- Pts w/ 1° & 2° Mobitz I: D/c home w/ f/u
- Pts w/ 2° Mobitz II & 3°: Admit all to Tele ward for cardiology consult & PPM

Pearls
- Avoid atropine for reversal of AV block as this can worsen conduction
- Have transcutaneous pacer attached & ready for use in high-risk pts
- Mobitz II is concerning b/c risk of progression to 3°

TACHYCARDIA/PALPITATIONS

Approach
- Follow ACLS protocols for anyone unstable or severely symptomatic (CP, SOB, AMS)
- Anticipate need for intubation & defibrillator early
- Always obtain ECG & rhythm strip
- Determine (1) rate, (2) wide or narrow QRS, (3) rhythm regular or irregular

Causes of Wide Complex Tachycardia	
	Tx
Ventricular tachycardia	Amiodarone, lidocaine, DCCV
SVT w/ *aberrancy (ie, BBB)	Adenosine, vagal maneuvers, DCCV
SVT w/ pre-excitation	Procainamide, DCCV
Tachycardia + PM	Treat cause of tachycardia, apply magnet if PM-mediated

*Causes of aberrancy: Bundle branch blocks (fixed, rate-related, Ashman's phenomenon), accessory pathways (ie, WPW), meds (ie, class Ia/Ic antiarrhythmics, TCAs), pseudo-STEMI, PM, hyperkalemia, hypothermia, cardiomyopathies, channelopathies.

Supraventricular Tachycardia
Approach
- Differentiate type based on ECG, rhythm strip, & response to adenosine/vagal maneuvers (see below)

Definition
- Rhythm arises above the ventricles (either atrium or AV jxn) w/ narrow QRS unless pre-excitation or aberrant conduction

History
- H/o pulmonary or cardiac dz → AT, MAT, AFL, AF, NPJT; o/w health adult → AVNRT, AVRT
- Gradual onset → ST, AT; abrupt onset → AVNRT, AVRT

Evaluation
- Consider CBC, TSH, tox screen, though in most cases, ECG/rhythm strip is sufficient

SVT Pathophysiologies		
	Type of SVT	Pathophysiology
Atrial	ST	Pain, fever, anxiety, hypovolemia, PE, medication, anemia, hyperthyroid
	AT	Originates in atria but not SA node; a/w COPD, CAD, EtOH, digoxin
	MAT	Originates in atria at ≥3 separate sites
	AFL	Atrial macroreentry, typically R atrium
	AF	Multiple irregular atrial impulses typically from pulmonary veins
AV jxn	AVNRT	Re-entrant pathway w/i AVN
	AVRT	Re-entrant pathway using AVN + accessory pathway b/w atria & ventricles
	NPJT	Originates at AV jxn, a/w myo/endocarditis, cardiac surgery, IMI, digoxin

From: NEJM 1995;332:162; 2006;354:1039.

Diagnosis by ECG, Vagal Maneuvers, and Adenosine (NEJM 2006;354:1039)	
Rate	ST: Typically <150 bpm AFL: Typically 150 bpm (2:1 AV block) AVNRT/AVRT: Typically >150 bpm
Rhythm	Irregular → AF, MAT
P wave	UPRIGHT before QRS: ST, AT, MAT Retrograde AFTER QRS: AVNRT (w/i QRS), AVRT (after QRS) FIBRILLATION or no P wave → AF SAWTOOTH appearance → AFL
Vagal/adenosine	Slows rate w/ ↑ AV block: ST, AT, MAT
Response	Terminates rhythm or no response: AVNRT, AVRT "Unmasks" sawtooth waves ↑ AV block → AFL

Treatment

- Cardiovert any unstable rhythm
- ST: Treat underlying condition
- AT/MAT: Treat underlying condition; consider AV nodal blocker
- AF/AFL: CCB, βB, dig, antiarrhythmic (amiodarone, lidocaine)
- AVNRT/AVRT: Vagal maneuvers, adenosine, CCB preferable to βB → avoid adenosine/ nodal agents if e/o pre-excitation (see WPW below)
- NPJT: CCB, βB, amiodarone

Disposition

- Most pts w/ ST, AVNRT, AVRT can be d/c home once rhythm is controlled if → asymptomatic & no acute underlying condition. Admission for other rhythms is variable, but often necessary due to underlying condition.
- Consult cardiology for any pt w/ unstable SVT & those difficult to control w/ standard tx

Pearl

- MAT is often misdiagnosed as AF. Look closely at P wave morphology.

Atrial Fibrillation and Atrial Flutter

Definition (JACC 2006;48:e149)

- AF is a supraventricular tachyarrhythmia characterized by uncoordinated atrial activity w/ consequent deterioration of mechanical function
- Can be 1st episode or recurrent (≥2 episodes) as well as paroxysmal (self-limited), persistent (>7 d), permanent (>1 y) &/or cardioversion has failed
- Valvular → rheumatic heart dz, or postvalve surgery
- Lone AF → <60 y/o & no e/o cardiac dz or HTN

Differential	
Pathophysiology	**Differential**
Other	Idiopathic (50%)
Cardiac	CHF, peri/myo/endocarditis, MI/ischemia, s/p cardiac surgery, HTN
Pulmonary	COPD, PNA, PE
Endo	Hyperthyroid, stress, infection, postop
Drugs	EtOH "holiday heart syndrome", cocaine, amphetamines, sympathomimetics, caffeine

History

- Abrupt vs. gradual onset (palpitations, DOE, fatigue presyncope/syncope, CP); recent illness, drug & alcohol use

Findings

- Irregularly irregular pulse; may be regular w/ AFL

Evaluation

- ECG, CBC, lytes, Ca, Mg, PO₄; CXR
- Consider cardiac markers (if active CAD is suspected); TSH, dig level if appropriate; echo (LA size, thrombus, valves, LV fxn)
- Consider outpatient Holter in pts w/ suggestive hx who arrive in NSR
- ECG in AF: Replacement of consistent P waves by rapid oscillating or fibrillatory waves that vary in amplitude, shape, & timing, a/w irregular, frequently rapid ventricular response rate
- ECG in AFL: Atrial rate 250–350 bmp w/ ventricular response rate typically 150 bpm presence of "sawtooth" flutter ("F") waves. Can be **typical** (spiky V1, negative in II, III, aVF, V5–V6) or **atypical** (appearance other than typical). F waves revealed via adenosine or vagal maneuvers. Most commonly 2:1 or 4:1 conduction.

Treatment

- Main objectives: Rate control, prevention of thromboembolism, & correction of rhythm
- When deciding on management strategies in the ED, several things to consider include:
  - a. Is the pt stable or unstable?
  - b. Is this 1st episode or recurrent episode, & is this part of a paroxysmal, persistent, or permanent duration paradigm?
  - c. If 1st-episode or paroxysmal, how long have sxs been present (ie, <48 h)?
  - d. What is the pt's stroke risk?
  - e. Does the pt have a cardiologist/PCP w/ whom you can make joint decision or poor f/u?

- **Rate control vs. rhythm control:** Numerous studies have sought to answer this question, but bottom line is that there appears to be no difference in symptomatic improvement, CHF, thromboembolic cx, severe bleeding, or mortality when comparing the 2 strategies (PIAF, *Lancet* 2000;356:1789; AFFIRM, *NEJM* 2002;347:1825; STAF, *J Am Coll Cardiol* 2003;41:1690; HOT CAFÉ, *CHEST* 2004;126:476); however, rhythm control seems to be a/w increased rates of hospitalization & adverse medication effects (PIAF, *Lancet* 2000;356:1789; AFFIRM, *NEJM* 2002;347:1825)
- *Note: majority of these studies included pts w/ persistent AF, thus may not be generalizable to ED pt presenting w/ 1st episode or paroxysmal AF
- Suggested initial tx algorithms (Adapted from guidelines: *Can J Cardiol* 2011;27(1):27; 2011;27(1):38; 2011;27(1):47; 2011;27:74; *Circulation* 2011;123(10):e269)

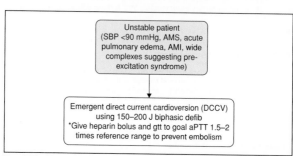

Figure 1.5 Unstable patient with afib. (Note: Mean energy level for successful cardioversion 50 J biphasic and 200 J monophasic [*Am J Cardiol* 2004;93:1495–1499]. There may be higher first-shock success for DVVC if initial energy used 200 J vs. 100 J [BEST-AF, *Heart* 2008;94:884–887]).

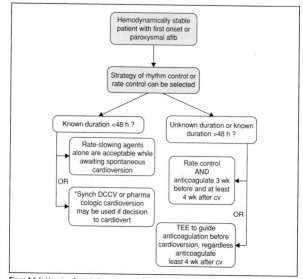

Figure 1.6 Stable patient, first episode or paroxysmal afib. Note: These patients may undergo cardioversion without anticoagulation, however, consider delaying DCCV and anticoagulate for 3 wk if high risk of stroke (ie, mechanical valve, RHD, recent CVA/TIA).

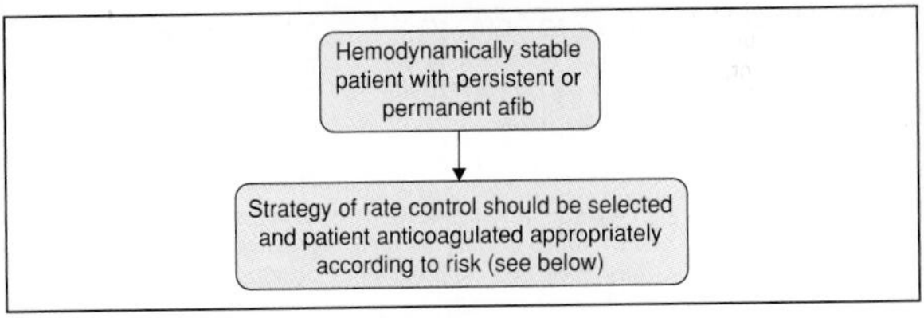

Figure 1.7 Stable patient, persistent or permanent afib.

- **Rate control:** βB or nondihydropyridine CCBs recommended as 1st-line therapy for rate control. CCB, however, should be avoided in pts w/ ADHF & AF.
- Digoxin can be added to therapy w/ βB or CCB in pts whose HR is not controlled
- Dronedarone may be added for additional rate control w/ uncontrolled ventricular rate despite above therapy
- IV administration of digoxin or amiodarone is recommended to control HR in pts w/ AF & HF
- Amiodarone for rate control should be reserved for exceptional cases in which other means are not feasible or insufficient
- IV procainamide, disopyramide, ibutilide, or amiodarone may be considered for HD stable pts w/ AF involving conduction over an accessory pathway. In this situation, IV CCB or digoxin should be avoided as they may paradoxically accelerate the ventricular response.

Rate Control Agents for Atrial Fibrillation/Atrial Flutter			
Medication		Initial Dose	Maint Dose
βB	Metoprolol	2.5–5 mg IV bolus q5min × 3	Start 25–100 mg PO BID
	Esmolol	500 mcg/kg IV q4min × 3	60–200 mcg/kg/min IV gtt
	Propranolol	0.15 mg/kg IV q5min × 5	Start 40 mg PO BID
CCB	Diltiazem	0.25 mg/kg IV × 1; may repeat 0.25–0.35 mg/kg IV after 15 min	Start 30 mg PO QID or 5–15 mg/h IV gtt
	Verapamil	0.075–0.15 mg/kg IV; may repeat dose after 15–30 min	Start 40–80 mg PO TID
Digoxin (onset in hours)		0.25 mg IV q2h, up to 1.5 mg	
Amiodarone		150 mg IV over 10 min	0.5–1 mg/min IV

- **Direct current cardioversion:** Recommended dose 150–200 J biphasic waveform
  - Mean energy level for successful cardioversion 50 J biphasic & 200 J monophasic (Am J Cardiol 2004;93:1495). There may be higher 1st-shock success for DVVC if initial energy used 200 J vs. 100 J (BEST-AF, Heart 2008;94:884).
  - Pretreatment w/ amiodarone, flecainide, ibutilide, propafenone, or sotalol can be used to enhance the success of DCCV & prevent recurrent AF.
- **Pharmacologic cardioversion:** Administration of flecainide, dofetilide, propafenone, or ibutilide is recommended for pharmacologic cardioversion
  - Procainamide has been shown to be effective in ED population w/ 58.3% cardioversion, w/ 91.7% success rate if followed by DCCV in nonresponders (CMEJ 2010;12(3):181)
  - Amiodarone is a reasonable option, but digoxin & sotalol may be harmful for cardioversion & are not recommended
  - βB or nondihydropyridine CCBs should be given before administering class I antiarrhythmic agents

Rhythm Control Agents for Atrial Fibrillation/Atrial Flutter			
Medication		Initial Dose	Special Considerations
Class Ia	Procainamide	15–17 mg/kg IV over 60 min	• Preferred w/ WPW • May cause hypotension
Class Ic	Propafenone	450 mg PO (<70 kg) 600 mg PO (>70 kg) 2 mg/kg IV	• May cause hypotension, bradycardia • CI in pts w/ ischemic HD, LV dysfxn, structurally abnl heart
	Flecainide	200 mg PO (<70 kg) 300 mg PO (>70 kg) 2 mg/kg IV	• May cause hypotension, bradycardia • ↓ dose in renal insuff • CI in pts w/ ischemic HD, LV dysfxn, structurally abnl heart

	Dofetilide	0.5 mg PO (eGFR >60) 0.25 mg PO (eGFR 40–60) 0.125 mg PO (GFR 20–40) CI if eGFR <20	• 2–3% risk torsades de pointes; CI long QT, bradycardia • Require hospitalization for initiation given QTc prolongation
Class III	Ibutilide	1 mg over 10 min (>60 kg) 0.01 mg/kg, 10 min (<60 kg) *May repeat once at same dose if doesn't terminate*	• CI in pts w/ hypokalemia, prolonged QTc, torsades de pointes
	Amiodarone	5–7 mg/kg IV over 30 min, then 1.2–1.8 g/day continuous IV infusion	• SE: Hepatotoxicity, hypothyroid, thyrotoxicosis, pneumonitis, pulmonary fibrosis, corneal microdeposits

- **Anticoagulation:** All pts w/ AF or AFL (paroxysmal, persistent, or permanent) should be stratified using a predictive index for stroke (ie, $CHADS_2$ or CHA_2DS_2-VASc) & for the risk of bleeding (ie, HAS-BLED) & most pts should receive anticoagulation
- Pts w/ very low risk of CVA ($CHADS_2$ = 0) should receive ASA 81–325 mg/d
- Pts w/ low risk of CVA ($CHADS_2$ = 1) should receive oral anticoagulation w/ either warfarin or dabigatran, but ASA is reasonable for some pts
- Pts w/ mod risk of CVA ($CHADS_2 \geq 2$) should receive oral anticoagulation w/ either warfarin or dabigatran
- Most pts should receive dabigatran 150 mg PO BID preferable to warfarin when anticoagulation indicated
- Newer effective oral anticoagulants include rivaroxaban 20 mg QD (ROCKET-AF, *NEJM* 2011;365:883) & apixaban 5 mg PO BID (ARISTOTLE, *NEJM* 2011;365:981)
- Anticoagulation not recommended for pts w/ lone AF

CHADS₂ Score for Estimating Stroke Risk in Patients with AF	
(*JAMA* 2001;285:2864)	
$CHADS_2$ Risk Criteria	**Score**
CHF	1
HTN	1
Age >75 y/o	1
Diabetes mellitus	1
Stroke or TIA (prior)	2
$CHADS_2$ Score	**Adjusted Stroke Rate%/y (95% CI)**
0	1.9% (1.2–3)
1	2.8% (2–3.8)
2	4% (3.1–5.1)
3	5.9% (4.6–7.3)
4	8.5% (6.3–11.1)
5	12.5% (8.2–17.5)
6	18.2% (10.5–27.4)

HAS-BLED Score for Estimating Major Bleeding Risk in Patients with AF	
(*CHEST* 2010;138:1093)	
Clinical Characteristic	**Score**
HTN (SBP >160 mmHg)	1
Abnl renal or liver fxn (1 pt each)**	1 or 2
Stroke	1
Bleeding	1
Labile INRs	1
Elderly (age >65 y/o)	1
Drugs or EtOH use (1 pt each)***	1 or 2

HAS-BLED Score	Major Bleed%/y*
0	1.13%
1	1.02%
2	1.88%
3	3.74%
4	8.70%
5	12.50%
6–9	Not reported

*Major bleeding defined as any bleeding requiring hospitalization &/or causing a decrease in Hgb of >2 g/L &/or requiring blood transfusion that was not a hemorrhagic stroke.
**Abnl renal fxn defined as chronic dialysis, renal transplant, or Cr >200 µmol/L (2.3 mg/dL). Abnl liver fxn defined as chronic hepatic dz (ie, cirrhosis), Tbili >2× ULN, in association w/ AST/ALT. ALP >3× ULN.
***Drugs included anti-plt agents & NSAIDs.

Disposition
- **Home:** Pts who convert to sinus, or are rate controlled, & anticoagulated if necessary
- All discharged pts should get close PCP or cardiology f/u
- **EDOU:** Depending on local clinical protocols
- **Admit:** Pts w/ acute underlying illness, ongoing sxs, or poor rate control

Pearls
- Risk of stroke is similar in all forms of AF/AFL (recurrent paroxysmal, persistent, & permanent AF, & AFL)
- Spontaneous cardioversion occurs w/i 24 h in 50–67% acute AF
- 5–8% elderly have recurrent AF
- Cairns JA, Connolly S, McMurtry S, et al. Canadian Cardiovascular Society atrial fibrillation guidelines 2010: Prevention of stroke and systemic thromboembolism in atrial fibrillation and flutter. Can J Cardiol 2011; 27:74–90.
- Fuster V, Ryden LE, Cannom DS, et al. 2011 ACCF/AHA/HRS focused updates incorporated into the ACC/AHA ESC 2006 guidelines for the management of patients with atrial fibrillation: A report of the American College of Cardiology Foundation/American Heart Association Task Force on Practice Guidelines. Circulation 2011; 123(10):e269–e367.
- Guidelines: Gillis AM, Skanes AC, CCS Atrial Fibrillation Guidelines Committee. Canadian Cardiovascular Society atrial fibrillation guidelines 2010: Implementing GRADE and achieving consensus. Can J Cardiol 2011;27(1):27–30.
- Gillis AM, Verma A, Talajic M, et al. Canadian Cardiovascular Society atrial fibrillation guidelines 2010: Rate and rhythm management. Can J Cardiol 2011;27(1):47–59.
- Steill IG, Macle L, CCS Atrial Fibrillation Guidelines Committee. Canadian Cardiovascular Society atrial fibrillation guidelines 2010: Management of recent-onset atrial fibrillation and flutter in the emergency department. Can J Cardiol 2011;27(1):38–46.

Pre-excitation
Definition
- **Accessory pathway:** A bypass tract that conducts impulses b/w atria
- **Wolff–Parkinson–White:** Accessory conduction pathway evident on resting ECG
- **Orthodromic AVRT:** Impulse travels down AV node (fast), then conducts retrograde, up the accessory pathway (slowly) → thus narrow-complex QRS
- **Antidromic AVRT:** Impulse travels down the accessory pathway (slowly), then conducts retrograde, up the AV node (fast) → thus wide-complex QRS

Evaluation
- ECG & rhythm strip
- Orthodromic AVRT: Narrow complex tachycardia
- Antidromic AVRT: WCT

Treatment
- AVRT: Vagal maneuvers, βBs, CCB
- AF/AFL w/ pre-excitation → cardiology consult, DC cardiovert, or use procainamide; βB & CCB are ineffective & can precipitate VF

Ventricular Tachycardia
Approach
- Determine if pt is stable or unstable → use ACLS protocol for any pt w/ unstable VT
- Differentiate VT from nonsustained VT (NSVT), & other causes of WCT (see above)
- Differentiate monomorphic from polymorphic VT

Definition
- NSVT: VT lasting <30 s

- SVT w/ aberrancy: VT look-alike b/c abnl conduction → WCT. Caused by fixed BBB, rate-related BBB, or accessory pathway
- Torsades de pointes: Polymorphic VT + prolonged QT

Causes
- **Monomorphic, structurally abnl heart:** Prior MI, CMP, arrhythmogenic RV dysplasia
- **Monomorphic, structurally nl heart:** Idiopathic VT
- **Polymorphic:** Ischemia, CMP, torsades de pointes, Brugada syndrome (see below)

History
- Palpitations, lightheadedness, CP, SOB, nausea, syncope, unresponsiveness; PMH: CAD, CMP, multiple CAD RFs, & FHx sudden death all ↑ risk VT

Evaluation
- ECG, rhythm strip, lytes, Ca, Mg, PO_4, cardiac markers; CXR; digoxin level if appropriate

Treatment
- **Unstable VT:** ACLS protocol
- **Stable VT:** Use either:
  - Lidocaine: 100 mg IV load, then 1–4 mg/min
  - Amiodarone: 150 mg IV load, then 1 mg/min
- **Polymorphic VT:** Magnesium 2–4 g IV bolus
- **Other:** Replete electrolytes (Ca, Mg, PO_4); treat coincident ischemia if present

Disposition
- Admit to cardiac step-down unit or cardiac ICU

Pearls
- Assume all WCT to be ventricular unless proven o/w
- Best clinical predictors that WCT is VT → prior MI, CHF, LV dysfxn (Am J Med 1998;84:53)

Brugada Criteria for WCT Suggesting VT (Circulation 1991;83:1649)	
Criterion	**ECG Appearance**
AV dissociation	Independent P waves, capture/fusion beats
Wide QRS	RBBB type: >140 ms LBBB type: >160 ms
Extreme axis deviation	—
Atypical QRS morphology for BBB	–QRS b/w +180° & –90° (–QRS lead I, & –QRS aVF) RBBB type: Absence of tall R′ in V1, r/S ratio <1 in V6 LBBB type: Onset to nadir >60–100 ms in V1, Q wave in V6
Concordance	Of QRS in precordial leads w/ same pattern & direction

Brugada Syndrome
Definition
- Incomplete RBBB w/ STE V1–V3 caused by alteration of the myocyte Na channel, a/w VT & sudden cardiac death

History
- Classically young, o/w healthy male, FHx sudden D; sxs: Presyncope, syncope, cardiac arrest

Evaluation
- ECG, electrolytes, Ca, Mg, PO_4

Treatment
- Tele; electrophysiology consult

Disposition
- If incidental finding, refer to cardiology for f/u. O/w, admit to Tele bed for EP study, possible ICD placement.

PACEMAKER AND AICD MALFUNCTION

Definition
- PM: Intracardiac device used for significant AV block &/or sinus node dysfxn
- AICD: Intracardiac device for the termination of VF/VT, & prevention of sudden cardiac death → for pts s/p VF/unstable VT arrest, persistent EF ≤30–35%, Brugada, or long QT syndrome (Circulation 2007;115:1170; NEJM 1997;337:1576)

- Biventricular pacing (cardiac resynchronization therapy): RA, RV, & coronary sinus leads → synchronize RV & LV function → ↓ CHF sxs & hospitalization, ↑ survival (NEJM 2004;350:2140; 2005;352:1539)

Approach
- Obtain an ECG & rhythm strip immediately
- Obtain the make & model of the device (most pts have a card, o/w obtain AP CXR → magnify device to obtain model number → internet search for type)
- Common PM codes: DDD (dual chamber paced, sensed, & response to sensed beat) & VVI (dual chamber paced, sensed, & inhibitory response to sensed beat)

Evaluation
- Magnet placed over device
- PM: Inhibits sensing, paces at fixed rate regardless of intrinsic cardiac activity
- AICD: Inhibits further firing, though not bradycardic pacing

Pacemaker Malfunction	
Definition	
Pathophysiology	**Differential**
Failure of output → no pacer spike despite indication to pace	Battery depletion
Failure to capture → pacing spikes *not* followed w/ depolarization	Lead fracture or dislodgement, ↑ pacer threshold, electrolyte abnormalities, local ischemia or scar
Oversensing → pacer spike despite *no* indication to pace	Lead fracture or dislodgement, sensing threshold too low
Undersensing → *no* pacer spike despite indication to pace	Lead fracture or dislodgement, sensing threshold too high
PM-mediated tachycardia	Re-entrant tachycardia in pts w/ D-paced PM, b/w the PM leads (act as an accessory pathway → anterograde conduction) & the AV node (retrograde conduction)

History
- Lightheadedness, palpitations, syncope

Findings
- ↑, ↓, &/or irregular HR, ↓ BP

Evaluation
- ECG, CXR (to visualize device & leads)

Treatment
- Transcutaneous pacing: For unstable pt
- **MAGNET: FOR PM-mediated tachycardia:** Magnet over the PM → paces @ 80 bpm OR OVERSENSING

Disposition
- Consult EP or device rep. for interrogation & reprogramming; to cath lab for lead/battery replacement

AICD Firing (JAMA 2006;296:2839; NEJM 2003;349:1836; JACC 2006;48:1064)	
Pt Sxs	**AICD Interrogation**
Pt-sensed AICD* firing	No firing
	Inappropriate firing
	Appropriate firing

*AICDs can also malfunction like PMs (see PM section above).

History
- **AICD firing:** Sudden jolt of pain
- **Premonitory sxs:** Palpitations, LH, dyspnea, CP
- **Precipitants:** Exercise, illness, noncompliance w/ antiarrhythmics, new meds

Evaluation
- ECG (ischemia, ↑ QT), CBC, Chem 7, cardiac markers, CXR

Treatment
- Treat 1°-illness, follow ACLS protocol for arrhythmia

Disposition
- Consult EP or device rep. for interrogation & reprogramming
- No firing (nl interrogation despite sxs): Look for other cause of sxs → d/c home
- Inappropriate firing (based on interrogation): Treat underlying condition; reprogram if necessary
- Appropriate firing (based on interrogation): Admit to Tele unit or CCU
  - Look for precipitants: VT, abnl electrolytes, ↑ QT, ischemia, medication noncompliance or abuse

Pearl
- If make/model # of device unknown, magnification of PA CXR will reveal device-sp code in small print.

COUGH

Pneumonia

Definitions (Clin Inf Dis 2016;63(5):575–582)
- Community-Acquired PNA (CAP): Occurs out of hosp or w/i 48 h of admx; no HCAP factors
- Healthcare-Associated PNA (HCAP): a/w hosp admx (2+ d) w/i last 90 d; residence in long-term care or nursing home; immunosuppression; family member w/ MDR organism; or any of the following w/i 30 d: IV abx, HD, home wound care
- Hospital- /Vent-Acquired PNA (HAP/VAP): Occurs >48 h after hosp admx or intubation

History
- Typical CAP (eg, Strep, Klebsiella, Haemophilus): Fever/chills, SOB, CP, cough, sputum
- Atypical CAP (eg, Mycoplasma): Low-grade fever, mild/mod SOB, CP, dry cough, GI sx
- Influenza: Fevers/chills, myalgias, malaise, MA, sore throat, dry cough
- Legionella: Severe PNA in elderly; a/w hyponatremia, GI sx
- Ask about risk factors for special organisms:
  - TB: Homeless, HIV+/immunosuppressed, IVDA, incarceration, travel to endemic region; present w/ blood-tinged sputum, night sweats, fevers, weight loss
  - PCP: Poorly controlled HIV (CD4 <200, Lymph <1 k); presents w/ subacute tachypnea
  - MDR organisms: IV abx w/i 90 d, chronic HD, immunosuppression, recent influenza (risk for MRSA), CF/bronchiectasis (pseudomonas), asplenia

Physical Exam
- Fever, tachycardia, tachypnea, hypoxia, rales, decreased breath sounds
- PNA less likely w/ nl VS & clear lungs, except in elderly, immunosuppressed

Evaluation (J Am Coll Radiol 2006;3:703–706, Clin Infect Dis 2007;44 Suppl 2:S27–S72)
- Who needs a CXR? Reserve for pts needing hospitalization, those w/ abnl VS or PEx, age extremes, numerous comorbidities, poor outpt f/u, high morbidity if PNA not detected
- CXR: Focal consolidation (typical); diffuse interstitial pattern (atypical); bat-wing pattern (PCP); hilar adenopathy, calcified or cavitary apical lesions (TB)
- CBC, Chem 7 +/– lactate (if suspecting sepsis), ABG & LDH (if PCP), BCx (if cavitary, parapneumonic eff., immunosupp/leukopenia, asplenia, liver dz, hx ETOH, failed outpt abx; ICU admx), Sputum cx (if cavitary, parapneumonic eff., hx severe lung dz, failed outpt abx, ICU admx), Influenza (in epidemics), Pneumococcal UAT (if asplenia, liver dz, immunosupp/leukopenia, parapneumonic eff.; Se 50–80%, Sp 90%), Legionella UAT (consider if recent travel, elderly, hypoNa, parapneumonic eff.; Se 80–95%, Sp 99%)

Treatment (Clin Infect Dis 2007;44 Suppl 2:S27–S72)	
Scenario/ Etiology	**Empiric Treatment Guidelines**
CAP, outpt	Healthy & no recent abx w/i 90 d: macrolide or doxycycline Comorbidities or recent abx: resp. fluoroquinolone OR (macrolide + [amoxicillin or amoxicillin/clav. or 2nd-gen cephalosporin])
CAP, inpt	Resp fluoroquinolone OR (macrolide + [ampicillin or 3rd-gen cephalosporin]) Consider pseudomonas & MRSA coverage if severe (eg, ICU). Legionella is covered by macrolide or fluoroquinolone.
MDR risk factors	Vancomycin + (antipseudomonal PCN or 3rd-gen cephalosporin or fluoroquinolone or carbapenem). Refer to local antibiogram.
Suspect PCP	PaO_2 >70:TMP-SMX DS 2 Tabs PO q8h OR (TMP 5 mg/kg PO TID + dapsone 100 mg PO QD) OR (clindamycin + primaquine) OR atovaquone. PaO_2 <70: (TMP-SMX [15 mg/kg of TMP component/kg] PO/IV q8h or [clindamycin + primaquine] or pentamidine) + (prednisone [40 mg BID] or methylprednisolone [40–60 IV Q6H] × 21 d); NNT for early steroids is 9 (Cochrane 2006:19;(3):CD006150).
Aspiration PNA	3rd-gen cephalosporin OR fluoroquinolone ± (clindamycin or metronidazole). If sick, b-lactam/b-lactamase inhibitor.
Influenza A & B (BMJ 2009;339:b5106)	Oseltamivir (75 mg PO BID × 7 d), zanamivir Tx only reduces sx by 1 d (given w/i the 48 h of onset) Tx if critically ill, extremes of age, lung dz (inc. asthma), morbid obesity, immunosuppressed, pregnant
Suspect TB	INH 5 mg/kg PO QD + Vit B_6 25–50 mg PO QD (neuropathy) + rifampin 10 mg/kg (max 600 mg) PO QD + pyrazinamide 15–30 mg/kg (max 2 g) PO QD + ethambutol 15–25 mg/kg (max 2.5 g) PO QD; ensure infectious dz f/u Airborne precautions, negative pressure room

Disposition
- CAP/HCAP: See *PNA Severity Index Score & CURB-65* (below), unless need for IV abx
- PCP: Inpt unless S$_p$O$_2$ >95% w/o desaturation on exertion
- TB: Inpt, report to Dept of Health

Pneumonia Severity Index *(NEJM 1997;336)*	
Variable	**Points Assigned**
Demographics	If male: (+age); if female, (+age − 10); nursing home resident (+10)
Comorbidities	Neoplastic dz (+30); liver dz (+20); CHF (+10); cerebrovascular dz (+10); renal dz (+10)
Physical exam	AMS (+20); HR ≥125 (+20); RR >30 (+20); SBP <90 (+15); temp <35°C or ≥40°C (+10)
Lab & radiographic findings	pH <7.35 (+30); BUN ≥30 mg/dL (9 mmol/L) (+20); Na <130 (+20); glucose ≥250 mg/dL (14 mmol/L) (+10); HCT <30 (+10); PaO$_2$ <60 (+10); pl eff. (+10)

PORT Score (Recommended Triage and Prognosis) Calculated from PSI			
Class	**Score**	**Mortality (%)**	**Disposition**
I	<50	<1	Outpt
II	≤70	<1	Outpt
III	71–90	2.8	Outpt/inpt (clinical judgment)
IV	91–130	8.2	Inpt
V	>130	29.2	ICU

CURB-65 Score *(Thorax 2003;58(5):377)*	
1 point each	**C**onfusion, **U**rea >20 mg/dL, **R**R >30, **S**BP <90, DBP <60, age >**65**
Score < 2	Low risk, consider outpt tx; Mortality 0.7% (if 0), 3.2% (if 1)
Score = 2	Short inpt hospitalization or close outpt supervision; Mortality 3%
Score > 2	Hospitalize, consider ICU; Mortality 17% (if 3), 41.5% (if 4), 57% (if 5)

Pearls
- Special considerations: IVDU/endocarditis (multifocal PNA, esp b/l), malignancy (postobstructive PNA), postinfluenza (MRSA PNA), recent elective surgery (asp PNA risk increases w/ duration of anesthesia, periop NG tube, age [*Arch Surg* 1998;133(2):194–198])
- In severe PNA, high-flow NC (vs. NIPPV) reduces 30 d mortality, & may reduce need for intubation (esp. if PaO$_2$:FiO$_2$ < 200) (*NEJM* 2015;372(23):2185–2196)
- Consider social factors if discharging pt w/ PNA (eg, f/u, ability to comply w/ regimen)

Acute Bronchitis
Etiology
- Most commonly viral: parainfluenza, adenovirus, rhinovirus, coronavirus, RSV, influenza
- Atypical bacteria ~5% of cases (*chlamydia p., mycoplasma, B. pertussis* esp. in epidemics)

History
- Cough >5 d (dry or wet), low-grade fever, myalgias, wheezing, often after URI sxs
- Consider pertussis: posttussive emesis, whoop, duration >1 wk (*JAMA* 2010;304(8):890)
- All-cause median duration of cough is 18 d; pertussis once called "100-day cough"

Physical Exam
- Fever uncommon (consider influenza or PNA); may have chest wall tenderness from muscle strain; lungs often clear but up to 40% have bronchospasm/wheeze

Evaluation
- CXR nl or bronchial wall thickening; mild leukocytosis
- Labs/CXR not routinely needed: Reserve for abnl VS, extremes of age, comorbidities

Treatment
- Supportive care, antipyretics, antitussive (e.g., Tessalon Perles 100 mg TID)
  - No good evidence for or against OTC expectorants, decongestants, or antihistamines (*Cochrane Database Syst Rev* 2012;8:CD001831)
- If wheezy or hx asthma: bronchodilator (albuterol MDI 2 puffs QID), can consider inhaled corticosteroids x 7 d (though no major data to support)
- Abx not routinely indicated (*Cochrane Database Syst Rev* 2012;CD000245)
  - Abx reduce duration of sx by <1 day (*NEJM* 2006;355(20):2125–2130)
  - Reserved for elderly, significant comorbidities, *high suspicion for pertussis*
  - Pertussis: Azithromycin 500 mg Day 1 then 250 mg QD × 4 d OR doxycycline 100 mg BID × 7 d; Abx limit transmission but minimal effect on sx duration (unless in first wk)
  - See *PNA* section for influenza tx guidelines

Disposition
- Discharge home w/ PCP f/u as needed; pts will likely recover in 2–3 wk

DYSPNEA (SHORTNESS OF BREATH)

Definition
- Difficult or labored breathing (acute or progressive) often due to primary pulm or cardiovascular etiologies, but carries broad ddx (e.g., endo, heme, tox, neuromuscular)
- Always assess for respiratory distress: RR >24 or <8, tripoding, accessory muscle use, unable to speak in full sentences, altered mental status (AMS), abnl chest movement

Approach to the Patient		
Etiology	**Features**	**Eval**
Common or Severe Cardiac Etiologies		
Myocardial ischemia	Hx: Exertional, but UA can present at rest. Often w/ pain, N/V, diaphoresis, LH	EKG, troponin, +/– stress
Arrhythmia • Supraventricular • Nonsustained VT	Hx: Can be paroxysmal or constant (AF). Sometimes w/ palpitations, CP, LH	EKG/Tele, troponin, lytes
Valve dz • Left heart (AV, MV) • Right heart (PV, TV)	Hx: Exertional, often indolent PE: Murmur, periph edema (RH), lung crackles (LH)	EKG, echo
Common or Severe Upper Airway Etiologies		
Airway obstruction • FB aspiration • Epiglottitis • Croup (pedi) • Angioedema • Abscess/hematoma	Hx: Often sudden, ask about vaccinations (epiglottitis) PE: Stridor, distress, pooled secretions (severe); check airway patency, neck ROM/ swelling	XR chest &/or neck CT Neck if considering abscess or hematoma Laryngoscopy/bronchoscopy Caution w/i exam if concern for epiglottitis
Common or Severe Pulmonary Etiologies		
Pulm. edema (2/2 CHF, left-sided valve dz, myocarditis, constrictive pericarditis, tamponade)	Hx: Exertional, orthopnea, PND, can have CP PE: Basilar crackles, LE edema/JVD (if RHF), murmur	CXR: edema, Kerley B lines, cephalization, eff. Lung u/s: B-lines BNP (insensitive in obese; *Int J Cardiol* 2014:176(3):611–617)
PTX (spontaneous [esp tall/thin or emphysema], traumatic, barotrauma [scuba, inh drugs])	Hx: Acute onset, w/ CP PE: Unequal breath sounds & chest rise; tracheal deviation, JVD if tension	CXR: can be subtle Lung u/s: absent lung slide
Pulm embolism	Hx: Often acute, can have pleuritic CP, s/sx of DVT; consider RFs PE: If massive, hypotension, JVD	D-dimer if low pretest prob CXR: wedge infarct EKG: right heart strain Bedside echo: R heart strain CTA chest or V/Q scan
Obstructive lung dz • Asthma • COPD • Bronchospasm (bronchitis, anaphylaxis) • Tracheomalacia (premature infants)	Hx: Chronic or acute irritants (allergens, URI, tobacco), hx atopy; assess freq & severity of exacerbations PE: Wheezing, prolonged expiration, accessory muscles, air movement	Decreased peak expiratory flow rate (PEFR) suggests obstructive etiology CXR (prn to r/o PNA): nl or hyperinflated (COPD)
Pl eff. (2/2 PNA, HF, cancer, cirrhosis, rarely other causes)	Hx: Slow onset, orthopnea (often due to atelectasis) PE: Diminished breath sounds & fremitus	CXR: blunted costophrenic angle, layering Lung u/s: hypoechoic fluid Diagnostic thoracentesis (use Light's criteria)
PNA	Hx: Fever, cough, +/– CP PE: Rales or rhonchi, tachypnea, tachycardia	CXR: +/– Infiltrate
Pneumonitis (drugs, XRT, environment exposure)	Hx: Fever, cough PE: Rales	CXR: +/– reticular or nodular opacities
Malignancy	Hx: Chronic cough, weight loss, hemoptysis, smoker PE: Cachexia, clubbing	CXR: +/– mass Low-dose CT chest

Other Etiologies	
Pathophysiology	Differential
Metabolic/endocrine	Hypermetabolic state (fever, thyrotoxicosis), metabolic acidosis from any cause w/ respiratory compensation (look for Kussmaul respirations), electrolyte derangements (Ca, Mg, P)
Hematologic	Anemia (heme malignancy, hemolysis, occult bleeding)
Toxins	Salicylate (respiratory alkalosis), organophosphate (bronchorrhea), CO (binds Hgb >O_2, inhibits O_2 delivery), cyanide (disrupts mitochondrial ox phosphorylation)
Mechanical	Abd distension (e.g., pregnancy, massive ascites), morbid obesity
Neuromuscular	Myasthenia gravis, Guillain-Barré, ALS, stroke, botulism, West Nile virus, phrenic nerve dysfxn (e.g., tumor infiltration, surgery)
Psychogenic	Anxiety/panic attack, somatization disorder

Asthma

Definition
- Chronic recurrent inflammatory disorder w/ airway hyperresponsiveness, bronchospasm, & reversible airway obstruction

Clinical Features
- Progressive wheezing, dyspnea, chest tightness, cough (esp nocturnal)
- Always assess sx frequency, severity, duration, home txs;
  - Evaluate for triggers: Cold air, exercise, URI, stress, allergens, meds (NSAIDs, βBs), respiratory irritants (perfumes, smoke, detergents, dander, dust)
- Assess asthma hx: Past txs, baseline PEFR, no. ED visits/yr, admx/yr, prior intubations

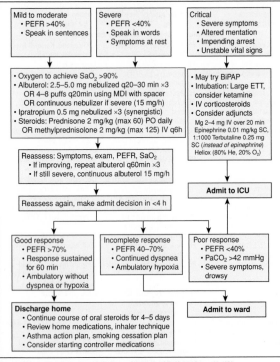

Figure 2.1 Treatment algorithm. From NHBLI Expert Panel Report 3, 2007. NIH Pub no. 08–4051.

Physical Exam
- Tachypnea, tachycardia, inspiratory/expiratory wheezes, prolonged expiration, decreased or no air movement, use of accessory muscles, tripoding, cyanosis

Evaluation
- CXR: Avoid in routine exacerbations; order to r/o PNA/PTX, elderly, comorbidities
- PEFR: Compare to pt's baseline if he/she is aware. Varies by age, gender, & height. Average adult female: 300–470; adult male: 400–660.
- ABGs are not routinely indicated to assess for severity, but normocarbia in severe asthma may be a sign of "tiring out," impending respiratory failure.

Pearls
- MDI w/ spacer as effective as nebulizers (but harder for ill pts) (NEJM 2010;363(8):755–764)
- Medium-dose inh budesonide Rx (21 d × 600–1200 mcg/d) at d/c in addition to PO corticosteroids decreases 21 d relapse by 48% (NEJM 2010;363(8):755–764)

Chronic Obstructive Pulmonary Disease (COPD)
Definition
- Progressive incompletely reversible airflow obstruction, w/ impaired gas exchange, usually w/ smoking hx. Formal dx needs PFTs (postbronchodilator FEV_1/FVC <70% predicted).
- Mild (FEV_1 ≥ 80%), Mod (FEV_1 50–80%), Sev (FEV_1 30–50%), Very sev (FEV_1 < 30%)

History
- Cough (worse than baseline), increased sputum (purulence & volume), dyspnea, wheeze
- Precipitants: Cold weather (inc incidence in winter months), infxn (viral > bacterial), cardiopulmonary dz, PE (16% of acute exacerbations; Chest 2016), med changes

Physical Exam
- Chronic bronchitis ("Blue Bloater"): Cough w/ inc. sputum production; cyanotic, plethoric, not in overt resp distress; scattered rhonchi & rales
- Emphysema ("Pink Puffer"): Thin, anxious, dyspneic, tachypneic; noncyanotic, tripoding, pursed-lip exhalation (for auto-PEEP), diminished breath sounds

Evaluation
- ECG for associated dysrhythmia (AF or MAT), cor pulmonale (P pulmonale: Big P in II)
- CXR to r/o PNA, PTX, eff., edema, malignancy
- Consider CTA Chest (2/3 of PEs in COPD are segmental or larger; Chest 2016)
- Blood gas to evaluate pH & P_aCO_2, BMP & CBC (esp if admitted)
- If chronic resp acidosis present, compare P_aCO_2 w/expected (calculated from HCO_3)
- Influenza (if epidemic), sputum cx (if severe COPD & PNA)
- Exacerbation severity: No resp failure (RR 20–30, no access muscles, no AMS, hypoxia FiO_2 <40%, nl P_aCO_2), Non-life-threatening acute resp failure (RR >30, +access muscles, no AMS, FiO_2 <40%, P_aCO_2 50–60), Life-threatening acute resp failure (same, but +AMS, FiO_2 >40%, $PaCO_2$ >60 or pH ≤7.25) (GOLD 2017 Report)

Treatment (GOLD 2017 Report)
- Titrate supplemental O_2 (goal S_pO_2 88–92%): Chronic hypoxemia inc. risk of O_2-induced hypoventilation (Crit Care 2012;16(5):323); ~2× mortality w/ high-flow O_2 (BMJ 2010;342:c5462)
- Albuterol (short-acting β-agonist): 2.5–5 mg neb q30min × 3, then q4h OR MDI w/ spacer
- Neb vs MDI (mild cases): no diff in sustained FEV_1 or admx (Cochrane 2016;(8):CD011826)
- Ipratropium bromide (anticholinergic): 0.5 mg nebulized q30min × 3 doses, then q4h (synergistic effect w/ albuterol, so give together)
- Steroids: Prednisone 40 mg PO QD (5–7 d) OR methylprednisolone (for severely ill pts)
- Abx recommended if increased sputum purulence & either increased SOB or sputum volume, OR life-threatening acute resp distress
  - Abx dec mortality 12% (NNT 8) & tx failure 31% (NNT 3) (Cochrane 2006;(2):CD004403)
  - Choice based on RFs (age >65, FEV_1 <50%, recent abx, heart dz); duration 5–7 d
  - Outpt w/o RFs: Macrolide, amoxicillin, doxycycline, or TMP/SMX
  - Outpt w/ RFs: Fluoroquinolone or amoxicillin/clavulanate
  - Inpt: Fluoroquinolone (esp if pseudomonas RF) OR (3rd-gen cephalosporin + Macrolide)
- Positive Pressure Ventilation (PPV):
  - Noninvasive PPV (BiPAP): resp acidosis, severe SOB or fatigue; watch for PTX w/PPV
  - Decreases mortality by 50% (NNT 8), intubation by 60% (NNT 3), tx failure by 50%, & hosp LOS by >3 d compared to usual care (Cochrane 2004;(3):CD004104)
  - Invasive (intubation): Not tolerating BiPAP, impending resp failure, CV instability, AMS

Disposition
- Home: Mild sxs, ambulatory S_pO_2 >90%, <Q4H bronchodilators, outpt f/u, home support
- Early f/u: dec. mortality; 20% pts not back at prior baseline by 2 mo (GOLD 2017 Report)
- Admx: Incomplete tx response, sig. below baseline, mx comorbidities, severe COPD / freq. exacerbations, elderly, poor home support (Am J Respir Crit Care Med 2013;187(4):347)

Acute Respiratory Distress Syndrome (ARDS)

Berlin Definition (JAMA 2012;307(23):2526–2533)

- Acute (sx < 1 wk) diffuse inflammatory lung injury, characterized by vascular leak, edema, & diffuse alveolar damage; imaging w/ b/l opacities, not fully 2/2 cardiac failure or fluid overload; PaO$_2$:FiO$_2$ 200–300 (mild), 100–200 (mod), <300 (sev) w/ PEEP ≥ 5 cm H$_2$O

Pathophysiology
- Impaired gas exchange, poor compliance (stiff lungs), intrapulmonary shunt

Etiology
- Direct lung injury: PNA, aspiration, near-drowning, hydrocarbons, inhalational injury, embolism (thrombotic, fat, air, amniotic)
- Systemic: Sepsis, shock, DIC, trauma, burns, transfusion, pancreatitis, meds

Clinical Features
- Rapid progressive dyspnea (<1 wk), cyanosis, crackles, & eventual respiratory failure

Evaluation
- Dx requires ABG (PaO$_2$:FiO$_2$ <300) & CXR w/ bilateral pulm edema
- May need TTE to r/o cardiac etiology, bronchoscopy to r/o diffuse alveolar hemorrhage

Treatment
- Supportive, focus on treating the underlying condition
- Lung-protective ventilation: dec 28 d mortality by 10% (NNT 10) (Cochrane 2007;(3):CD003844).
- Minimize barotrauma: low TV (<6 mg/kg), keep P$_{Plat}$ <30
- Avoid hyperoxia: wean FiO$_2$, maintain high PEEP to keep alveoli open.
- Avoid excess fluids: (CVP goal 4–6 cm if CVC present) (NEJM 2006;354(24):2564–2575)
- Excess volume initially may negate any subsequent benefit from conservative fluid management in ICU (Crit Care Med 2016;44(4):782–789)
- Refractory hypoxia: Best PEEP trial, paralysis, inh prostacyclin, prone positioning, ECMO
- No consensus on role of steroids; most meta-analyses show no mortality benefit

Upper Airway Obstruction/Foreign Body (FB)

History
- Acute FB aspiration: May be witnessed but often hx is unclear in adults
  - RFs: Extremes of age, neuro disorders, syncope, szs, alcohol or sedative abuse
  - DDx: angioedema, infectious etiology (eg, epiglottitis), soft tissue abscess/hematoma
- Subacute (eg, malignancy, expanding goiter): Often a delayed Dx (eg, wheezing unresponsive to bronchodilators)

Physical Exam
- General appearance: May arrive cyanotic & in respiratory arrest if total obstruction
- In breathing pt, respiratory exam depends on degree & location of obstruction: dec air movement, stridor, wheezing, secretion intolerance. Do not underestimate pt distress.

Evaluation
- CXR, XR neck rarely shows FB. Diagnostic & therapeutic flex bronchoscopy is standard.

Treatment
- If still breathing: Airway equipment, including cricothyrotomy kit, at bedside. Prepare for transfer to OR to remove FB in a controlled environment (bronchoscopy or DL).
- If not breathing: Attempt direct laryngoscopic visualization & removal of FB w/ forceps. If unsuccessful, perform surgical airway.
- If FB moves inferior to vocal cords but still occluding, push object into 1 lung by pressure from Ambu bag/ETT; once intubated, position ETT to ventilate contralateral lung.

Disposition
- Flex bronchoscopy successful in 90% cases (Respir Care 2015;60(10):1438–1448)
- If object is safely removed & pt stable, can discharge home

HEMOPTYSIS

Definition
- Expectoration of blood or blood-stained sputum from below the vocal cords
- "Massive" hemoptysis: no defined volume (generally >500 cc/d or >100 cc/h), but any volume inhibiting breathing should be treated similarly; high mortality 2/2 asphyxiation
  - Bronchial arteries (high pressure) > pulm arteries (low pressure) > alveoli

Differential	
Pathophysiology	**Differential**
Pulm	COPD, CF, bronchiectasis, pulm HTN, PE, AVM, lung trauma
Cardiac	Pulm edema (eg, 2/2 CHF, mitral valve pathology)
Infectious	Acute bronchitis (#1 cause), PNA, TB, abscess, fungal infxn
Neoplastic	Malignancy (primary or met), carcinoid
Autoimmune	Goodpasture's (anti-BM), granulomatosis polyangiitis (ANCA+)
Other	Recent instrumentation, tracheoarterial fistula (recent thoracic/ vasc surgery), FB aspiration, inh cocaine, Osler–Weber–Rendu (telangiectasias), spontaneous (coagulopathy),

Approach to Patient

History
* Onset (sudden vs. progressive); quantity of blood; differentiate from GI or ENT source
* ROS: Fever, SOB, CP, weight loss, epistaxis (granulomatosis polyangiitis, coagulopathy)
* Identify hx or RFs for COPD, PE, TB, CHF, cancer, autoimmune dz, coagulopathy

Physical Exam
* Assess airway first, if compromised, proceed directly to stabilizing airway
* Lungs: May show signs of COPD, PNA, edema
* Cardiac: for signs of CHF or valve dz
* Skin: Evaluate for evidence of bleeding &/or telangiectasias

Evaluation
* Labs: CBC, PT, PTT; type & screen. Consider AFB, BNP, D-dimer, UA (Goodpasture, granulomatosis polyangiitis) based on clinical scenario
* Imaging: CXR if unstable; chest CT if stable (much more helpful); ±bronchoscopy

Treatment
* Airway: HOB >45°; lean to side of bleeding (if known), suction, supplemental O_2 prn
  * If intubation necessary: double suction, large-bore ETT (consider advancing ETT into unaffected lung; double-lumen ETT if skilled operator), urgent bronchoscopy
* Definitive management: Minor hemoptysis can usually be managed conservatively, but if massive requires bronchoscopy or IR embolization, surgical resection if all else fails

Disposition
* Healthy, minimal bleeding: Get CXR; if negative: Home, outpt f/u
* High-risk pt, minor bleeding: Get CT, consider admit for observation, bronchoscopy
* Massive: ICU, consult pulmonology, interventional radiology, thoracic surgery

ABDOMINAL PAIN

Approach

Assess nature of pain: Location, acute or chronic, constant or intermittent, relation to eating, associated sxs such as fever, nausea, vomiting, dysuria, change in bowel habits

Always ask about previous abd surgeries

Labs depend on presentation. Consider CBC, BMP, UA, LFTs, lipase, hCG, lactate

In the elderly, low threshold to evaluate for AAA w/ bedside US & ACS w/ EKG

Abdominal Pain Differential	
Location	**Differential**
RUQ	Cholelithiasis, acute cholecystitis, cholangitis, acute hepatitis, perforated duodenal ulcer, RLL pneumonia, pulmonary embolism (PE)
LUQ	Gastritis/PUD, splenic enlargement/rupture/infarction, LLL pneumonia, PE
Epigastric	Gastritis/PUD, pancreatitis, MI, myocarditis (see *Cardiology*), GERD
Lower Quadrants	Ruptured ectopic pregnancy, ovarian cyst/torsion, PID/TOA, endometriosis, kidney stone, incarcerated/strangulated hernia
RLQ	Appendicitis, Meckel's diverticulum, psoas abscess
LLQ	Diverticulitis
Diffuse	Early appendicitis, mesenteric ischemia, gastroenteritis, peritonitis, AAA, SBO, large bowel obstruction/volvulus, spontaneous bacterial peritonitis, IBD, colitis, DKA, sickle cell crisis, irritable bowel syndrome, anaphylaxis, colon ischemia, constipation

RIGHT UPPER QUADRANT PAIN

Emerg Med Clin North Am. 2011;29:293)

Biliary Etiologies	
Dx	**Definition**
Cholelithiasis	The presence of stones in the gallbladder
Biliary Colic	Intermittent obstruction of cystic duct or ampulla of Vater
Choledocholithiasis	Full obstruction of the CBD by a stone
Cholecystitis	Acute inflammation of the gallbladder due to obstruction in cystic duct, often a stone
Cholangitis	Infection of the CBD, 80% caused by stone

Cholelithiasis

Presentation

Intermittent epigastric &/or RUQ pain, +N/V, a/w fatty meals

Pain may radiate around to the back or to the R scapula

In biliary colic, sxs generally resolve completely in b/w episodes (minutes to hours)

Mild RUQ tenderness but no fever or Murphy's sign

In choledocholithiasis & cholecystitis, sxs will become constant

Evaluation

Nl labs in biliary colic

RUQ U/S spec/sens is 90–95% for stones.

Treatment

NSAIDs, opiate analgesics, antiemetics; elective surgical management

Disposition

If pain controlled, d/c home w/ surgery f/u to consider cholecystectomy

If persistent pain, consider posisiblity of impacted stone in GB neck/impending cholecystitis

Pearls

Acutely, biliary colic presents w/ diffuse upper abd pain before localizing to the RUQ

RFs for gallstones include female gender, increasing age & parity, & obesity

Choledocholithiasis

Presentation

Biliary colic that becomes constant; late presentation may be a/w jaundice

Mild RUQ tenderness but no fever or Murphy's sign

Evaluation
- Obstructive LFT pattern, U/S shows dilated CBD >6 mm

Treatment
- ERCP-guided stone removal +/− cholecystectomy

Disposition
- Admit medicine. Usually initially managed by GI.

Cholecystitis
Presentation
- Persistent RUQ pain w/ N/V; may be accompanied by fever
- In elderly, delayed presentation w/ fever & poorly localized abd pain
- RUQ tenderness; Murphy's sign (arrest of inspiration w/ RUQ palpation), or Sonographic Murphy's sign (pain w/ palpation of visualized gallbladder w/ U/S probe); fever

Evaluation
- CBC (elevated WBC ± left shift), LFTs (may be elevated but are often nl), RUQ US: The presence of stones, thickened gallbladder wall (>3 mm), & pericholecystic fluid has a PPV of >90%, but early presentation may lack US findings
- HIDA scan: May be considered if US is equivocal; high sens/spec for GB duct obstruction

Treatment
- 2nd- or 3rd-generation cephalosporin (E. coli, Enterococcus, Klebsiella) broaden coverage if septic
- Surgical consult for cholecystectomy; may do percutaneous drain if poor surgical candidate

Disposition
- Admit for surgical management

Cholangitis
Presentation
- Charcot's triad: RUQ pain, jaundice, fever (present in 70% of pts)
- Reynold's pentad: Charcot's triad +shock & MS changes (present in 15% of pts)

Evaluation
- Labs: ↑ WBC, ↑ LFTs, ↑ alk phos, positive blood cultures
- US/CT not very sens; can be suggestive
- ERCP is diagnostic & can be therapeutic if obstructing stone is found

Treatment
- Broad-spectrum abx for gram-negative enterics (eg, E. coli, Enterobacter, Pseudomonas): Piperacillin/tazobactam OR ampicillin/sulbactam OR ticarcillin/clavulanate OR ertapenem OR metronidazole + (ceftriaxone OR ciprofloxacin)

Disposition
- Admission to medicine for IV abx ± ERCP w/ surgery consultation

Pearls
- 80% pts respond w/ conservative mgmt & abx w/ elective biliary drainage
- 20% require urgent ERCP biliary decompression, percutaneous drainage, or surgery
- 5% mortality

EPIGASTRIC PAIN

Pancreatitis
(Tenner S, Baillie J, DeWitt J, et al. American College of Gastroenterology Guideline: Management of acute pancreatitis. Am J of Gastroenterology. 2013;108:1400.)

Etiology
- Alcohol (25–30%), gallstones (40–70%), idiopathic, hypertriglyceridemia (TG >1000), hypercalcemia, drugs (thiazides, furosemide, sulfa, ACE-I, protease inhibitors, estrogen, acetaminophen, steroids), obstructive tumors, infection (EBV, CMV, HIV, HAV, HBV, coxsackievirus, mumps, rubella, echovirus), trauma, post-ERCP, ischemic

Presentation
- Epigastric pain radiating through to the back, nausea, vomiting
- Often h/o previous pancreatitis, alcohol abuse, gallstones
- A/w smoking, type 2 diabetes mellitus
- May be ill appearing, tachycardic, epigastric ttp, guarding, ↓ bowel sounds (adynamic ileus)

Evaluation
- Increased lipase >3× nl (amylase is not specific)

- If severe: ↑ WBC, ↑ BUN (>20 or rising), ↑ HCT (>44% or rising), ↑ creatinine
- CT scan: 100% spec but low sens. Not required; should be obtained only to r/o cx (acute fluid collection, pseudocyst, necrosis, abscess), esp after 24–48 h if no improvement
- Abd U/S: Used to evaluate for gallstones, CBD dilatation, or pseudocyst
- CXR: Pleural effusions & pulmonary infiltrates are a/w severe dz

Treatment
- Aggressive IV fluids (LR preferred); NPO initially, but early enteral nutrition if tolerated
- IV analgesia, antiemetics
- Prophylactic abx have unclear benefit; may use for severe necrotizing pancreatitis
- Delayed cholecystecomty for gallstone pancreatitis
- IR drainage for persistent or infected fluid collection,

Disposition
- Admission for supportive care if severe or not tolerating PO
- Atlanta criteria: In mild dz, there is absence of organ failure & local cxs, which are present in severe dz. Organ failure defined as GI bleeding, shock, PaO_2 ≤60%, creatinine ≥2.

LOWER QUADRANT/PELVIC PAIN

Appendicitis
(*Lancet.* 2015;386:1278)

History
- Classically, dull vague periumbilical pain → migrates to RLQ, localizes & becomes sharp
- Nausea, vomiting, anorexia, fever
- Greatest at 10–30 y of age but can occur at any time

Physical Findings
- RLQ (McBurney's point) tenderness, localized rebound, & guarding
- Psoas sign: Pain w/ active flexion against resistance or passive extension of the right leg
- Obturator sign: Pain w/ internal rotation of the flexed right hip
- Rovsing sign: RLQ pain w/ palpation of the LLQ

Evaluation
- Labs: Leukocytosis (not sens or spec); cannot r/o w/ nl WBC. Check hCG.
- US: Less sens than CT but high spec. Consider esp in children young (thin) adults
- Abd CT (92% sens)—secondary signs of appendicitis (eg, fat stranding) less visible in thin pts
- MRI is a useful modality in pregnancy
- Alvarado score uses signs, sxs & lab values to place pts in low risk (1–4 points), intermediate risk (5–6) & high risk (7–10) groups. High sens/low spec.
- In cases w/ strong clinical e/o appendicitis & low suspicion of alternate etiology, it may be reasonable to proceed to OR w/o imaging

Alvarado Score for Acute Appendictis	
RLQ tenderness	+2
Elevated temp >99.1	+1
Rebound tenderness	+1
Migration of pain to RLQ	+1
Anorexia	+1
Nausea or vomitin	+1
Leukocytosis >10 K	+2
Leukocyte left shift	+1

Management
- Abx: Cefoxitin, cefotetan, fluoroquinolone/metronidazole, OR piperacillin–tazobactam
- Admission to surgical service. Traditionally surgically removed; treatment w/ abx alone a/w high readmission rate (25–30%) for surgery w/i 1 year

Pearl
- Pts at extremes of age are more likely to have atypical presentations & present w/ perforated appendicitis.

Hernia
(*NEJM.* 2015;372:756)

Definition
- Defect in the abd wall that allows protrusion of abd contents
- Incarcerated hernia: Cannot be reduced
- Strangulated hernia: Incarcerated hernia w/ vascular compromise (ischemia)

History
- Bulging mass in abd wall (eg, umbilical, epigastric), inguinal region, or scrotum, or inner thigh (femoral); worse w/ increased intraabdominal pressure
- Inguinal hernias are either direct or indirect; medial or lateral to the inferior epigastric vessels, respectively

Physical Findings
- Bulge &/or palpable defect in abd wall or groin
- Strangulated: Tenderness, fever, skin discoloration, or associated peritonitis

Evaluation
- If concern for strangulated hernia, consider CBC, lactate, pre-op labs
- CT scan required if concern for strangulated hernia

Management
- Attempt reduction w/ generous analgesia/anxiolysis, pt in Trendelenburg
- If easily reduced, d/c w/ analgesic, stool softener, & surgery f/u
- If not reducible or if strangulated, consult surgery for operative intervention

Pearl
- Be cautious about reducing a hernia that has been irreducible by the pt for more than 12 h & is difficult to reduce in the ED b/c bowel may be compromised.

Diverticulitis
(*BMJ.* 2006;332:271)

Definition
- Inflammation of (colonic) diverticulum
- Complicated diverticulitis: Associated perforation, obstruction, abscess, or fistula

Presentation
- LLQ pain, fever, nausea, change in bowel habits, urinary sxs
- Mild LLQ tenderness, 50% of pts have heme-positive stool
- Complicated may have peritonitis, septic shock

Evaluation
- Clinical Dx if mild sxs & typical presentation
- Labs: Increased WBC
- CT to confirm dx or if concern for complicated diverticulitis. May see pericolonic stranding, abscess or contained free air if micro perforation

Treatment
- Mild: PO metronidazole + (cipro or TMP-SMX) for 7–10 days
- Severe: NPO, IV fluids, IV ampicillin–sulbactam OR piperacillin–tazobactam OR ceftriaxone/metronidazole OR quinolone/metronidazole OR carbapenem
- Most complicated diverticulitis can be managed medically +/– IR drainage
- Surgery is required if medical therapy fails, large free air is present, or for large abscess that can't be drained percutaneously. Elective surgery may be recommended for & recurrent dz (≥2 episodes)

Disposition
- If mild, d/c w/ abx, antiemetic, analgesia & PCP or general surgery f/u. If severe, admit.

Pearl
- Consider diverticulitis in older pts w/ urinary sxs but unremarkable or equivocal urine sediment

---

DIFFUSE PAIN

Abdominal Aortic Aneurysm
(Hirsch AT, Haskal ZJ, Hertzer NR, et al. ACC/AHA 2005 Practice Guidelines for the management of patients with peripheral arterial disease. *Circulation.* 2006;113:e463.)

Definition
- Dilation of the abd aorta (true aneurysm, involves all layers of the vessel wall).

History
- Older pt w/ low back pain, abd pain, or flank pain (may mimic renal colic), syncope/hypotension

Physical Findings
- Pulsatile mass (often not present), early satiety due to duodenal compression
- Ruptured/leaking AAA: Hypotension, abd tenderness, decreased femoral pulses, mottling

Evaluation
- Abd CT if hemodynamically stable
- Bedside US may reveal enlarged aorta & free fluid

Treatment
- Stable, nonruptured: Surgical or endovascular repair required if >5.5 cm (1%/y risk of rupture if >5 cm) or rapidly growing; usually arranged as outpt
- Ruptured/leaking: Immediate surgical repair, allow permissive hypotension (SBP 90s)

Disposition
- Direct to OR/IR if unstable

Pearls
- Larger the AAA the greater the risk for rupture
- Rupture into RP can temporarily tamponade, intraperitoneal rupture is rapidly fatal, can also rupture into GI tract (aortoabdominal fistula)
- RFs: Smoking, HTN, hyperlipidemia, CAD, PVD, age ≥65 y, male (5×), FH
- 50% mortality for AAA if ruptured at presentation

Small Bowel Obstruction
(Acad Emerg Med. 2013:20:528)

Definition
- Mechanical obstruction of nl intestinal transit leading to proximal bowel dilation

History
- Diffuse, colicky abd pain, nausea/vomiting, abd distension, h/o abd surgeries/prior obstructions/hernia, obstipation (not passing gas)

Physical Findings
- Diffuse abd tenderness, distension, high-pitched bowel sounds

Evaluation
- Supine & upright abd x-rays (~75% sens): Multiple air–fluid levels, >3 cm small bowel dilation, more than 3 mm small bowel wall thickening
- Bedside US (~90% sens): >2.5-cm dilated loops of bowel, back & forth peristalsis
- Abd CT (~87% sens) can be diagnostic & used to characterize the obstruction (level, severity, cause)

Treatment
- NPO, bowel rest, gastric decompression w/ NGT placement
- IV fluids, analgesia, antiemetics
- Surgical consultation—most cases managed conservatively

Disposition
- Admission
- Direct to OR if high risk (e.g., closed-loop obstruction, impending perforation, e/o bowel ischemia)

Large Bowel Obstruction/Volvulus
(J Gastrointest Surg. 2013;17:2007)

Definition
- Mechanical obstruction of the large bowel usually caused by cancer (most commonly), volvulus (twisting of the large bowel on itself), intussusception, fecal impaction

History
- Insidious onset of diffuse, colicky abd pain, distention, constipation, N/V

Physical Findings
- Diffuse abd tenderness, distension, bowel sounds present early

Evaluation
- Supine & upright abd x-rays: Dilated large bowel (84% sens), but cannot identify underlying cause
- Abd CT: Can be helpful to distinguish from pseuo-obstruction

Treatment
- IV fluids & correction of electrolyte abnormalities
- NGT for proximal decompression
- Surgical consultation for likely operative reduction (particularly for cecal volvulus)

Disposition
- Surgical admission

Pearls
- Sigmoid volvulus most common in ill, debilitated, elderly pts, or pts w/ psychiatric/neurologic disorders
- Cecal volvulus common in young adults, classically marathon runners

Perforated Viscus
(Surgical Clin North Am. 2014;94:471)

Definition
- Perforation of hollow viscus leading to abd free air, intraluminal spillage

History
- Acute onset, severe abd pain, worse w/ movement
- May be consequence of bowel obstruction, diverticulitis, cancer, or other primary GI pathology

Physical Findings
- Acute peritonitis: Rigidity, tap tenderness, rebound, hypotension, sepsis

Evaluation
- Supine & upright abd x-rays: May show pneumoperitoneum
- Abd CT: Definitive study but not required for operative management

Treatment
- Immediate surgical consult
- Broad spectrum abx to cover polymicrobial infection (enteric GNR, GPC, anaerobes)

Disposition
- Surgical admission

Pearl
- Findings may be masked in pts who are elderly or chronically immunosupressed

Mesenteric Ischemia
(Curr Gastroenterol Rep. 2008;10:341)

Definition
- Insufficient perfusion to the intestine
- Etiologies: arterial embolism (40–50%, typically SMA), arterial thrombosis (25–30%, a/w severe atherosclerosis), nonocclusive mesenteric ischemia (20%, low cardiac output state), mesenteric venous thrombosis (10–15%, a/w clotting disorders)

History
- RFs: Age >60, recent MI, AF, vascular dz (coronary, peripheral), CHF (↓ forward flow)
- May have h/o prior abd angina: Postprandial pain, food aversion
- Acute presentation w/ abd pain, anorexia, vomiting, bloody stools

Physical Findings
- Ill appearing, pain out of proportion to exam, tachycardia, fever, occult blood in stools. Late signs include peritonitis, shock.

Evaluation
- Early surgical eval
- Labs: May see ↑ WBC, ↑ HCT, AG acidosis, ↑ lactate, ↑ amylase, ↑ LDH
- Abd x-ray: Nl prior to infarction, "thumbprinting" of the intestinal mucosa later
- Abd CT: Colonic dilation, bowel wall thickening, pneumatosis of the bowel wall
- CT angiography: More sens than CT alone

Treatment
- IV fluids
- Broad spectrum abx
- Surgical consultation
- Anticoagulation for venous thrombosis & embolic dz
- IR for thrombolysis or embolectomy
- OR for resection of dead/nonviable gut

Disposition
- Surgical admission vs. IR/OR

Pearl
- 20–70% morality; improved if dx made prior to infarct

Colon Ischemia (Ischemic Colitis)

(Curr Gastroenterol Rep. 2015;17:45)

Definition
- Nonocclusive microvascular dz of the colon, secondary to hypoperfusion & reperfusion injury

History
- Crampy abd pain over segment of colon involved (typically left), blood in stool, diarrhea, recent surgery, or illness

Physical Findings
- Tenderness over affected colon usually mild, peritoneal findings suggest perforation

Evaluation
- Labs: WBC, BUN, creatinine, LDH may be high but all nonspecific
- Abdominal CT: Nonspecific mesenteric fat stranding, bowel wall thickening, abnormal colon wall enhancement

Treatment
- Supportive care, bowel rest, hydration, pain management, abx for severe dz

Spontaneous Bacterial Peritonitis

(Wiest R, Krag A, Gerbes A. Spontaneous bacterial peritonitis: recent guidelines and beyond. Gut. 2012;61:297.)

Definition
- Infection of the ascitic fluid in pts w/ severe chronic liver dz

History
- Fever, abd pain, new or worsening ascites, hepatic encephalopathy

Physical Findings
- Stigmata of liver failure, diffuse abd pain, ascites

Evaluation
- Labs: ↑ Bili, ↓ platelets increase likelihood of dz. Coags, platelets prior to paracentesis
- Paracentesis: >250 PMN, blood:ascites pH gradient >0.1, culture

Treatment
- Abx: Cefotaxime 2 g IV OR levofloxacin 750 mg IV. Carbapenem if nosocomial, recent abx or long-term ppx abx.
- Albumin 1.5 g/kg at Dx & 1 g/kg for 3 d shows survival benefit

Disposition
- Medical admission

Pearls
- Caused by bacteria that translocate from gut. 70% GNR (E. coli, Klebsiella), 30% GPC (S. pneumoniae, Enterococcus)
- Occurs in 20% of cirrhotics
- Clinical signs unreliable; have low threshold for paracentesis in admitted pt w/ ascites. Delayed paracentesis >12 h a/w higher mortality. (Am J Gastroenterology. 2014;109:1436)

INFLAMMATORY BOWEL DISEASE
(ULCERATIVE COLITIS AND CROHN'S DISEASE)

(Lancet. 2007;369:1641)

Definition
- Ulcerative colitis (UC): Inflammation of the colonic mucosa
- Crohn's dz (CD): Transmural inflammation of the GI tract

Inflammatory Bowel Disorder (Ulcerative Colitis and Crohn's Disease)		
	Ulcerative Colitis	**Crohn's Dz**
Clinical features	Fever, bloody diarrhea, tenesmus, urgency, painful BMs	Fever, abd pain, diarrhea (less often bloody)
GI involvement	Exclusively colon (mostly rectal), continuous lesions limited to submucosa, friable mucosa; irregular, shallow ulcers; pseudopolyps; crypt abscesses; loss of haustral markings	Colon & jejunum, but can extend to esophagus; transmural involvement; cobblestone mucosa; granulomas; skip lesions
GI cx	Toxic megacolon (>8 cm, usually transverse colon), colon cancer	Strictures, fistulas, perianal dz

History
- Women >men typically presents in 2nd or 3rd decade, weight loss, vomiting, abd pain/diarrhea (grossly bloody in UC) that flares w/ emotional stress, infections, withdrawal from steroids

Physical Findings
- Diffuse abd tenderness (focal RLQ tenderness in CD), heme-positive stools 20% of pts have extraintestinal sxs, perianal dz (seen in CD); fissures, fistulas, abscess

Common Extraintestinal Features	
Arthritic	Ankylosing spondylitis, tendinitis, arthritis
Intraabdominal	Primary sclerosing cholangitis, pancreatitis, nephrolithiasis
Dermatologic	Pyoderma gangrenosum, erythema nodosum
Ophthalmic	Uveitis, episcleritis

Evaluation
- Labs: Low HCT (from chronic blood loss), increased WBC, hypokalemia (from diarrhea)
- Plain abd x-ray: If perforation, obstruction, or toxic megacolon suspected
- Abd CT: May r/o cx (eg, abscess, obstruction, fistula)
- Outpt colonoscopy: If Dx not known & once acute flare resolved

Treatment
- IV fluids, bowel rest, surgical consult, steroids, ± 5 ASA agents (mesalamine, sulfasalazine)

Disposition
- Admit for severe dz or acute cx

NAUSEA AND VOMITING

(Emerg Med Clin North Am. 2011;29:211)

Approach
- Common sxs of many dz processes (eg, intra-abd dz, metabolic derangements, toxic ingestions, neurologic dz)
- Careful attention to ROS, PMH, previous abd surgeries
- Labs: Consider CBC, BMP, UA, LFTs, lipase, hCG
- Treat underlying cause: Antiemetics (eg, ondansetron, promethazine), IVF if not taking PO

Nausea & Vomiting Differential			
Abdominal/GU	Toxicologic	Neurologic	Metabolic/Other
Obstruction (gastric outlet, small bowel, large bowel)	Alcohol intoxication or withdrawal	Vertigo (cerebellar, vertebrobasilar, vestibular)	Systemic infection
Infections (appendicitis, cholecystitis, pyelonephritis)	Other drugs of abuse	Meningitis	Dehydration
Gastroenteritis, food poisoning	Intentional ingestions	Increased intracranial pressure	Hypoglycemia, hyperglycemia
Gastritis/ulcers	Chemotherapy or medication-related	Intracranial bleed	Hyponatremia
Ischemia, perforation	Caustic ingestions	Migraine	Acidosis (DKA, AKA)
Torsion (testicular or ovarian)		Tumors	Cardiac ischemia
Kidney stones			Pregnancy

Gastroenteritis
- **Definition:** Irritation of the GI tract causing vomiting & diarrhea usually caused by infections (viruses, bacteria, bacterial toxins, parasites) or due to medications or diet
- **History:** Vomiting & diarrhea, crampy abd pain, ±fever

- **Physical Findings:** Nl exam or mild diffuse abd ttp, tachycardia, dehydration
- **Evaluation:** Consider BMP if clinical concern for significant electrolyte derangement. Stool culture if systemically ill, fever, recent abx, exposure to treatable pathogen.
- **Management:** Supportive care, antiemetics. IVF if not taking PO. Home when tolerating PO. Abx & antimotility agents generally not indicated
- **Pearl:** Viral & bacterial toxins (food poisoning) are most common, typically resolve w/o tx in 48H

GASTROINTESTINAL BLEED

(*Emerg Med Clinics North Am.* 2016;34:309)

Approach
- Hemodynamically unstable pts should get 2 large-bore IVs (14–18 gauge), early transfusion of PRBC as well as FFP & Vit K if impaired coagulation
- ROS, PMH, previous GIB, alcohol use, liver dz
- Labs: CBC, BMP, LFTs, lipase, coagulation studies, lactate, type & screen. BUN/Cr ratio >30 indicates upper GI source

GI Bleed Differential	
Location	**Differential**
UGIB (bleeding proximal to the ligament of Treitz)	PUD, gastritis, variceal bleed (esophageal & gastric), Mallory–Weiss tear, aortoenteric fistula, gastric cancer
LGIB (bleeding distal to the ligament of Treitz)	Diverticulosis, angiodysplasia, colon cancer, ischemic bowel, IBD, infectious diarrhea, FB, Meckel's diverticulum, anal fissure, hemorrhoids

UPPER GI BLEED

Approach
- Glasgow–Blatchford score was designed to predict need for transfusion or urgent endoscopy. A score of zero identifies low-risk pts who can safely be discharged w/ outpt f/u (*JAMA* 2012;307:1072; *Lancet* 2000;356:1318).

Criteria for Glasgow–Blatchford Score of 0	
Hemoglobin	>12 g/dL (men) or >11.9 (women)
Systolic BP	>109 mmHg
Heart rate	<100
BUN	<18.2 mg/dL
No melena, syncope, heart failure, or liver dz	—

Bleeding Peptic Ulcer Disease (PUD) or Gastritis
(*NEJM.* 2016;374:2367)

Definition
- Inflammation or ulceration of the stomach or duodenal lining caused primarily by *H. pylori* infection, NSAIDs, (15–30%), alcohol

History
- Bloody or coffee ground emesis; dark, tarry stool

Physical Findings
- Epigastric tenderness, melena or heme-positive stool

Evaluation
- Labs: CBC, LFTs, coagulation panel, elevated BUN; *H. pylori* serology (90% sens)
- NG tube not routinely indicated

Treatment
- IVF resuscitation, PRBC if Hgb <7 or hypotensive, IV proton pump inhibitor ↓ need for endoscopic therapy but does not ↓ bleeding or mortality
- Emergent EGD if hemodynamically unstable

Disposition
- If ongoing bleeding, Blatchford >0, high risk: Admit for EGD

Variceal Bleeds
(*Hepatology.* 2007;46:922)

History
- Bright red hematemesis, diffuse abd pain, nausea, h/o portal hypertension

Physical Findings
- Stigmata of liver failure (jaundice, spider angiomas, ascites, caput medusae), Ill-appearing hypotension, tachycardia, melena

Evaluation
- Labs: CBC, LFTs, coagulation panel, type & cross

Treatment
- Place 2 large bore IVs, initiate IV fluid resuscitation, PRBC if Hgb <7 or active bleeding
- Octreotide bolus & drip; IV PPI
- Antibiotic prophylaxis (ceftriaxone or levofloxacin) increases survival
- Emergent EGD if hemodynamically unstable, may need emergent TIPS if still bleeding
- Balloon tamponade w/ Minnesota or Blakemore tube if exsanguinating (after intubation)

Disposition
- Usually ICU admission, pts can decompensate quickly

Mallory–Weiss Tear
Definition
- Tears in the mucosal membrane of the distal esophagus caused by vomiting. A/w heavy alcohol use.

History
- Specks of bright red blood in emesis or mild hematemesis after forceful retching

Physical Findings
- Most have no physical findings, mild tachycardia

Evaluation
- Upright CXR if hemodynamically unstable to evaluate for subcutaneous or mediastinal air for Boerhaave syndrome (complete esophageal rupture)

Treatment
- Antiemetics, PO challenge

Disposition
- D/c w/ outpt EGD

Pearl
- Boerhaave syndrome can result from emesis but usually pts are ill-appearing w/ shock & require surgical management. Consider water-soluble swallow study if high suspicion.

Aortoenteric Fistula
(Hirsch AT, Haskal ZJ, Hertzer NR, et al. ACC/AHA 2005 Practice Guidelines for the management of patients with peripheral arterial disease. *Circulation.* 2006;113:e463.)

Definition
- Fistula b/w the aorta & GI tract, most commonly in duodenum

History
- H/o AAA, aortic graft (usually >5 y), may have sentinel bleed or large-volume GIB

Physical Findings
- Rapid GIB, hemodynamic collapse

Evaluation
- CBC, type & cross, emergent surgical consult, CT scan if stable

Treatment
- IV fluid resuscitation, PRBC if indicated
- Surgical repair

Disposition
- Surgical ICU admission

Pearl
- Mortality directly related to time to the OR

(Crit Care Clin. 2016;32:241)

Diverticular Bleeding
- **History:** Painless bright red rectal bleeding often initiated by urge to defecate
- **Physical Findings:** Nl abd exam, BRBPR, no etiology found on rectal exam
- **Evaluation:** Labs: CBC, LFTs, coagulation panel, type & cross
- **Treatment:** Usually self-limited. IV fluid resuscitation, PRBC if indicated
- **Disposition:** Admit for colonoscopy

Colorectal Cancer

History
- Chronic blood in stool, change in bowel habits, anorexia, weight loss, light-headedness

Physical Findings
- Pale, heme occult positive stools

Evaluation
- Labs: CBC, LFTs, coags; CT if concern for obstruction or significant bleeding

Treatment
- IV fluid resuscitation, PRBC if indicated
- Surgical consultation if significant bleeding (rare)

Disposition
- If stable, d/c for outpt colonoscopy/oncology w/u

Colonic Angiodysplasia
- **Definition:** Enlarged, fragile blood vessels, usually in cecum or proximal ascending colon (10–20% of LGIB)
- **History:** >60 y/o, small frequent bleeds. Usually coagulopathy or NSAID use precipitates bleed.
- **Physical Findings:** nl abd exam, BRBPR, or heme occult positive stools
- **Evaluation:** CBC, coagulation panel
- **Treatment:** IV fluid resuscitation, PRBC if indicated; endoscopic cautery or IR embolization
- **Disposition:** Admit for observation & colonoscopy

DIFFICULTY SWALLOWING

(Nat Rev Gastroenterol Hepatol. 2015;12:259)

Definition
- Dysphagia is difficulty swallowing, odynophagia is pain w/ swallowing

Approach
- Nature: Time course, sudden or progressive, localization (oropharyngeal vs. esophageal)
- ROS, PMH, hx, or FH of GI disorders or neurologic disorders
- Labs: CBC, BMP
- Studies: Barium swallow or EGD for structural/mechanical lesions; motility studies

Dysphagia Differential	
Dysphagia	**Differential**
Solids (mechanical obstruction)	Esophageal ring (intermittent), eosinophilic esophagitis (intermittent), esophageal cancer (progressive), oral/pharyngeal abscess (4d), neck cancer
Solids & liquids (motility disorder)	Spasm (intermittent), scleroderma (progressive), achalasia (progressive), neurologic (eg, myasthenia, ALS)
Odynophagia	Reflux esophagitis, infection (candida, herpes), radiation, chemotherapy

Esophageal Food Impaction/Foreign Bodies
(Curr Gastroenterol Rep. 2013;15:317)

Definition
- Food or FB stuck in esophagus (70% lodge at the lower esophageal sphincter)

History
- Sensation of food (often meat) or FB stuck in the esophagus, retching, unable to swallow secretions. A/w esophageal stricture, esophageal ring, or eosinophilic esophagitis

Physical Findings
- Odynophagia, neck or chest pain, respiratory distress, drooling, retching

Evaluation
- CXR (may show dilated esophagus w/ air–fluid level or FB)

Treatment
- Airway management
- Historically glucagon given however no data to support its use. Effervescents, benzos are also often used.
- Endoscopy if a dangerous object is present (batteries, sharp object), or FB doesn't pass w/i 12–24 h

Disposition
- If tolerating PO, d/c w/ outpt EGD

DIARRHEA

(Emerg Med Clin North Am. 2011;29:211)

Definition
- Frequent, watery stools. Specifically, >3 loose stools/d OR >200 g stool/d.
- Acute ≤14 d, persistent 14–30 d, chronic >30 d

Approach
- Nature: Bloody, mucus present, duration, frequency, volume; recent travel or abx
- Labs: Consider BMP for electrolyte derangement; consider CBC, LFTs, heme occult

Diarrhea Differential	
Causes	**Differential**
Infectious	**ACUTE** Viruses: Norovirus, rotavirus, adenovirus, CMV Preformed toxins (food poisoning <24 h): *S. aureus, B. cereus* Toxins formed after colonization: *E. coli* (ETEC), *C. difficile, C. perfringens* Invasive bacteria (generally +fecal WBC, +blood): *E. coli* (EIEC, EHEC), *Salmonella, Shigella, Campylobacter, Yersinia, V. parahaemolyticus* Parasites: *Giardia* (–blood), *E. histolytica* (+blood) **CHRONIC** *Giardia, E. histolytica, C. difficile*
Medications - ↑ secretion - ↑ motility - ↑ cell turnover	Abx, antacids, lactulose, sorbitol, chemotherapy, colchicine, gold
Inflammatory - Fever - Hematochezia - Abd pain	IBD, radiation enteritis, ischemic colitis, diverticulitis
Malabsorption - Chronic - ↓ sx w/ fasting - ↑ osmotic gap - ↑ fecal fat - Vitamin deficient	Bile salt deficiency (cirrhosis, cholestasis, ileal dz, bacterial overgrowth), pancreatic insufficiency, mucosal abnormalities (celiac sprue, tropical sprue, Whipple dz), lactose intolerance
Secretory - nl osmotic gap- - ↓ sx w/ fasting - Nocturnal sx	Hormonal (VIP, carcinoid tumor, medullary cancer of the thyroid, Zollinger–Ellison, glucagon, thyroxine), laxative abuse, neoplasm
Motility	IBS, scleroderma, hyperthyroidism, diabetic autonomic neuropathy

Infectious Diarrhea
(NEJM. 2014:370:1532)

History
- Diarrhea ± blood/fever, recent ingestion of meats/poultry/dairy/shellfish/sea food/ unrefrigerated food, sick contacts, recent travel (last 6 mo), antibiotic use
- Invasive bacterial enteritis is a clinical Dx: Fever, blood in stool, tenesmus, abd pain

Physical Findings
- Dehydration, mild abd tenderness. If invasive: Heme-positive stool, fever.

Evaluation
- Labs: Increased WBC (*Salmonella*), low WBC (*Shigella*), eosinophilia (parasites) hypokalemia, metabolic acidosis
- Stool culture, fecal WBC & O&P appropriate if ill appearing, severe diarrhea, extremes of age, chronic, or immunocompromised

Treatment
- IV fluid resuscitation if needed, electrolyte repletion
- Abx: TMP-SMX, ciprofloxacin or azithromycin (recent travel, ill appearing, fever, immunocompromised), OR metronidazole (*C. difficile*, *Giardia*, *E. histolytica*)
- Antimotility agents may be used for traveler's diarrhea
- Constipating diet (BRAT: Bananas, rice, applesauce, toast) for a short time

Disposition
- Admit if unable to keep up w/ volume loss or toxic

Pearl
- Significant abd pain in not common & should be evaluated further

Diarrhea Epidemiology	
Pathogen	**Most Common Cause of...**
Norovirus	Infectious diarrhea in adults
Campylobacter	Bacterial diarrhea
Staphylococcus aureus	Toxin-related diarrhea
Giardia	Parasitic diarrhea in US (backpackers, freshwater)
Enterotoxigenic *Escherichia coli*	Traveler's diarrhea

Diarrhea Pathogen Characteristics	
Pathogen	**Characteristics**
Campylobacter	Duration 5–7 d. Fever, vomiting, abd pain. RFs: Day care, food (dairy, meats, poultry), exposure to young dogs & cats, summer months Cx: Bacteremia, meningitis, cholecystitis, pancreatitis Reiter syndrome
Salmonella	Duration 2–7 d. Fever, vomiting, abd pain. RFs: Food (dairy, meats, eggs), exposure to turtles, comorbidities (esp sickle cell anemia) Cx: Enteric fever (*S. typhi*), bacteremia, meningitis, osteomyelitis, Reiter syndrome Controversy regarding whether antimicrobial tx prolongs carrier state
Shigella	Duration 2–5 d. High fever, abd pain, no vomiting. Marked bandemia. RFs: Day care, swimming pools, summer & fall Cx: HUS, febrile szs in infants
Yersinia	Duration up to 1 mo. Fever, vomiting, abd pain. RFs: Food (pork), winter Cx: Appendicitis, terminal ileitis, intussusception, toxic megacolon, cholangitis
Preformed toxin-mediated (*Staphylococcus*, *Bacillus*)	Duration 1–2 d. Onset w/i 6 h. RFs: *Staphylococcus* (dairy, meats, custard, mayonnaise); *Bacillus* (reheated fried rice)
Enterotoxic *Escherichia coli*	Duration 3–5 d. Fever, vomiting, abd pain. RFs: Foreign travel

Pathogen	Characteristics
Enterohemorrhagic *Escherichia coli*	Duration 3–6 d. Fever, no vomiting, abd pain. RFs: Ground beef Cx: HUS. Controversy over role of abx in increasing risk of HUS.
Clostridium perfringens	Duration 1 d. No fever, vomiting, abd pain. RFs: Food (meats, pork, vegetables)
Clostridium difficile	Variable duration. Fever, no vomiting, abd pain. RFs: Hospitalization, antibiotic use Cx: Fulminant colitis (2–3%), toxic megacolon (colonic dilation >6 cm), bowel perforation
Vibrio parahaemolyticus	Duration 5–7 d. No fever, vomiting, abd pain. RFs: Seafood (esp raw)
Giardia	Duration >7 d. No fever, vomiting, or abd pain. RFs: Contaminated water (backpackers) Cx: Chronic diarrhea
Entamoeba	Duration 7–14 d. No fever, vomiting, no abd pain. RFs: Contaminated water Cx: Liver abscess

RFs, risk factors; Cx, complications.

Irritable Bowel Syndrome
(*BMJ*. 2015;350:h1622)

Definition: Disorder of the colon: Causes cramping, bloating, diarrhea, constipation (F > M)

History: Recurrent abd pain >3 d/mo over the last 3 mo. Plus 2 or more of the following: Improvement w/ defecation, onset w/ change in frequency of stools, onset w/ change in form of stools. No constitutional sxs.

Physical Findings: May have mild lower abd tenderness, heme-negative stools

Treatment: Fiber for constipation, antimotility for diarrhea, antispasmodics (Bentyl) for pain

Disposition: D/c, outpt management

Pearl: Dx of exclusion. Unlikely if age of onset >35 or associated constitutional sxs.

CONSTIPATION

(*JAMA*. 2016;315:185)

Definition
- Reduced frequency of stool (<3/wk), &/or difficult passage of hard stool

Approach
- Nature: Duration, severity, character of stool, pain, fever, medication use, prior episodes

Constipation Differential	
Etiology	Differential
Functional	Slow transit (dietary, dehydration, immobility), pelvic floor disorders, IBS
Obstruction	Cancer, stricture, rectal FB
Medication	Opiates, anticholinergics, iron, CCBs, AEDs, antidepressants
Neurologic	Parkinson's, MS, spinal cord lesion, stroke
Metabolic	DM, hypothyroid, hypokalemia, panhypopituitary, hypercalcemia, pregnancy

Simple Constipation (Including Stool Impaction)
History
- Poor diet, decreased fluid/fiber intake, decreased mobility, constipating medications

Physical Findings
- Firm stool in the rectal vault, palpable stool on abd exam, minimal abd ttp

Evaluation
- Abd x-ray or CT if need to r/o obstruction, or to confirm dx in high-risk pt

Treatment
- Manual disimpaction if needed
- Colace, magnesium citrate, enema (esp in elderly), bisacodyl (oral or suppository)
- Natural bulking agents (Metamucil) when constipation resolves

Disposition
• Home

Rectal Foreign Body
(Surgical Clin of North Am. 2010;90:173)

Physical Findings
• FB in rectum on exam or anoscopy, peritonitis if perforation

Evaluation
• Abd x-ray to eval location/shape & presence of pneumoperitoneum

Treatment
• Removal w/ forceps traction while the pt bears down. Impacted object may cause proximal vacuum suction; can pass foley around object to break vacuum seal & use balloon to pull back on object.
• Removal in OR if unsuccessful or if sharp object w/ risk of perforation

Disposition
• Home if removed

Pearl
• Procedural sedation may be needed to sufficiently dilate anus to remove FB in ED

JAUNDICE

(Prim Care. 2011;38:469)

Definition
• Yellowing of the skin as a result of elevated bilirubin (>3 mg/dL)

Approach
• Duration, associated pain, fever, recent travel, h/o liver dz or alcohol abuse
• Labs: CBC, BMP, UA, LFTs, lipase, ±ammonia if MS changes, paracentesis if ascites

Jaundice Differential		
Hyperbilirubinemia	**Predominant Bilirubin**	**Differential**
Prehepatic: Increased bilirubin production or impaired conjugation	Unconjugated (indirect)	Hemolysis, hematoma resorption, prolonged fasting, Crigler–Najjar syndrome, Gilbert syndrome
Hepatocellular	Mixed, mostly conjugated	Infectious hepatitis, hepatotoxins, autoimmune, alcoholic (AST:ALT >2:1), drugs (eg, tylenol, amiodarone, statins), metabolic disorders (Wilson, Reye), hemochromatosis, α_1-antitrypsin deficiency, ischemic ("shock liver," AST/ALT >1000 + ↑ LDH), nonalcoholic fatty liver dz
Intrahepatic (nonobstructive): Impaired excretion of conjugated bilirubin	Conjugated (direct)	Cholestatic jaundice of pregnancy, Dubin–Johnson syndrome, rotor syndrome, primary biliary cirrhosis, sarcoidosis, graft-versus-host dz
Extrahepatic (obstructive): Impaired excretion of conjugated bilirubin	Conjugated (direct)	Cholecystitis, choledocholithiasis, cholangitis, pancreatitis, carcinoma (ampulla, gallbladder, pancreas, CBD), biliary stricture (postsurgical), sclerosing cholangitis

Viral Hepatitis			
Dz	**Transmission**	**Serologic Pattern**	**Comments**
Hepatitis A	Fecal-oral, contaminated food/water	Acute: IgM anti-HAV Prior: IgG anti-HAV	Incubation 2–6 wk, self-limiting, tx is supportive

Dz	Transmission	Serologic Pattern	Comments
Acute Hepatitis B[a]	Blood, sex, perianal	IgM anti-HBc: Acute HBeAg: Active infection HBsAg: May appear before sxs	Incubation 1–6 mo, 70% acute infections subclinical, 30% jaundice, 1% fulminant failure, acute tx is supportive, <10% persist to chronic hepatitis B
Chronic Hepatitis B[a]	Blood, sex, perianal	IgG anti-HBc	Major cause of hepatocellular cancer (10–390 × increased risk), tx: INF-α-2b, PEG INF-α-2b, lamivudine, adefovir, telbivudine, entecavir
Acute Hepatitis C	Blood, sex	HCV viral load	Incubation 2 wk–5 mo, 75% acute infections subclinical, 25% jaundice, 50–80% persist to chronic
Chronic Hepatitis C	Blood, sex	HCV & anti-HCV	Major cause of cirrhosis (20–30%), 2–3% of cirrhotics develop HCC, tx: PEG INF-α-2b + ribavirin
Hepatitis D	Blood, sex	Anti-HDV	Exists only in association w/ hepatitis B, faster progression to cirrhosis
Hepatitis E	Fecal–oral (travel)	IgM anti-HEV	Self-limiting, mortality 10–20% in pregnancy

[a]Implies secondary (Dienstag JL, Delemos AS. "Viral Hepatitis." In: Bennett JE, ed. *Mandell, Douglas and Bennett's Principles and Practice of Infectious Diseases*. 8th ed. Philadelphia, PA: Saunders; 2015:1439–1468.)

Cirrhosis
(*Lancet*. 2014;383:1749)

Definition
- Fibrosis & nodular regeneration resulting from hepatocellular injury
- Major etiologies include viral hepatitis (esp HCV), alcoholism, nonalcoholic steatohepatitis

History
- Abd pain, jaundice, pruritus, abd distension

Physical Findings
- Liver: Enlarged palpable liver or shrunken nodular
- Signs of liver failure: Jaundice, spider angioma, palmar erythema, gynecomastia, asterixis, encephalopathy
- Signs of portal HTN: Splenomegaly, ascites, caput medusae

Evaluation
- New onset: LFTs, BMP, CBC (for anemia, thrombocytopenia), INR (to evaluate synthetic function), abd US if pain, tenderness, or fever present to r/o acute biliary dz or if concern for Budd–Chiari, paracentesis if new-onset ascites
- Exacerbation/decompensation of known cirrhosis: CBC, BMP, INR, ammonia. Paracentesis to r/o SBP if fever, abd pain, new hepatic encephalopathy, GIB, significant leukocytosis.

Treatment
- Directed at treating cultures
- Hepatic encephalopathy (failure of liver to detoxify ammonia & other agents): Protein restriction, lactulose (goal 2–4 stools/d)

Disposition
- Admit if decompensated (increasing ascites/edema despite compliance w/ outpt regimen), pulmonary edema, renal failure, hypotensive, encephalopathic, febrile

Pearl
- Cxs: Portal HTN (ascites, varices), encephalopathy, hepatorenal syndrome, hepatopulmonary syndrome, infections (relative immunosuppression), HCC

Acute Liver Failure
(*NEJM*. 2013;369:2525)

Definition
- Acute hepatic dz often w/ coagulopathy & encephalopathy
- Fulminant liver failure is when encephalopathy occurs <8 wk since onset of 1st sx

- Etiologies: Viral hepatitis (A, B, E), drugs (acetaminophen), acute ischemic injury in critically ill pts, neoplastic infiltration, acute Budd–Chiari, mushroom ingestion, Wilson's dz

History
- Abd pain, jaundice, toxic ingestion, nausea, vomiting, malaise, confusion

Physical Findings
- Jaundice, abd tenderness, enlarged liver, encephalopathy, pulmonary edema, GIB (decreased clotting factors, DIC)

Evaluation
- Labs: CBC (anemia, thrombocytopenia), PT/INR, BMP (electrolytes, renal function), acetaminophen level, viral serologies

Treatment
- Treat underlying causes (eg, acetaminophen w/ NAC)
- If etiology unclear have low threshold for NAC regardless of acetaminophen level
- Abx: Broad-spectrum (Vancomycin + 3rd-generation cephalosporin)
- Coagulopathy/GIB: Vit K, FFP, platelets, cryoprecipitate if active hemorrhage
- Cerebral edema: Consider ICP monitoring, hypertonic saline/mannitol, avoid fever
- Transplantation improves survival but not universally available

Disposition
- Admit medicine. ICU if fulminant, hypotensive, or otherwise unstable.

RECTAL PAIN (PROCTALGIA)

(Medical Clin of North Am. 2014;98:609)

Approach
- Nature: Duration, consistency of stools, bleeding, fevers

Proctalgia Differential	
Bleeding	Cryptitis (inflammation of epithelial pockets), hemorrhoids, anal fissure, proctitis (inflammation of the rectal mucosa)
No bleeding	Anorectal abscess, anal fistula, anorectal FB, proctalgia fugax (idiopathic severe brief rectal pain), pilonidal dz

Anal Fissure
- **Definition:** Superficial tear of the anoderm that begins just below the dentate line
- **History:** H/o passage of hard stools, sharp pain w/ defecation, blood on toilet paper
- **Physical Findings:** Visible fissure, painful. If not midline, eval for cancer, HIV, IBD, STDs.
- **Management:** Sitz baths (warm baths 15 min 3×/d), high-fiber diet, lidocaine jelly, topical nitroglycerin ointment, topical diltiazem gel

Hemorrhoids
Definition
- Dilated or bulging veins of the rectum & anus. Internal hemorrhoids may prolapse & become incarcerated (irreducible) or strangulated (ischemic).

History
- Bright red-coated stool/toilet paper/dripping into the bowl, pain w/ defecation, h/o hard stools, constipation, prolonged sitting

Physical Findings
- External hemorrhoids are visible on eversion of the anal orifice, internal hemorrhoids may be palpable & are only visible w/ anoscopy

Evaluation
- CBC only if significant blood loss suspected or concerning underlying condition

Management
- Outpt w/ stool softener (Colace, Senna), Sitz baths (15 min TID & after BMs), suppositories for symptomatic relief
- Acute thrombosis (<48 h since onset of pain) can be excised at bedside in ED
- If prolapsed hemorrhoid is incarcerated w/ signs of strangulation, consult surgery

Pearl
- Hemorrhoidal bleeding rarely a cause of significant anemia

FEVER

Background
- Temp >100.4°F/38°C
- Caused by response to bacteria, viruses, inflammation; ↑ metabolic rate, meds
- Distinct from hyperthermia (caused by exogenous factors)

Approach
- Careful hx: COLDER, associated sxs (N/V, diarrhea, cough, abd pain, rash, AMS)
- Eval directed by pt hx & sx localization
- Assess VS for significant abnormalities that may indicate serious infection (↓ BP, ↑ HR)
- If immunosuppressed (HIV/AIDS, elderly, malnourished, chronic steroids, DM) or neutropenic, more intensive eval & testing: CBC, Chem, UA & cx, CXR; consider blood cx & admission
- Intermittent/relapsing fever, FUO, or occurring after foreign travel: Consider travel-related infectious etiologies, endocarditis

Fever Differential	
Pathophysiology	**Differential**
Cardiac	Endocarditis, myocarditis (1j)
Pulmonary	Pneumonia (2b), bronchitis (2b), empyema, TB (2b), PE
GI	Intra-abd abscess, cholangitis (3a), diverticulitis (3a), appendicitis (3a), hepatitis (3g), cholecystitis
GU	UTI (6a), pyelonephritis (6b), PID (7e)
Neurologic	Meningitis (5d), subarachnoid hemorrhage, TBI, dysautonomia
ENT	Pharyngitis (13b), sinusitis (13), otitis
Toxicology	Neuroleptic malignant syndrome (10l), malignant hyperthermia (10l)
Environmental	Hyperthermia (10k), drug-induced, vector-borne & zoonotic diseases (4h), parasitic infections (4l), Rocky Mountain spotted fever (8a)
Infectious	Mononucleosis (4f), TB (2b), HIV (4g), rheumatic fever, viral infections (4f)
Hematologic	DVT (1b), PE (1b), sickle cell (11e)
Orthopedic	Osteomyelitis (19k), septic arthritis (12c)
Oncologic	Malignancy (11), neutropenic fever, tumor lysis syndrome
Immunologic	Autoimmune, Mediterranean fever, vasculitis, sarcoid

ENDOCARDITIS

(NEJM. 2013;369:785)

History
- RFs: IVDU, congenital or acquired valvular dz, prosthetic valves, structural heart dz, HD, indwelling venous catheters, cardiac surgery, bacteremia, HIV, previous endocarditis
- Dx difficult 2/2 nonspecific sx (lethargy, weak, anorexia, low-grade temp), or negative w/u

Findings
- Fever (80%), new murmur (48%), CHF, splenomegaly (11%), petechiae
- Classic physical exam findings
  - Roth spots (2%): Exudative, edematous retinal lesions w/ central clearing
  - Osler nodes (3%): Violaceous tender nodules on toes & fingers
  - Janeway lesions (5%): Nontender, blanching, macular plaques on soles & palms
  - Splinter hemorrhages (8%): Nonblanching, linear, reddish-brown under nails
- Septic emboli (mitral valve vegetations)

Diagnosis

Modified Duke Criteria	
Classification	**Requirements for Dx**
Definite	Microorganism on culture or histology of vegetation/cardiac abscess OR Clinical criteria: 2 major, 1 major & 3 minor, or 5 minor
Possible	1 major & 1 minor, or 3 minor

Criteria	Evidence
Major	≥2 positive blood cultures, endocardial involvement, vegetation, new valvular regurgitation
Minor	Predisposing cardiac dz, IVDU, or other RFs, fever, vascular phenomena (septic infarcts, ICH, Janeway lesions), immune phenomena (glomerulonephritis, Osler's nodes, Roth's spots, RF), positive blood culture not meeting major criteria

Evaluation
- EKG, CBC, Chem, coags; CXR, ↑ ESR/CRP (nonspecific), at least 3 sets blood cx
- Typically *Staph aureus* or *Strep* species, also *Enterococcus*, *Candida* (prosthetic). Up to 10% never have organism identified
- Echo for vegetations or valve ring abscesses; TEE more sens than TTE

Treatment
- Hemodynamic stabilization if valve rupture, can present w/ acute pulm edema cultures
- Immediate abx in suspected cases, preferably after blood cultures (see table)

Disposition
- Admit w/ continuous telemetry & IV abx, ICU if hemodynamic compromise

Pearls
- Infection of endothelium of heart (including but not limited to valves)
- Consider cardiac surgery consultation for heart failure, uncontrolled infection or prevention of embolic events
- Mortality w/ native valve dz: ~25%; prosthetic valve higher
  - Worse prognosis if involves aortic valve, DM, *S. aureus* (30–40%)
  - Left-sided endocarditis (mitral 41%, aortic valve 31%) most common
  - IVDU: Tricuspid valve endocarditis; rheumatic valve dz: Mitral, then aortic valve

Antimicrobial Treatment of Bacterial Endocarditis	
Hx	**Antibiotic**
Native valve	Ampicillin-sulbactam 3 g IV q6h or Amoxicillin-clavulanate 3 g IV q6h + gentamicin 1 mg/kg IV q8h Vancomycin 15 mg/kg IV BID + gentamicin 1 mg/kg IV q8h + ciprofloxacin 400 mg IV BID (for patients allergic to beta-lactams)
Prosthetic valve (<12 mo post-op)	Vancomycin 15 mg/kg IV BID + gentamicin 1 mg/kg IV q8h + rifampin 600 mg PO BID
Prosthetic valve (≥12 mo post-op)	Same as native valve

ABSCESS

Approach
- ↓ activity of infiltrated local anesthetic agents b/c of the low pH of abscess area; consider regional nerve or field blocks + IV procedural sedation/analgesia
- Gram stain & wound cx rarely necessary for skin or perirectal abscesses
  - Cx from intra-abd, spinal, or epidural abscesses usually sent from OR to guide therapy
  - Pharyngeal abscess cx can also help tailor antibiotic therapy
- In diabetic, immunocompromised, w/ systemic sxs, septic, obtain labs & blood cultures, start IVF & abx & admit for IV abx

SOFT TISSUE

Cutaneous Abscess
(*NEJM.* 2014;370:1039)

History
- ↑ pain, tenderness & induration, usually w/o h/o fever or systemic tox
- Disruption of skin from trauma or penetrating injury, often pt cannot recall injury
- H/o IVDA/skin popping, prior MRSA abscesses

Findings
- Exquisitely tender, soft, fluctuant mass surrounded by erythema
- Most commonly *Staph* species, often polymicrobial

Evaluation
- Blood work rarely needed unless appear systemically ill; US may help w/ localization
- Culture from abscess only if tx w/ abx, severe infection, systemic illnesses, failed initial tx

Treatment
- Traditionally no abx indicated in healthy hosts unless cellulitis, systemic illness, immunosuppression, failed I&D. However, RCT of 1247 pts showed higher cure rate (80.5% v 73.6%) as well as lower rates of subsequent I&Ds, skin infections at new sites & infections in household members. *(NEJM. 2016;374:823)*
- I&D w/ regional nerve or field block ± procedural sedation
  - Create elliptical incision to prevent premature wound closure, deep enough to drain cavity. Follow tension lines to minimize scarring.
  - Break up loculations in abscess cavity w/ hemostat
  - Consider packing w/ 1/4-in gauze × 48 h (24 h if cosmetically important) for large abscesses
- Tx cellulitis if indicated (see *Cellulitis* section below)

Disposition
- D/c w/ wound care instructions, 2-d f/u
- Warm soaks TID × 2–3 d after removal of packing to allow continued wound drainage

Pearls
- Can develop essentially anywhere: Furuncle, acne, skin breakdown, insect bites
- Routine packing of abscesses after I&D is controversial

Paronychia
(J Hand Surgery. 2012;37:1068)

History
- Pain & swelling lateral to nail edge; abscess beneath eponychial fold
- Usually secondary to contaminated nail care instruments, hang nail, or trauma

Findings
- Purulent collection lateral to nail bed w/ minimal surrounding erythema
- Most commonly *S. aureus, S. pyogenes, Pseudomonas* or *Proteus.*

Evaluation
- No labs necessary

Treatment
- Oral antibiotics (cephalexin, clindamycin, amoxicillin + clavulanate) may be used
- Digital block w/ 1% lidocaine with or without epinephrine in each web space of affected digit
- #11 blade scalpel to lift cuticle from nail on affected side & express purulent material

Disposition
- D/c w/ wound care instructions, 2 d f/u
- Warm soaks to finger TID × 2–3 d to allow complete drainage

Pearls
- Often h/o manicure/pedicure, nail biting
- If recurrent or chronic paronychia, consider *Candida* infection
- May spread to pulp space of finger (felon) or deep spaces of hand, tendon if neglected

Pilonidal Cyst
(Emerg Med Clin North Am. 2016;34:251)

History
- Painful, tender abscess in midline pit between upper part of the gluteal clefts, often in obese or hirsute individuals
- More prevalent in males; fever & systemic tox very rare

Findings
- Painful, localized abscess in natal cleavage/midline sacrococcygeal region, 4–5 cm posterior to anal opening; surrounding erythema & fluctuance
- Mixed flora: *Staph* or *Strep* species, anaerobic cocci, mixed aerobic & anaerobic flora

Evaluation
- No labs necessary unless systemically ill

Treatment
- Same as for cutaneous abscess, I&D
- Antibiotics if overlying cellulitis, immunosuppressed or systemically ill
- Surgical referral for excision of follicle & sinus tract after acute episode subsides

Disposition
- D/c w/ wound care instructions, 2-d wound care f/u

Pearl
- Thought to be caused by hair penetrating into subcutaneous tissues creating abscess

Bartholin Gland Cyst/Abscess
(Best Pract Res Clin Obstet Gynaecol. 2009;23:661)

History
- Severe localized pain in labia caused by obstructed Bartholin duct
- Difficulty walking & sitting secondary to pain
- Fever & signs of systemic tox are rare

Findings
- Painful, tender, cystic mass on inferior lateral margin of vaginal introitus, often w/ purulent drainage from sinus tract
- Typically mixed vaginal flora (*Bacteroides, E. coli, S. aureus,* gonorrhea, chlamydia)

Evaluation
- Culture for chlamydia, gonorrhea

Treatment
- I&D through mucosal surface, place Word catheter ×48 h
- Sitz baths TID for the 1st 2–3 d to assist drainage
- Gyn f/u for consideration of marsupialization to prevent recurrence

Disposition
- D/c w/ wound care instructions, 2-d wound care f/u

Pearl
- Recurrence rate still 5–15% after marsupialization; consider gyn malignancy

---

PERIRECTAL ABSCESSES

(Emerg Med Clin North Am. 2016;34:251)

History
- Pain & swelling in rectal area w/ defecation & often w/ sitting down or walking
- High fever & signs of systemic tox are rare
- Pts often have h/o IBD, obesity, DM, hemorrhoids, or rectal trauma.

Findings
- Rectal exam essential to ensure abscess localized outside of anal sphincter & to identify upper extent of abscess
- Typically mixed flora (*E. coli* species, *Enterococcus, Bacteroides* species, *S. aureus*)

Evaluation
- Lab studies unnecessary unless systemically ill
- DM or immunocompromised should have Chem, CBC
- CT/MRI if concern for intersphincteric or supralevator or postanal abscess or fistula

Treatment
- ED I&D of superficial abscesses outside the anal verge w/ visible indurated area
- Pain control; I&D extremely painful, procedural sedation often needed
- If abscess is only identified on rectal exam & no induration visible, refer to surgery for I&D under general anesthesia
  - DM or immunocompromised pts should undergo I&D in OR to ensure full drainage
- Pack w/ Vaseline gauze ×48 h, Sitz baths TID for 1st 2–3 d to assist drainage
- No abx for healthy host w/ superficial abscess
- Consider abx for immunocompromised, prosthetic device/valve, incomplete I&D
  - Levofloxacin 500 mg QD (ampicillin 1 g + gentamicin 80 mg q8h) + metronidazole 500 mg q8h, consider vancomycin

Disposition
- D/c w/ wound care instructions, 2-d wound care f/u
- Admit diabetic & immunocompromised for IV abx

Pearls

- 50–75% treated w/ I&D or spontaneous drainage will develop chronic anal fistula
- Consider adding stool softeners

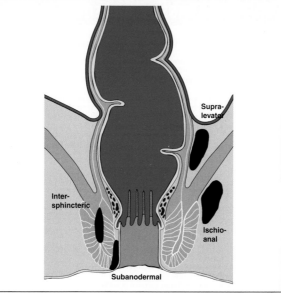

Figure 4.1

INTRACRANIAL ABSCESS

(NEJM. 2014;371:447)

History

- Caused by contiguous spread (sinus, ear, dental), hematogenous seeding from distant infection, (endocarditis) or post-CNS surgery/penetrating trauma. Often predisposing factor such as underlying disease (eg, HIV, transplant patients)
- HA (most common), ± fever, meningismus, photophobia, sz (25%), vomiting, AMS frequently absent, may have CN palsy, gait disorder
- Subacute time course (vs. meningitis or encephalitis)

Findings

- Focal neuro deficits, low-grade fever, obtundation (mass effect), sz, AMS, nuchal rigidity, papilledema
- Wide variety of organisms depending on method of entry, 1/3 polymicrobial

Evaluation

- Blood cultures, CBC (WBC nonspecific), Chem, coags
- CT scan w/ & w/o IV contrast; MRI to help differentiate abscess from tumor
- Avoid LP if any concern for high ICP as may cause brain herniation

Treatment

- Emergency neurosurgical consult for drainage in OR; airway management, sz tx
- Early IV abx w/ good CSF penetration, tailored to likely pathogen
- Start broad-spectrum IV abx: Ceftriaxone 2 g + vancomycin 1 g + metronidazole 500 mg; consider adding coverage for toxoplasmosis, tuberculosis in immunocompromised
- Corticosteroids ONLY for tx of cerebral edema: Decadron 10 mg IV × 1 then 4 mg q6h

Disposition

- Neurosurgical intervention for operative washout, 6–8 wk IV abx then prolonged PO abx

Pearls

- Mortality 15%, unless abscess ruptures into ventricular system (mortality 27–85%)
- Morbidity from residual neuro deficits, new sz from scar tissue or neuropsych Δ (30%)

SOFT TISSUE INFECTIONS

Approach

- Careful hx, associated sxs (V/D, cough, abd pain, AMS), progression
- Check blood sugar if diabetic
- Assess VS for significant abnormalities that may indicate serious infection (↓ BP, ↑ HR)
- If immunosuppressed (HIV/AIDS, elderly, malnourished, chronic steroids) or neutropenic, more intensive eval & testing: CBC, Chem, UA & cx, CXR; consider blood cx & admission
- If recent foreign travel: Consider travel-related infectious etiologies

Soft Tissue Infections Differential	
Pathophysiology	**Differential**
Dermatology	Subcutaneous cellulitis, erysipelas, impetigo (8a), SSSS, TSS, necrotizing fasciitis, abscess (4d), hidradenitis suppurativa, cat scratch (4h)
GU	Fournier gangrene
Ophthalmology	Periorbital cellulitis, orbital cellulitis
ENT	Ludwig angina
Vector-borne	Rocky Mountain spotted fever (8a), Lyme (8a)
Bioterrorism	Anthrax (4n)

DERMATOLOGIC

Cellulitis
(JAMA. 2016;316:325)

History

- Often no h/o broken skin; ± local trauma, recent surgery, FB
- May report fever, chills, malaise
- RF: Edema/lymphedema (facilitates bacterial growth)

Findings

- Warm, blanching erythema & tenderness to palpation, mild to moderate swelling
- May lead to dilated/edematous lymphatics (peau d'orange), bulla formation or linear streaking/lymphangitis
- ± distal skin disruption (eg, tinea pedis b/w toes w/ cellulitis of anterior shin)

Evaluation

- If elevated BS, check Chem, UA; rule out abscess clinically or with bedside ultrasound
- Consider blood cultures, CBC w/ differential, chemistries, CRP, CPK in systemically ill pts
- Bacterial cultures of inflamed area not indicated; only 10–50% positive
- Most often caused by *Strep pyogenes* or *S. aureus* (including MRSA); can be from metastatic seeding

Treatment

- If LE cellulitis, recommend rest & elevation × 48 h, crutches if needed
- Typically aim to treat *Strep* & MSSA, but if purulent, MRSA coverage should be added. Duration of therapy 5–10 d outpt. IV therapy changed to oral after 48 h afebrile & regression from skin markings.
- Mild cellulitis:
  - Nonpurulent: Cephalexin, PCN VK, amoxicillin/clavulanate
  - Purulent: ADD trimethoprim-sulfamethoxazole, doxycycline, OR minocycline
  - PCN allergic: Clindamycin
- Moderate nonpurulent cellulitis (+ ≥2 SIRS criteria − T >38°C or <36°C, HR >90, RR >20, WBC >12 or <4):
  - Nonpurulent: IV cefazolin, IV ceftriaxone, IV PCN G, if PCN allergy clindamycin
  - Purulent: IV vancomycin, IV clindamycin or linezolid
- Severe nonpurulent (≥2 SIRS PLUS hypotension, immunocompromised or rapid disease progression):
  - Nonpurulent: IV vancomycin + IV piperacillin/tazobactam, IV imipenem, IV meropenem
  - Purulent: vancomycin, clindamycin, linezolid, daptomycin, tigecycline
- Pain control w/ NSAID/APAP; if severe pain, consider necrotizing infection

- Wound debridement if infected, contaminated, or devitalized wound
  - Surgery consult if aggressive/necrotizing infection/gas in soft tissue

Disposition
- D/c w/ PO abx & 24–48 h f/u, strict return instructions
- Admit if signs of systemic infection, DM, immunocompromise, failure of outpt tx

Pearls
- Due to inflammation of dermal & subcutaneous tissue due to nonsuppurative bacteria, infection does not involve fascia or muscles
- Consider Doppler vascular studies in single limb w/ diffuse swelling, posterior calf or medial thigh to rule out DVT
- Mark border w/ permanent ink, write time & date
- Mimics: Stasis dermatitis (more likely if bilateral), hematoma (consider if h/o trauma), gout (consider if over joint)

Erysipelas
(Am J Med. 2010;123:414)

History
- Rapidly expanding, well-demarcated, painful plaque a/w swelling
- Extremes of age, obesity, DM, CHF, postop, nephrotic syndrome at higher risk
- Acute onset of fever, chills, malaise

Findings
- Skin painful superficial, indurated, raised; erythema w/ sharply demarcated border
- Irregular erythema w/ lymphangitis, may see desquamation, dimpling, vesicles, LAD
- Mostly found on lower extremities, sometimes on face, typically malar or "butterfly" pattern

Evaluation
- None indicated unless toxic appearing

Treatment
- Dicloxacillin, cephalexin, if c/f MRSA trimethoprim-sulfamethoxazole, doxycycline, clindamycin
- PCN allergic: Levofloxacin

Disposition
- D/c w/ PO abx & analgesics, elevate affected area, 24–48 h f/u, strict return instructions

Pearls
- Typically caused by group A β-hemolytic streptococcus; involves upper dermis & superficial lymphatics
- More superficial than cellulitis. Infection involving the ear "Milian's ear sign" unique to erysipelas because ear does not contain deeper dermis tissues

Staphylococcal Scalded Skin Syndrome (SSSS)
(Am J Med. 2010;123:505)

History
- Young children <5 yr, fairly rapid progression of prodromal sore throat, conjunctivitis, fever, malaise to painful red skin w/ sloughing
- Rare in adults, a/w chronic illness, immunosuppression, & renal failure

Findings
- No mucous membrane involvement (vs. TEN)
- Erythematous cellulitis followed by acute exfoliation: Bullae, vesicles → large sheets of skin loss resulting in scalded-appearing skin
- General malaise, fever, irritability, tenderness to palpation, does not appear severely ill

Evaluation
- None indicated unless systemically ill
- Positive Nikolsky sign (epidermis separates when pressure applied)

Treatment
- Similar to burns (IVF, topical wound care, burn consult)
- Vancomycin is antibiotic of choice

Disposition
- Admit for burn care, IVF; consider ICU

Pearls
- Caused by exfoliative exotoxins of S. aureus, reports of MRSA
- Separation of epidermal layers vs. more severe TEN (necrosis at level of basement membrane)
- Prognosis: Children (<5% mortality) often w/o significant scarring; adults (60% mortality)

Toxic Shock Syndrome (TSS)
(Lancet Infect Dis. 2009;9:281)

History
- Multiple sxs: Prodrome, pain at site of infection (out of proportion to findings), fever, GI upset, myalgia, confusion, lethargy, sore throat
- Recent surgery, infrequently changed packing (tampons, nasal packing), disruption of skin, commonly no source found

Findings
- Clinical Dx w/ findings from all organ systems:
  - Staph TSS: Temp >38.9°C, rash (diffuse macular erythroderma including palms/soles), desquamation (1–2 wk after onset), hypotension, multisystem involvement (≥3 GI, muscular, mucous membranes, renal, hepatic, hematological, CNS), cultures negative except for blood culture for *S. aureus*
  - Strep TSS: Culture positive for Strep (blood, CSF, tissue biopsy, throat, vagina, sputum); hypotension, multisystem involvement (≥2 renal impairment, coagulopathy, hepatic involvement, ARDS, generalized erythematous macular rash, soft tissue necrosis)

Evaluation
- CBC w/ differential, Chem, UA, LFTs, coags, cultures (blood, urine, throat, sputum, CSF)

Treatment
- Remove tampon or packing if still in place, drain abscesses if present; surgical debridement of necrotizing fasciitis or myositis; burn care
- Aggressive resuscitation, pressors if needed
- Abx may not have impact (toxin-mediated process); tx any identified source
- Staph: nafcillin, vancomycin, clarithromycin, linezolid + clindamycin (to suppress bacterial toxin synthesis)
- Strep: PCN G + clindamycin OR linezolid
- IVIG (blocks T-cell activation by superantigens) may be added if no clinical response to aggressive supportive therapy in first 6 h of treatment

Disposition
- ICU admission

Pearls
- Rate ↓ w/ ↓ in use of superabsorbent tampons
- Caused by inflammatory response to superantigen from toxin-producing Gram-positive organisms (*S. aureus*, *S. pyogenes*)
  - *Strep*: Usually after surgery or trauma; scarlet fever-like rash; 30–44% mortality, fulminant. Blood cultures positive ~60% of cases.
  - *Staph*: More indolent, 0–20% mortality. Blood cultures positive <5% of cases.

Necrotizing Soft Tissue Infections
(Crit Care Clin. 2013;29:795)

History
- Often diabetic, IVDU, obesity, EtOH abuse or nutritionally compromised
- Sudden onset of pain & swelling which progresses to anesthesia

Findings
- Cellulitis, skin discoloration/ecchymosis or gangrene, edema, spectrum of sensation from anesthesia to pain out of proportion
- Hemodynamic instability, crepitance (subcutaneous air due to gas-forming organisms), bullae & skin necrosis are rare but should trigger emergent surgical debridement
- Can progress to involvement of deeper layers, causing myositis or myonecrosis

LRINEC Score	
Points	**Lab Indicators**
4	CRP ≥150 mg/L
1	WBC 15–25/mm^3 (2 points if >25 mm^3)
1	Hgb 11–13.5 g/dL, (2 points if <11 g/dL)
2	Na <135 mmol/L (135 mEq/L)
2	Cr >1.6 mg/dL
1	Glucose >180 mg/dL
Score of ≥6	Sens 92.9%, spec 91.6% for necrotizing fasciitis

(Wong CH, Khin LW, Heng KS, et al. The LRINEC (Laboratory Risk Indicator for Necrotizing Fasciitis) score: a tool for distinguishing necrotizing fasciitis from other soft tissue infections. *Crit Care Med.* 2004;32:1535.)

Evaluation
- CBC w/ differential, Chem, UA, CRP, coags
- Plain radiographs less sens than CT/MRI in eval of gas w/i soft tissue

Treatment
- Early surgical consult for debridement (definitive tx); hemodynamic support
- Early & broad spectrum IV abx
  - Piperacillin/tazobactam 3.3 g IV q6–8h + clindamycin 600–900 mg IV q8h + ciprofloxacin 400 mg IV q12h + vancomycin 15–20mg/kg IV q12h (if c/f MRSA)
- Consider hyperbaric oxygen tx, IVIG after debridement (both controversial)

Disposition
- ICU admission for surgical debridement

Pearls
- Mortality 16–46%, fatal if untreated
- Mostly *S. pyogenes* (group A), *Clostridium*, *S. aureus*, or mixed Gram + & − bacteria, anaerobes

---

GENITOURINARY

Fournier Gangrene
(*Surgeon.* 2013;11:222)

History
- Men (10:1), >50 yo, diabetic, chronic EtOH abuse, immunocompromised
- Recent h/o instrumentation/surgery, urethral strictures or calculi, hemorrhoids, perirectal abscess, malignancies
- Fever, lethargy prodrome
- Rapidly progressing scrotal swelling, pain, erythema, warmth, possible purulent drainage

Findings
- Intensely tender, swollen, warm scrotum w/o clear fluctuance, pruritic genitalia
- Fever, chills, systemic sxs (tachycardia, ↓ BP), ± crepitus, drainage
- Deep-space infection is often vastly greater than skin involvement would suggest

Evaluation
- CBC w/ differential, Chem, blood & urine cx, CRP, coags
- X-rays may show subcutaneous air; CT will show extent of infection & necrosis

Treatment
- Urology or general surgery consult for wide debridement & drainage
- Hemodynamic support & resuscitation w/ IVF, pressors
- Broad-spectrum abx: Vancomycin, Unasyn, Zosyn, clindamycin; Td prophylaxis
- Consider hyperbaric oxygen tx. IVIG after debridement.

Disposition
- ICU admission for surgical debridement, transfer for hyperbaric oxygen therapy

Pearls
- Mortality 3–67%; early surgical debridement most strongly correlated w/ outcome
- Polymicrobial (*E. coli*, Proteus, Enterococcus, *Bacteroides*, & other anaerobes) necrotizing infection of perineum, scrotum, & penis characterized by obliterative endarteritis of the subcutaneous arteries resulting in gangrene
- Rapid destruction of fascial planes

OPHTHALMOLOGIC

(*Dis Mon.* 2017 Feb;63(2):30–32)

Periorbital/Preseptal Cellulitis
History
- Recent infection of sinuses, periorbital skin, trauma to periorbital area, insect bites

Findings
- Unilateral eyelid swelling, erythema, warmth, discoloration of skin
- Injected sclera, conjunctival ecchymosis
- No pain w/ extraocular movements, no proptosis, normal pupillary reaction & vision

Evaluation
- CBC w/ differential, blood cultures, CT scan of orbits to evaluate for orbital extension

Treatment
- Head elevation
- Abx: Ceftriaxone or Unasyn 3 g IV q6h (if need admission) or cephalexin, dicloxacillin, clindamycin or Augmentin 500 mg PO TID × 10 d if d/c

Disposition
- Admit if appears systemically ill or has other comorbidities
- O/w d/c w/ close ophthalmology f/u (2 d)

Pearls
- Infection of soft tissue of eyelids & periocular region anterior to orbital septum
- Most often caused by *Staph & Strep*, rarely *H. influenza* since vaccine
- Distinguish from orbital cellulitis: No pain w/ EOM or proptosis in periorbital cellulitis

Orbital Cellulitis
History
- Orbital pain increased w/ extraocular movements, ↓ vision
- Recent infection of sinuses, periorbital skin, trauma to periorbital area, facial trauma

Findings
- Fever, HA, rhinorrhea, malaise
- Proptosis & ophthalmoplegia are cardinal signs
  - Unilateral eyelid swelling, erythema, warmth, discoloration of skin
  - Injected sclera, chemosis
  - Tenderness on gentle globe palpation, ↑ IOP
  - ↓ visual acuity, relative afferent pupillary defect, visual field abnormalities

Evaluation
- CBC w/ differential, CT scan of orbits, soft tissue aspirate if possible, blood cultures

Treatment
- Ophthalmology consult, head elevation
- Aggressive tx w/ immediate broad spectrum IV abx

Disposition
- Admission for abx

Pearls
- Infection of soft tissues of orbit posterior to orbital septum
- Most common: *Strep, Staph, H. influenzae*, polymicrobial
- Cx: Meningitis, brain abscess, death, cavernous sinus thrombosis (bilateral involvement, rapidly worsening, congestion of veins of face or conjunctiva)

OTOLARYNGOLOGIC

Ludwig Angina
(Am J Med. 2011;124:115)

History
- A/w dental infection, mandible fractures, tongue piercings
- Typically males, a/w DM< HIV, malnutrition, alcoholism

Findings
- Fever, malaise, neck swelling, trismus, drooling, pain with tongue movement, stridor
- Swelling of submandibular/sublingual space feels hard & "board like" or woody

Evaluation
- CBC w/ differential, Chem, UA, blood cultures, coags
- CT scan head & neck

Treatment
- If severe swelling, aggressively ↑ infection, or airway threatening, endotracheal intubation may be difficult, fiberoptic nasotracheal intubation may be the best initial approach w/ cricothyrotomy as backup
- Consultation w/ otolaryngologist for admission
- Broad spectrum IV antibiotics (clindamycin, unasyn, zosyn)

Disposition
- Admit to ICU for IV abx, airway watch

Pearls
- Rapidly spreading bilateral cellulitis of submandibular space a/w displacement of tongue causing life-threatening airway obstruction
- Polymicrobial, includes group A strep, also *Staph, Fusobacterium, Bacteroides*
- Surgical debridement was tx in preantibiotic era; now only if unresponsive to IV abx or e/o purulent collections

VIRAL INFECTIONS

Viral Infections Differential	
Pathophysiology	**Differential**
Cardiac	Myocarditis (1j), pericarditis
Pulmonary	Pneumonia (2b), URI/bronchitis (2b)
GI	Hepatitis (3g), gastroenteritis (3b), EVD
Dermatology	Herpes zoster (8a), rubella (8a), measles (8a), roseola (8a), Herpes simplex (8a)
ENT	Pharyngitis (13b), sinusitis (13), diphtheria (13b), croup (13b), conjunctivitis (13d), mononucleosis
Other	HIV, rabies

EBOLA VIRUS DISEASE (EVD)

(Crit Care. 2016;20:217)

History
- Fever, chills, myalgias, malaise, then 5 d later GI symptoms such as severe watery diarrhea, nausea/vomiting, abd pain. Other symptoms like chest pain, SOB, HA, confusion may also develop. Bleeding is not universally present, mild bleeding (30%), frank hemorrhage is uncommon.
- 2–21 d incubation period
- Recent travel to country with outbreak (primarily West Africa, check CDC website for current updates)

Findings
- Fever, abd pain
- Diffuse erythematous maculopapular rash may develop day 5–7
- Pts with fatal disease typically die day 6–16 from complications including MSOF, sepsis

Evaluation
- CBC (leukopenia, lymphopenia, late elevated neutrophils, thrombocytopenia), ↑amylase, ↑AST/ALT, ↑PT/PTT, ↑fibrinogen, UA (proteinuria)
- RT-PCR assay specific for ebola

Treatment
- Supportive care of complications such as hypovolemia, electrolyte abnormalities, hematologic abnormalities, hypoxia, MSOF, septic shock, DIC
- Volume repletion, pressors as needed, pain control, nutritional support

Disposition
- Strick contact isolation, prevent contact or splashes with blood & body fluids, equipment & surfaces

Pearls
- Can be confused with more common diseases (malaria, typhoid, PNA, meningitis)
- Enters through mucous membranes, breaks in skin or parenterally

INFECTIOUS MONONUCLEOSIS

(NEJM. 2010;362:1993)

History
- Fever, pharyngitis, lymphadenopathy, HA, rash, nonspecific sxs
- 4–6 wk incubation period, 1–2 wk prodrome: Fatigue, malaise, myalgias, low-grade temp

Findings
- Low-grade temp, pharyngitis, tonsillitis
- Tender & firm LAD for 1–2 wk, most often postcervical nodes, but can be generalized
- Rash: Papular erythematous on UE, erythema nodosum, erythema multiforme
- Splenomegaly; severe abd pain uncommon, may indicate splenic rupture
- May have petechiae, jaundice, hepatomegaly, periorbital edema

Evaluation
- CBC: ↑ WBC, ↑ atypical lymphocytes, ↓ platelets, ↑ LFTs (bilirubin, AST, ALT); monospot test
- Consider rapid strep if clinical ambiguity

Treatment
- Supportive, rest, analgesics, antipyretics
- Corticosteroids if airway edema

Disposition
- Admission rarely indicated; close PCP f/u
- Advise to avoid contact sports or vigorous exercise × 1 mo to prevent splenic rupture

Pearls
- Represents syndrome response to EBV (90% of people have EBV); most cases of mono caused by EBV but most EBV infections do not result in mono
- Secondary etiology: CMV
- Transmission through saliva; infects epithelial cells of oropharynx & salivary glands
- B lymphocytes become infected → allows viral entry into bloodstream
- Self-limited; usually spontaneous resolution in 3–4 wk, complete in several months

---

HIV/AIDS

(Emerg Med Clin North Am. 2008;26:367)

History
- Fever, fatigue, night sweats, pharyngitis, diarrhea, myalgia/arthralgias, HA, flu-like sxs

Findings
- Generalized maculopapular rash, oral ulcers (thrush), fever, lymphadenopathy

Evaluation
- CBC: Leukopenia, thrombocytopenia, ↑ LFTs
- ELISA to test for HIV Ab; if + confirm w/ Western blot (VL >100 K in acute infection)
- PCR to detect viral load, CD4 count

Treatment
- Counseling pre- & post-HIV testing

Disposition
- D/c unless systemically ill, ID f/u for antiretroviral tx

Pearls
- Transmitted through sexual contact (70%), IVDU; mother-to-child transmission possible during pregnancy or birth
- Untreated HIV → AIDS (CD4 <200) w/ life expectancy of 2–3 yr

Opportunistic Infection Prophylaxis		
Infection	Indication	Prophylaxis
TB	+PPD (>5 mm) or high-risk exposure	Isoniazid + Vit B6 × 9 mo
PCP PNA	CD4 <200 or thrush	Bactrim QD OR dapsone 100 QD OR Atovaquone 1500 QD OR Pentamidine 300 q4wk
Toxoplasmosis	CD4 <100 AND + toxoplasma serology	Bactrim QD OR dapsone 200 QD + pyrimethamine 75 QD + leucovorin 25 qwk
MAC	CD4 <50	Azithromycin 1200 qwk OR clarithromycin 500 BID

Complications of HIV/AIDS	
CD4 Count	Cx
<500	Kaposi sarcoma, lymphoma, oral hairy leukopenia Candidiasis: Oral, esophageal, vaginal Recurrent bacterial infections Pulmonary & extrapulmonary TB HSV, VZV
<200	PCP PNA, *Toxoplasma, Bartonella, Cryptococcus, Histoplasma,* Coccidioides, HIV encephalopathy
<50–100	CMV, MAC Disseminated *Bartonella,* invasive aspergillosis CNS lymphoma, PML

Organ Involvement of HIV/AIDS

Organ	Manifestation/Etiology
Constitutional	Fevers: Bacterial, MAC, CMV, PCP, TB, lymphoma, drug rxn, endocarditis
Dermatologic	Kaposi sarcoma, lymphoma, VZV, HSV, HPV, *Molluscum contagiosum*
Ophthalmologic	CMV retinitis
Oral	Oral hairy leukopenia, Kaposi sarcoma, thrush, aphthous ulcers
Cardiac	Dilated cardiomyopathy, endocarditis, myocarditis, CAD, pericardial effusion, LVH
Pulmonary	PCP PNA, TB, fungal PNA (aspergillosis, *Cryptococcus*, etc.), CMV
GI	Oral candida, hairy leukoplakia, esophagitis, enterocolitis, GIB (CMV, Kaposi, lymphoma), proctitis, hepatitis, diarrhea (*Cryptosporidium*, *Isospora*)
Renal	Nephropathy (drugs), HIV-associated nephropathy
Hematologic	Anemia (chronic dz), leukopenia, thrombocytopenia
Oncologic	NH & CNS lymphoma, Kaposi sarcoma, cervical cancer
Endocrine	Hypogonadism, metabolic syndrome, adrenal insufficiency, HIV wasting syndrome
Neurologic	Meningitis: *Cryptococcus*, bacterial, viral, TB, cocci, histoplasmosis Neurosyphilis: Meningitis, CN palsy, dementia Mass (toxoplasmosis), AIDS dementia, myelopathy, peripheral neuropathy, HIV encephalopathy, progressive multifocal leukoencephalopathy

Antiretroviral Drugs Reactions

Drug Class	Drugs	Rxn
Nucleoside reverse transcriptase inhibitors	Zidovudine (AZT) Didanosine Stavudine Zalcitabine	Bone marrow suppression (AZT) pancreatitis (didanosine) Peripheral neuropathy
Nonnucleoside reverse transcriptase inhibitors	Nevirapine Efavirenz	Steven–Johnson syndrome
Protease inhibitors	Indinavir Atazanavir	N/V, diarrhea, hyperlipidemia, hyperglycemia, fat redistribution

RABIES

(*Curr Infect Dis Rep.* 2016;18:38)

History
- Exposure to rabid (agitated, drooling, unprovoked attack) mammal (dog, cat, bat, raccoon)
- Prodrome lasts 2–10 d; nonspecific: fatigue, loss of appetite, HA, anxiety, irritability, fever

Findings
- Encephalitic (80%) & paralytic (20%) rabies, affects brain & spinal cord respectively
  - Encephalitic form: hypersalivation, sweating, piloerection, hydrophobia, impaired consciousness → quadriparesis → death
  - Paralytic form: weakness in bitten limb, progression to quadriparesis & facial weakness, urinary incontinence → neurologic progression → death
  - Dog-acquired cases: hydrophobia, aerophobia, encephalopathy
  - Bat-acquired cases: symptoms at exposure site, abnl neuro findings (tremor, myoclonus, CN exam, motor/sensory exam)

Evaluation
- Neutralizing anti-rabies virus AB in serum (if not vaccinated), RABV antigen in tissues, RABV RNA in saliva or CSF
- CSF: pleocytosis, ↑ protein; Ab titer diagnostic, regardless of vaccine status
- Imaging (head CT, MRI) used to evaluate for other causes of encephalopathy

Treatment
- Supportive, palliative. Universally fatal within 14 d of initial symptoms
- No proven medical tx has been shown to be effective
- Therapeutic coma (ketamine, benzo's) & antiviral therapy (amantadine, ribavirin) rarely a/w survival

Disposition
- ICU admission if neuro or resp sxs w/ inpt ID consult
- Notify public health department & animal control center
- Identify others at risk & initiate postexposure prophylaxis if indicated

Pearls
- Caused by *Lyssavirus* in family *Rhabdoviridae* transmitted by animal bites
- IP is variable, typically 20–90 d but ranges from days to 1 year
- Dogs are the most commonly infected animals worldwide, but very rare in US & Canada
- Rabies PEP
  - Wound care (soap, water, irrigation w/ povidone–iodine solution), debridement of devitalized tissue, secondary closure, update Tetanus vaccination
  - If domestic dog or cat bite, determine vaccination status of animal from owner. If animal can be observed, start PEP only if animal develops symptoms
  - Assess rabies risk & need for human rabies immune globulin (HRIG) & human diploid cell vaccine (HDCV)
  - HRIG: 20 IU/kg; as much as possible at exposure site, remaining administered at distant site (eg, deltoid)
  - HDCV: 1 mL dose in deltoid in ED. F/u doses given days 3, 7, 14
  - HDCV 5th dose on day 28 if immunocompromised
  - Do not stop rabies immunization b/c of mild rxn to vaccine doses
  - Rabies cases from nonbite exposures > from known bite exposures; consider prophylaxis for any contact w/ high-risk animals (eg, bats, skunks, raccoons, coyotes, foxes)

SYPHILIS

(*Lancet.* 2017;389:1550–1557)

History
- Primary syphilis: hallmark is a chancre – painless, usually solitary, indurated, clean-based ulcerative lesion 2–3 wk after contact infected lesion.
- Secondary syphilis: painless, macular rash of 1–2 cm, lesions on palms & soles; but can vary in appearance (thus the "great imitator"). May be a/w malaise, myalgia, HA (syphilitic meningitis), sore throat.
- Latent disease
- Tertiary syphilis – late neurosyphilis (general paresis, tabes dorsalis), cardiovascular syphilis (aneurysm of ascending aorta, AV insufficiency, CAD), gummatous syphilis (reactive, granulomatous processes)

Findings
- Primary syphilis: chancre, ± nontender LAD
- Secondary syphilis: painless rash may be associated with fever, LAD, HSM, hepatitis
- Tertiary syphilis: General paresis causes progressive dementia, seizures, psychiatric syndromes. Tabes dorsalis "lightening" radicular pains, ataxia, Argyll Robertson pupil (small, do not react to light but accommodate), loss of reflexes, impaired vibratory sense.

Evaluation
- Treponemal test (eg, RPR, VDRL) → nontreponemal assay to confirm (eg, FT-ABS, TP-PA)
- Reactive CSF VDRL is diagnostic of neurosyphilis

Treatment
- Early (primary, secondary, or early latent): benzathine PCN G 2.4 million units IM ×1 OR doxycycline 100 mg PO BID × 14 d
- Late/unknown duration latent syphilis: benzathine PCN G 2.4 million units IM wk × 3 wk OR doxycycline 100 mg BID × 28 d
- Neurosyphilis: PCN G 3–4 million units IV q4H × 10–14d
- After treatment 30–50% patients have Jarisch–Herxheimer reaction (fever, myalgia, worsening skin rash). Will self-resolve, can tx with IVF, antipyretics.

Disposition
- Pts with neurosyphilis or cardiovascular syphilis should be admitted for antibiotics.

Pearls
- Caused by *Treponema pallidum*
- Increases risk of HIV infection; HIV incidence up to 20% in the decade after syphilis Dx
- Spread through direct lesion contact, small proportion through blood transfer

TETANUS

(Crit Care. 2014;18:217)

History
- Acute onset hypertonia, painful muscular contractions esp. the masseter ("lockjaw")
  → generalized muscle spasms/rigidity, dysphagia
- RFs: Inadequate vaccination status, chronic wound, IVDU

Findings
- Spasms of muscles in close proximity to site of injury, cephalic, lockjaw, risus sardonicus
  (characteristic grimace) tetanic sz, respiratory failure
- Autonomic Dysfxn: BP ↑ or ↓, dysrhythmias, cardiac arrest
- Cx include fractures & dislocations

Evaluation
- No spec tests available; clinical Dx

Treatment
- Heavy sedation (benzos, propofol) & paralysis supported by artificial ventilation
- Magnesium sulfate has been used to control muscle spasms
- Intrathecal, intramuscular antitetanus immunoglobulin hastens clinical improvement
- Abx: Metronidazole, PCN G, or doxycycline

Disposition
- ICU admission

Pearls
- *C. tetani* is obligate anaerobe, gram-positive spore forming bacillus, resistant to heat, desiccation, & disinfectants
- DTaP (diphtheria, tetanus, pertussis; inactivated) vaccine given at 2, 4, & 6 mo, booster given b/w 15–18 mo & at 4–6 yr; booster recommended q10y or if dirty wound
- Mortality 30–45%; if received tetanus toxoid at sometime in life mortality 6%
- Slow recovery over 2–4 mo, usually complete resolution of sxs

Prevention

Tetanus Postexposure Prophylaxis Guide		
Wound	**Vaccination Hx**	**Prophylaxis**
Minor, clean	<3 doses of tetanus toxoid, >10 yr since last dose or unknown immunization status	Td toxoid booster
All other wounds	<3 doses of tetanus toxoid, >5 yr since last dose or unknown immunization status	Td toxoid booster
	<3 doses of tetanus toxoid, or unknown immunization status	Tetanus immune globulin (250 mg or 500 IU IM)

- Clean & debride wound as needed
- Pts who have not completed primary immunization series should repeat Td booster in 4–8 wk & 6–12 mo

SCABIES

(Prim Care. 2015;42:661)

History
- Persistent pruritus, worse at night. Sometimes multiple family members involved
- Common in overcrowding, poor hygiene, elderly, homeless. More common in winter (survive longer on fomites, more crowded living)

Findings
- Small, pruritic, erythematous papules. Typically, web spaces between fingers & toes, flexor aspects of wrists, under armpits, around umbilicus, under knees, around nipples, genital region
- Burrow from mites: elevated thin red or gray line
- Secondary skin infections may also be present

Evaluation

- Clinical Dx. Other Dx tests (skin scrapings, shave biopsy, tape test, etc.) may increase certainty but negative results do not rule out

Treatment

- Permethrin 5% cream, 2 applications 1 wk apart OR oral ivermectin 200 µg/kg, 2 applications 2 wk apart
- Second line: crotamiton 10% cream, lindane 1% lotion
- Symptomatic relief, tx 2° infections & household members, clean clothes/linens

Disposition

- D/c w/ instructions for household to be treated, decontaminate clothing, bedding
- Exclude from school until treated, topical permethrin usually effective w/i 12 h

Pearls

- Caused by female mite, S. scabiei
- Delayed type IV hypersensitivity rxn to mite proteins (from saliva, feces, eggs, mite itself), symptoms initially develop 3–4 wk after exposure, then 1–2 d after re-exposure
- Skin-to-skin contact, indirect contact through bedding or clothing

VECTOR-BORNE INFECTIONS

Vector-borne Infections Differential	
Pathophysiology	**Differential**
Tick-borne	Lyme, Rocky Mountain spotted fever, ehrlichiosis, babesiosis
Mosquito-borne	Malaria, yellow fever, dengue fever, West Nile, eastern equine encephalitis

TICK-BORNE DISEASES

Lyme Disease (*Borrelia burgdorferi*)
(*NEJM*. 2014;371:684)

History

- 1/3 recall h/o tick bite. Often by *I. scapularis* (deer tick) in endemic area b/w May & August, or of exposure to wooded areas, incubation period 3–31 d.
- Tick must be attached for >36 h to cause infection
- Erythema migrans (typical "bull's eye" rash w/ central clearing, but can be uniform or enhanced central erythema w/o clearing; can last 3–4 wk if untreated); malaise, fatigue

Findings

- Progression can result in polyarthritis (late), cardiac conduction dz, neurologic sequelae
- Rash: Erythema migrans (absent in 20–40%)
- Lyme carditis – AV block &/or myopericarditis
- Lyme meningitis; does not present as classic bacterial meningitis
  - Early: HA, Bell's palsy, radiculoneuritis, erythema migrans
  - Late: Neurocognitive Dysfxn (ie, encephalopathy)

Evaluation

- Testing not recommended for pts w/ only erythema migrans, poor sensitivity
- For pts w/ nonerythema migrans presentations: First antibody screen assay (EIA), if positive, obtain immunoblot. Both results positive required to confirm Dx.
- ECG to assess for HB, CSF may be considered in pts w/ neurologic involvement

Treatment

- Tick removal: Using forceps or tweezers, grasp the tick as close to skin as possible, pull upward w/ steady pressure. Disinfect site, save tick for identification.
- See table, consider Rheum consult
- Avoid doxycycline in pregnant pts

Dispositions

- D/c w/ abx regimen, PCP f/u unless has symptomatic AV block/syncope

Pearls

- Deer tick tiny (head of pin) vs. dog tick (larger, more, common, don't transmit Lyme)
- Most common tick-borne dz in US; 90% of cases in MA, CT, RI, NY, NJ, PA, MN, WI, CA

ED Intervention of Lyme		
Sxs/Findings	Onset After Bite	Tx
Asymptomatic exposure	W/i 72 h	Doxycycline 200 mg PO ×1
EM rash, nonspecific viral syndrome (fever, fatigue, malaise), regional LAD	Few days–1 mo	Doxycycline 100 mg PO BID or amoxicillin 500 mg PO TID or cefuroxime 500 mg PO BID × 14 d
CN palsy w/o meningitis, asymptomatic carditis	Days–10 mo	Ceftriaxone 2 g IV QD × 14 d, up to 21 d for Lyme carditis
Musculoskeletal (arthritis), neurologic (encephalitis, meningitis, neuropathy), symptomatic carditis	Months–years	Arthritis alone: PO regimen as above × 28 d Neurologic sxs/findings: Ceftriaxone 2 g IV QD × 14–28 d

Rocky Mountain Spotted Fever (Rickettsia Rickettsii)
(Lancet Infect Dis. 2007;7:724)

History
- Tick exposure. IP 2–14 d.
- Sudden high fever, malaise, HA, myalgia, anorexia, N/V, abd pain, photophobia
- Rash 2–5 d after fever

Findings
- Multisystem dz; Temp >102°F, may be ↓ BP on presentation
- Rash (85–90%): Petechial rash typically starts at wrist & ankles; may be diffuse at onset. Typically moves out (palms & soles) then in (arms, legs, & trunk). By end of first week, rash is maculopapular with central petechiae, spares face. ~10% have no rash
- Multiple systems can be involved: Cardiac (myocarditis), pulmonary (cough, PNA), GI (abd pain, N/V, hepatomegaly), renal (ARF), CNS (meningismus, photophobia, confusion), ocular (conjunctivitis, retinal hemorrhage, arterial occlusion), muscular (CK elevation)

Evaluation
- IFA assay most commonly used, cannot distinguish between rickettsial diseases
- Ab not detectable until 7–10 d after disease onset
- CBC (thrombocytopenia, anemia), Chem (hyponatremia, ↑ BUN), LFTs, coags, blood cx
- CXR if appear toxic or abnl lung findings
- CT or MRI for AMS may show infarction, edema, meningeal enhancement
- CSF may show pleocytosis, nl glucose, elevated protein

Treatment
- Intubation if indicated, resuscitation; dialysis, fluids, PRBC + platelets if indicated
- Abx: Tetracyclines (doxycycline), chloramphenicol

Disposition
- Most require hospitalization, consider ICU (rapid progression)

Pearls
- R. rickettsii obligate intracellular bacterium spread by ticks to human endothelial cells causing small, medium vessel vasculitis
- Found in US (primarily MD, VA, NC, SC, OK, TN, AR), also western Canada, western & central Mexico, & South America
- Mortality 5% treated, 20% untreated

Ehrlichiosis and Anaplasmosis
(Prim Care. 2013;40:619)

History
- Travel to endemic area in spring/early summer, tick bite; 5–14 d incubation
- Fever, myalgia, HA, malaise, cough, chills, rash (10–30%)

Findings
- Fever, LAD (<25%), maculopapular, petechial, or macular rash on UE/trunk

Evaluation
- CBC (↓ WBC, ↓ plat), ↑ LFT, LDH, ↑ ESR; blood cultures not helpful
- PCR most sens during acute infection, serologies, peripheral smear
- CT/LP if severe HA to R/O meningitis, may show pleocytosis, mildly elevated protein

Treatment
- Analgesics, resuscitation, abx: Doxycycline 100 mg IV/PO BID × 10 d

Disposition
- Admit as needed for supportive tx

Pearls
- Obligate intracellular gram-negative bacteria; *Anaplasma* infects granulocytes (HGA), *Ehrlichia* targets monocytes (HME); distinct epidemiologically but same clinical picture
- HGA—American deer tick; found in NE & Midwest US in summer
- HME—American dog tick, lone star tick; found in SE & south-central US, April–September

Babesiosis
(*NEJM.* 2012;366:2397)

History
- Travel to endemic areas b/w May & September, tick bite; 1–4 wk incubation
- Usually asymptomatic in healthy host; affects elderly, immunocompromised, asplenic
- Fever, weakness, fatigue, HA, photophobia, AMS, cough, SOB, N/V, abd pain, arthralgias, chills, myalgias, anorexia, cough

Findings
- Fevers, rigors, hepatosplenomegaly, pharyngeal erythema, jaundice, retinopathy

Evaluation
- CBC (hemolytic anemia), ↓ haptoglobin, ↑ LFTs, ↑ LDH, ↑ reticulocytes, ↓ platelets, UA (proteinuria or hematuria)
- Wright or Giemsa peripheral blood smear; PCR, immunofluorescence Ab testing
- Serial blood smear may show parasites

Treatment
- Resuscitation, symptomatic tx, airway management
- Early abx: Atovaquone IV + azithromycin IV OR clindamycin PO or IV + quinine PO
- RBC exchange transfusion if parasite load >10%, severe anemia, end-organ Dysfxn

Disposition
- Admit for ongoing supportive therapy, abx
- Most pts recover spontaneously in 1–2 wk, fatigue may continue for months

Pearls
- Protozoan parasite *Babesia* transmitted by tick or blood transfusion from infected individual
- Peak in May–October; found in Europe & US (MA, NY, RI, CT, upper Midwest, Northwest)
- Mortality 10% (US), 50% (Europe); if symptomatic

MOSQUITO-BORNE DISEASES

Malaria
(WHO Guidelines for the Treatment of Malaria. 3rd ed. 2015.)

History
- Travel to Central & South America, Sub-Saharan Africa, India, SE Asia, Middle East, Caribbean, South Central Asia; incubation period 7–30 d, may present months after
- Paroxysmal chills, sweats, & high fevers q48–72h
- Fever, cough, fatigue, myalgias, malaise; less common anorexia, N/V, diarrhea, HA

Findings
- Fever, hypotension, tachycardia, may see jaundice, signs of anemia, splenomegaly, icterus
- Severe malaria: AMS, ≥2 szs, pulm edema, HD unstable, >40°C, DIC, severe anemia, renal failure, hypoglycemia, hyperparasitemia, acidosis, hyperbilirubinemia
- Cerebral malaria: AMS, meningitis, szs, encephalopathy; 15–20% mortality even w/ tx

Evaluation
- CBC, Chem, haptoglobin, UA, blood cx, thick & thin blood smear, rapid antigen tests
  - Triad of thrombocytopenia, ↑ LDH, atypical lymphocytes
- Head CT/LP if AMS or encephalopathy to look for cerebral malaria
- CXR if signs of pulm edema

Treatment

- Airway management, IV access & IV fluid resuscitation, infectious dz consultation
- Prophylaxis regimen often recommended; depends on region of travel
  - Use DEET & insect repellent, bed nets w/ permethrin, long-sleeved clothing
- Tx regimen dependent on geography, which species, & severity of dz
- Watch QT interval when giving antimalarials

Disposition

- Admit if suspected or confirmed, if child, pregnant, or immunodeficient
- ICU if end-organ sxs noted, signs of cerebral malaria
- Thin & thick blood smears should be performed qwk × 4 after d/c to ensure resolution

Pearls

- *Plasmodium (ovale, vivax, malariae, falciparum)* cause malaria, transmitted through bite of infected female *Anopheles* mosquito, causing systemic infection of erythrocytes
  - *P. falciparum* most severe: Can cause cerebral malaria, pulm edema, renal failure, anemia; highest occurrence in Sub-Saharan Africa
  - *P. vivax* & *P. ovale* produce dormant form in liver, usually causes uncomplicated malaria
- 2 million deaths annually, majority in kids <5 y/o, ~90% in rural Sub-Saharan Africa
- Sickle cell trait, thalassemia, Hemoglobin C disease & G6PD deficiency are protective
- Pregnant women up to 10× more likely to contract & develop severe malaria, ↑ M&M

Yellow Fever
(Clin Infect Dis. 2007;44:850)

History

- Travel to endemic area (Sub-Saharan Africa [90%] & South America), incubation 3–6 d
- Mild form sudden fever HA → more severe cases with high fever, chills, HA, myalgias, lumbosacral pain, anorexia, N/V, dizziness → 10–25% have severe recurrence 2 d later with multiple organ systems involved (GI, renal, cardiac, hematologic)

Findings

- High fever, relative bradycardia, N/V, epigastric tenderness
  - Severe cases: ↑ fever, HA, N/V, abd pain, somnolence, jaundice, hematologic complications (eg, hematemesis, melena, petechiae, epistaxis)
- Late: ↓ BP, shock, confusion, coma, DIC, hemorrhage
- Liver is the most affected organ: Hepatocellular damage (steatosis, necrosis); bleeding
- Kidney is also affected: Renal insufficiency, albuminuria, ATN
- Cardiac: Fatty infiltration of myocardium → myocarditis & arrhythmias

Evaluation

- CBC (leukopenia, thrombocytopenia), ↑ LFTs, abnl coags, ↑ BUN/Cr, fibrinogen (DIC), ↓ ESR, serology, viral IgG, IgM

Treatment

- Resuscitation, supportive, symptomatic tx; no antiviral meds approved
- Live attenuated vaccine available for prevention, extremely effective

Disposition

- Admit for supportive care

Pearls

- *Flavivirus* transmitted by *A. aegypti* mosquito during tropical wet & early dry season, causes viral hemorrhagic fever
- Up to 20–50% mortality in symptomatic patients
- Mandated reporting to WHO, local health dept

Dengue Fever
(NEJM. 2012;366:1423)

History

- Travel to endemic areas: Mostly SE Asia, Central America, Western Pacific, sometimes from Eastern Mediterranean, Africa
- Sxs begin after 3–7 d incubation
- High fever: Abrupt onset × 1–7 d, biphasic, w/ HA, vomiting, myalgia, joint pain
- Rash: Characteristically bright red blanching petechiae, usually 1st on lower limbs & chest → morbilliform, maculopapular & sparing palms & soles → desquamation

Findings

- Hemorrhagic fever (DHF) or shock syndrome (DSS) occur during 2nd infection by different dengue virus

- Fever, ↓ BP, rash, LAD, hemorrhage (petechiae, purpura, epistaxis, GIB, menorrhagia)
- DHF: High fever, hepatomegaly, hypotension, DIC; begins w/ sudden ↑ in temp & flu sxs

Evaluation
- CBC (↑ Hct, ↓ plat, ↓ WBC), Chem (↑ BUN), ↑ LFTs, guaiac, DIC panel, ELISA, lactate
- CXR, head CT (if AMS), US, viral culture, dengue antigen tests, PCR, viral serologies

Treatment
- Aggressive supportive therapy, IVF, fluid status important 2/2 to plasma leakage, blood transfusions for severe bleeding

Disposition
- Admit for supportive tx

Pearls
- Caused by dengue virus (*Flavivirus*) infection, transmitted by A. aegypti mosquitoes
- Called "break-bone fever" due to acute onset severe HA, muscle & joint pains
- Benign acute febrile illness that can cause bleeding or DIC in small # of cases but can lead to lethal DHF

West Nile Disease
(*MMWR*. 2014;63:521)

History
- Outdoor exposures in area of outbreak during summer months, 2–14 d incubation
- Most infections asymptomatic. Symptomatic pts have fever, HA, malaise, myalgia, GI symptoms, rash.
- <1% have neuroinvasive Dx (meningitis, encephalitis, flaccid paralysis)

Findings
- Low-grade fever, hepatomegaly, splenomegaly, generalized LAD
- Rash: Erythematous maculopapular
- CNS: AMS, confusion, coma, meningismus, papilledema, CN abnormalities, flaccid paralysis, sz, ataxia, tremor, involuntary movements

Evaluation
- CBC (↓ WBC, ↓ lymphocytes, anemia), Chem (↓ Na), ↑ LFTs; ↑ lipase, viral IgM Ab
- CSF: Mild ↑ protein, mild ↑ leukocyte, nl glucose, serologies
- Brain MRI may be normal or show signal abnormalities in brainstem, basal ganglia, thalamus, anterior spinal cord

Treatment
- Supportive care, airway management, resuscitation
- Limited evidence for interferon & IVIG in case series & reports

Disposition
- Admit for supportive tx, may need rehabilitation from neuro cx

Pearls
- *Flavivirus* transmitted by several types of mosquito to horses, dogs, birds; crosses the blood–brain barrier to infect nervous system
- Has been reported throughout the world
- Excellent prognosis unless elderly or w/ other comorbid factors

Eastern Equine Encephalitis
(*MMWR*. 2006;55:697)

History
- Outdoor exposure to area of outbreak in summer or early fall
- Fevers, chills, malaise, weakness, HA, myalgias; progression to confusion, coma, N/V

Findings
- Similar to any other encephalitis; fever, tachycardia, tachypnea
- Neuro: Papilledema, sz, nuchal rigidity, focal neuro abn, CN abnormalities, spastic paralysis

Evaluation
- CBC (↑ WBC), Chem (↓ Na), serologies (IgM), viral isolation from CSF, blood, tissue
- Head CT: Punctuate/intraventricular hemorrhage, focal edema, meningeal enhancement
- MRI, LP: CSF shows ↑ protein, ↑ RBC, ↑ WBC

Treatment
- Supportive care, airway management, resuscitation, corticosteroids, & anticonvulsants

Disposition
- Admit, likely to ICU; will need extensive rehab

Pearls
- *Arbovirus* transmitted subcutaneously by mosquito, birds serve as primary reservoir; virus causes acute inflammatory process mainly involving meninges
- Primarily found in North America (east of MS river; MI, MA, NY, NJ, NC, SC, FL, LA, GA); wooded areas near freshwater swamps, marshes; less commonly Central/South America
- Poor prognosis: 33–70% mortality in a few days, 90% morbidity, only 10% fully recover

Chikungunya
(*Lancet.* 2012;379:662)

History
- IP 1–12 d. Sudden onset fever with joint pain, HA, photophobia, rash

Findings
- Polyarthralgia (can last months–years), joint swelling, fever, transient maculopapular rash

Evaluation
- CBC, viral PCR, serologies, r/o other possible culprits (eg, dengue)

Treatment
- NSAIDs for joint pain, supportive care

Disposition
- Admit as needed for supportive care

Pearls
- Caused by alphavirus transmitted by *Aedes* mosquitos
- Joint pain can last years
- Found in tropical/subtropical regions (African, Indian Ocean Islands, Asia)

Zika Virus Disease
(*NEJM.* 2016;374:1552)

History
- Asymptomatic or mild Dx (fever, arthritis/arthralgia, rash, conjunctivitis, HA, myalgia)

Findings
- Fever, macular or popular rash, conjunctivitis

Evaluation
- Consider CBC, viral testing

Treatment
- Supportive care

Disposition
- Home

Pearls
- Caused by Flavivirus transmitted by *Aedes* mosquitos
- Found in Southern US, central America, South America, Southeast Asia
- Temporal & geographic relationship with neurologic complications in adults such as Guillain–Barré syndrome, meningoencephalitis, as well as association with birth defects such as microcephaly. (*Lancet.* 2016;388:898)

BIOTERRORISM

(*NEJM.* 2015;372:954)

Background
- Characterized by low visibility, high potency, accessibility, easy delivery
- Only small amount of agent needed to kill large numbers of people
- Only plague, smallpox, & viral hemorrhagic fevers spread from person to person

Approach

- Take protective measures: Universal precautions w/ HEPA filter masks, decontaminate pt including remove clothing, shower w/ soap & water
- Isolation (negative pressure room) of affected, proper disposal of corpses

ANTHRAX (BACILLUS ANTHRACIS)

History

- Contact w/ infected goats, sheep, cattle, horses, swine, 1–6 d incubation period
- Most commonly cutaneous infection, also respiratory or GI; not human to human
- Fever, malaise, HA, cough, weakness, SOB, pruritus, N/V, diarrhea, abd pain
- Less likely than influenza to have sore throat or rhinorrhea

Findings

- Dependent on route of inoculation
- Cutaneous (most common): Incubation 1–12 d; starts as small papule → vesicle containing serosanguineous fluid (1–2 d) → vesicle rupture leaves painless necrotic lesion w/ surrounding edema → massive edema
- Ulcer base develops 1–5 cm black eschar; after 2–3 wk separates & leaves scar
- Inhalational: Incubation 1–6 d; initial nonspecific sxs w/ cough × 2–3 d → sudden onset respiratory distress (dyspnea, stridor, cyanosis, ↑ CP, diaphoresis) → rapid onset shock & death in 24–36 h
- GI: From ingestion of infected meat; incubation 2–5 d; local oral/tonsillar ulcer, dysphagia & respiratory distress → abd pain, hematemesis, massive ascites, diarrhea
- Injectional: Characterized by skin lesions seen in "skin popping" drug users, may progress rapidly & require surgical debridement or may disseminate.

Evaluation

- Blood cultures; Gram stain or culture confirms cutaneous anthrax, serologies, rapid antianthrax antibody test can be performed w/i 1 h
- Difficult to diagnose inhalational or GI anthrax
- CXR (inhalational): Mediastinal widening, pleural effusion, e/o ARDS

Treatment

- Early abx for cutaneous Dx: PCN, doxycycline, ciprofloxacin IV. Multiple abx if systemic/ extensive dz.
- Raxibacumab injection recently FDA approved for inhalational anthrax
- Prophylaxis: Ciprofloxacin or doxycycline PO; anthrax vaccine
- Corticosteroids may be useful in severe edema, meningitis

Disposition

- Consider admission based on clinical findings

Pearls

- Large, aerobic, gram-positive, spore-forming, nonmotile, pyogenic B. anthracis
- Found in animals in South & Central America, Southern & Eastern Europe, Africa, Asia, Caribbean, Middle East
- Death from respiratory failure, overwhelming bacteremia, septic shock, meningitis
- Mortality variable: Cutaneous <1%, inhalational 45–92%, GI 25–60%, injectional 34%

PLAGUE (YERSINIA PESTIS)

History

- Contact w/ rat flea; 99% cases in SE Asia (Vietnam), rarely Southwest United States
- Acute onset high fevers, LAD, myalgias, cough, SOB, CP, hemoptysis, sore throat, GI sx

Findings

- Bacilli spread to lymph nodes → supportive lymphadenitis, producing bubo → spread to other organs (spleen, liver, lungs, skin) & septic shock if untreated
- Bubonic (85–90%): Incubation 1–8 d; buboes emerge in groin, axilla, or cervical regions w/ f/C/HA, N/V, AMS, cough → buboes visible in 24 h, severely painful
- Septicemia (10–15%): Result of hematogenous dissemination of bubonic plague
- Pneumonic (1%): From inhalation of aerosols or hematogenous dissemination; productive cough w/ blood-tinged sputum, rales, decreased breath sounds

Evaluation

- Presence of painful bubo; Gram stain of bubo aspirate; blood, sputum, & CSF cultures, lymph node aspiration
- CXR (pneumonic): Bilateral alveolar infiltrates, consolidation

Treatment

- Isolate pts for 1st 48 h after tx; if pneumonic plague, isolate for 4 d
- Levofloxacin recently approved
- Streptomycin 15 mg/kg IM BID × 10 d ± doxycycline 200 mg IV × 1
- Alternative regimens: Chloramphenicol, gentamicin, Bactrim, ciprofloxacin
- Septicemia plague: Same as for other causes of sepsis
- Prophylaxis: Doxycyclin or ciprofloxacin PO × 7 d; use insecticides, reduce rodent populations

Disposition
- Admission, isolation

Pearls
- *Y. pestis*: Gram-negative nonmotile nonsporulating coccobacillus; can remain viable for days → weeks in water, moist soil, grain, buried bodies; reservoir: Rodents
- Mortality variable: Untreated bubonic 50%, Septic/pneumonic ~100%; tx reduced mortality to 10–15% overall

SMALLPOX (VARIOLA)

History
- High fever, HA rigors, malaise, myalgias, vomiting, abd pain, back pain, rash

Findings
- Virus multiplies in respiratory tract
- Incubation 10–14 d, spreads hematogenously → regional lymph nodes, blood vessels → skin changes
  - 2 types: Major (30% mortality), minor (<1% mortality)
- 2–3 d after initial sxs, exanthema on face, hands, forearms → trunk & lower extremities
- Skin exanthem: Macules → papules (day 2) → vesicles (day 5) → umbilicated pustules (day 8); pustules form scabs after 8–14 d; death in 2nd wk from toxemia (mortality 25%)

Evaluation
- Clinical Dx; centrifugal distribution, lesions all in same stage of development, PCR

Treatment
- Isolation, hemodynamic support, skin care, vaccination w/i 4 d of exposure (after fever, before rash)

Disposition
- Isolation × 17 d; pts most infectious on day 3–6 after onset of fever, remain infectious until all scabs separated

Pearls
- Variola virus: Highly infectious by aerosol, environmentally stable, prolonged infectivity
- Transmitted through respiratory droplets, bodily fluids
- Last occurrence in Somalia in 1977; routine vaccination stopped in 1972

BOTULISM

History
- 6 H after inhalation pt would have descending paralysis, CN dysfunction (diplopia, dysphagia, ptosis) progresses to ventilatory failure

Evaluation
- Clinical Dx, confirmed with mouse bioassays through culture

Treatment
- Antitoxin (equine derived), available exclusively from CDC
- Respiratory support, mechanical ventilation

Disposition
- ICU

Pearls
- Not contagious
- Inhalational or gastrointestinal form could be used as weapon. Other forms occur (infantile, wound, iatrogenic).

ALTERED MENTAL STATUS

Approach

- **Definition:** Any transient or fixed change in cognition &/or arousability including but not limited to disorientation, memory impairment, behavioral changes, hallucinations
- "AMS" can describe a wide spectrum of clinical severity & be 2/2 diverse causes (see table); encompasses mild confusional states → delirium → coma, or dementia
- **Approach:** Dictated by clinical severity of AMS; if unconscious or severely altered:
  - Immediate IV access, telemetry, ABCs, O_2 for hypoxia (caution if hx severe COPD)
  - Bedside glucose measurement: If low, give immediate 1–2 amps $D_{50}W$
  - If concern for narcotic o/d or h/o opiate meds: Naloxone 0.4–2.0 mg IV/IM/IN
  - If h/o ETOH abuse or malnutrition: empiric thiamine 100 mg IV (can give $D_{50}W$ first if hypoglycemia; replete thiamine before prolonged dextrose 2/2 risk of Wernicke's)
- **History:** Start by assessing baseline MS, degree of change, acuity/timing of change, any circumstances surrounding AMS (Δ meds, intoxication/substance use, trauma), PMH
  - Eyewitness accounts helpful: Contact eyewitness if not present with patient
- **Exam:** Assess for focal neurologic sxs (if present, consider CVA, ICH, space-occupying lesion), pupil exam (toxidrome, ↑ ICP/herniation), skin exam (diaphoresis may suggest tox; dehydration may suggest lyte d/o), asterixis (CO_2 or NH_3 excess), clonus
- **Evaluation:** All patients should get CBC, Chem 10, LFTs, UA, Tox screen, ECG, ± hcg; Consider CXR (esp if unable to give hx), TSH, VBG, NH_3, Drug levels, CO (esp if unwitnessed at home), Head CT, LP

Organic Causes of Acute Altered Mental Status	
Category	**Differential**
Intracranial	**Ischemia:** CVA (can cause AMS if large ± swelling, brainstem) **Hemorrhage:** Epidural (if trauma), SDH (can be atraumatic), SAH (traumatic or aneurysmal), IPH (2/2 neoplasm, HTN, AVM) **Seizure (complex):** Sz, post-ictal, or consider nonconvulsive status **Space-occupying lesion:** Neoplasm, Abscess (esp IVDU, HIV) **Other:** HTN encephalopathy, PRES, concussion (traumatic), diffuse axonal injury (traumatic), anoxic brain injury (esp if s/p ↓ O_2 or ↓ BP)
Metabolic	**Metabolic:** Acidosis, ↑ CO_2, ↓ O_2, electrolyte Δ (Na, Ca), uremia, NH_3 **Endocrine:** ↓ glucose, ↑ glucose (HHS, DKA), adrenal, thyroid (↑/↓) **Nutritional:** Wernicke's, B_{12} deficiency
Infectious	Sepsis, occult infection (esp in elderly: PNA, UTI, skin), fever-related delirium, meningitis/encephalitis, rarely neurosyphilis
Substances	**Depressants:** Opioids, antipsychotics, sedative-hypnotics (eg, benzos), antihistamines, anticholinergics, alcohols (inc. toxic alcohols) **Stimulants:** Sympathomimetic agents, hallucinogens, w/d states
Medications	Psychotropic meds most often at fault, but always consider polypharmacy **Serotonin syndrome** (SSRI, NSRI, Linezolid, triptans, dextromethorphan, meperidine, methadone, tramadol, ecstasy) **Neuroleptic malignant syndrome** (antipsychotics)
Trauma	Burns, electrocution, systemic inflammatory response, fat embolism, occult trauma (eg, abuse/neglect)
Environment	CO, cyanide

Physical Exam Clues in the Patient with Altered Mental Status		
Exam Finding		**Etiology**
VS	↑ Temp	Infxn, thyroid storm, adrenergic stim (drug o/d, w/d), SS/NMS
	↓ Temp	Environmental, hypothyroidism, sepsis
	↑ RR	Metabolic acidosis (DKA), stimulant, aspirin OD
	↓ RR	Narcotic o/d, CNS insult
	↑ HR	Fever, sepsis, dehydration, thyroid storm, OD (stimulant, TCA, aspirin, theophylline, anticholinergic), acidosis
	↓ HR	Heart block, ingestion (BB, CCB, digoxin), ↑ ICP
	↑ BP	HTN emergency, preeclampsia, adrenergic stim (drug o/d, w/d), PRES, ↑ ICP, pain
	↓ BP	Shock, sepsis, hemorrhage, toxins, GIB, adrenal crisis
Eyes	Miosis	Opioid ingestion, clonidine
	Mydriasis	Sympathomimetic or anticholinergic toxidrome
	Asymmetric	Intracranial process w/ mass effect or herniation
	Papilledema	↑ ICP

Delirium

- **Definition:** Acute state of temporary or fluctuating disturbance of consciousness (eg, impaired cognition, perception disturbances, reduced attention, hypo- or hyperactivity) that is caused by an organic medical condition or medication/drug (ie, *not psychiatric*)
- Can have many causes (see table above); w/u & tx dependent on causal etiology
- Delirium (vs. dementia or psych) suggested by: Age <12 or >40, visual hallucinations (vs. auditory), acute onset, exam abnormalities
- Dispo: Admit all pts not at baseline MS or with recent unexplained AMS; delirium in ED may independently predict 6-mo mortality (*Ann Emerg Med* 2010;56(3):244–252)

Dementia

- **Definition:** Progressive, unremitting decline in cognitive function due to a variety of causes (Alzheimer's, vascular, Lewy-body, etc.), classically marked by decline in short- & eventually long-term memory, but advanced cases may have behavioral chgs (hypo- or hyperactive, agitation) or even nonverbal.
- Much more subacute than delirium, though can predispose pts to delirium from otherwise occult pathology (eg, UTI, PNA) due to poor cognitive reserve; 50% of elderly pts w/ delirium have some degree of underlying dementia (*Ann Emerg Med* 2010;56(3):261–269)
- Important to screen for elder abuse (e/o physical trauma, neglect); EA is underdiagnosed but especially important in pts w/ dementia 2/2 inc risk of caregiver fatigue

Dementia Differential	
System	Differential
Degenerative	Alzheimer's, Parkinson's, Huntington's, Pick's dz
Vascular	Multi-infarct dementia
Infectious	Neurosyphilis, Creutzfeldt–Jakob dz, HIV
Inflammatory	Lupus, demyelinating dz
Neoplastic	Primary CNS tumor, metastatic dz, paraneoplastic syndromes
Traumatic	TBI, SDH, anoxic brain injury
Toxic	Alcohol, medications, heavy metals
Metabolic	B₁₂/folate deficiency, thyroid, Wilson dz, lipid storage dz
Psychiatric	Depression
Hydrocephalus	NPH, noncommunicating hydrocephalus

HEADACHE

Approach

- Must differentiate life-threatening HA (minority) from benign HAs (majority)
- **History:** Essential to describe timing/acuity of onset, location, quality, radiation/movement, severity, & associated sx (fever, photophobia, emesis, vision chg, eye pain, neck pain, focal neuro sx, chg in speech or cognition, sinus congestion), circumstances surrounding onset (trauma, med chgs, environment)
- **PMH:** Always ask about HA hx (if present: obtain detailed info regarding how current HA is similar/different), IVDU, immunosupp, & current/recent meds (eg, A/C)
- **Red flags** requiring neuroimaging: Sudden/rapid onset (<1 h to peak), exertional onset, worst of life, AMS, 1st severe HA >age 35, fever, neck stiffness, immunosupp, daily HA, no similar prior HAs, abnl neuro exam, meningismus, papilledema

Headache Differential	
Pathophysiology	Differential
Primary HA	Migraine, tension, cluster, trigeminal neuralgia, analgesia rebound
Trauma	ICH (SAH, SDH, EDH, IPH), postconcussive syndrome
CNS Infection	Meningitis, encephalitis, abscess
Vascular	HTN emergency, aneurysm/AVM growth, cerebral venous sinus thrombosis, carotid/vertebral art. dissection, temporal arteritis, preeclampsia; HA rarely presenting complaint w/ CVA
Neoplastic	Malignancy (primary or metastatic), benign (eg, meningioma)
CSF d/o (↑↓ ICP)	Hydrocephalus, pseudotumor cerebri, dural leak/post-LP (↓ CSF)
Otolaryngologic	Sinusitis, TMJ syndrome, mastoiditis
Ophthalmologic	Glaucoma, Myopia/Presbyopia/Hyperopia/Astigmatism
Environmental	CO poisoning (Ch. 10), noxious aerosols

PRIMARY HEADACHE SYNDROMES

Migraine Headache & Variants

History, Physical Exam, & Evaluation
- **HX:** Slow in onset (over hours), unilateral throbbing or pulsatile, often w/ N/V (>50%), photophobia; visual or sensory aura/prodrome may precede HA (15%); duration 4–72 h
  - Migraine variants discussed below
- Classically have migraine hx; beware of assuming migraine if first time & age >35
- **EXAM:** Nl neuro exam (except in migraine variants)
- **DX:** No studies or consults routinely indicated unless need to exclude other cause (eg, CT, LP, MRI) as in the case of severe or prolonged sx (see *Migraine Variants*)

Treatment
- Abortive: Most effective if given w/i 15 m of onset; often involves combo tx w/ IVF, NSAIDs, APAP, antiemetic (check QTc; common options inc prochlorperazine, metoclopramide; give w/ diphenhydramine to ↓ extrapyramidal sxs); additional options include triptans & DHE (both c/i in preg & CAD), & dexamethasone
- Prophylaxis: Indicated if >2/mo, duration > 24 h, major lifestyle disruption, failure of abortive tx; Options include AEDs, BB, TCAs, CCBs, SSRIs, behavioral/environmental chgs

Disposition
- Most pts able to return home within hours; may need Observation Unit if protracted

Migraine Variants
- Migraine variants are rare but can resemble other concerning conditions; often strong h/o similar events in the past, but if not, requires involved w/u to r/o other more serious dx
- **Hemiplegic migraine:** HA a/w hemiplegia (± paresthesias); hemiplegia may resolve w/i hrs or persist days; HA may be subtle but classically pts have h/o similar prior sx
- **Basilar migraine:** HA w/ dizziness/vertigo, ± ataxia, N/V, tinnitus, AMS
- **Abdominal migraine:** Paroxysmal mid-abd pain a/w N/V, often w/o HA; strong h/o prior similar episodes & +FH; ddx inc. cyclic vomiting syndrome; more common in Peds
- **Ocular migraine:** Gradual loss of vision in one eye 2/2 transient vasospasm of retinal arteries; often h/o prior similar episodes & +FH; avoid triptans & DHE
- **Status migrainosus:** Migraine HA >72 h

Pearl
- Migraine HA are independent RF for ischemic CVA (RR 1.64) & silent CVA (avoid triptans/DHE) (*Neurol Sci* 2017;38(1):33–40)

Tension Headache

History, Physical Exam, & Evaluation
- **HX:** Dull, aching or throbbing "vice-like" pressure HA w/ gradual onset, bilateral frontal &/or occipito-nuchal; rarely w/ N/V or prodrome; duration 30 min to 7 d; a/w insomnia, stress, anxiety, or depression
- **EXAM:** Normal neuro exam, no true photophobia
- **DX:** No studies or consults routinely indicated (unless need to exclude other cause)

Treatment
- NSAIDs or APAP, neck massage & heat, relaxation techniques, *not* narcotics

Disposition
- Most patients can go home within hours; if chronic HA, refer to HA specialist

Cluster Headache

History, Physical Exam, & Evaluation
- **HX:** Sudden onset unilateral, paroxysmal, sharp, stabbing severe temporal/periorbital HA that may awaken from sleep; ± ipsilateral lacrimation, flushing, rhinorrhea or nasal congestion, conj injection or Horner syndrome (30% of pts); occur in clusters of short (15–180 min) episodes (1 QOD to >8/d) for up to 6–8 wk; more common in men
- **EXAM:** Normal neuro exam or +Horner's; may have +lacrimation, flushing, conj injection
- **DX:** No studies or consults routinely indicated (unless need to exclude other cause)

Treatment
- Abortive: High-flow O_2 (12–15 L/min) by mask, sumatriptan (CI in pregnancy or CAD), intranasal lidocaine, NSAIDs.
- Prophylaxis: Prednisone 60 mg ×10 d then taper, ± verapamil or valproic acid

Pearl
- Make sure to distinguish from acute angle-closure glaucoma

Trigeminal Neuralgia

History, Physical Exam, & Evaluation

- **HX:** Unilateral paroxysmal pain in sensory distribution of CN V, commonly involves the maxillary (V2) or mandibular (V3) branches; ± brief facial spasm or tic ("tic douloureux"); may be triggered by light touch or vibration, shaving, face washing, chewing
- **EXAM:** No e/o CN dysfxn or other neurologic abnlty
- **DX:** Can be treated w/o w/u if characteristic hx; MRI if atypical features present (neuro deficit, age <40). Refer to neurology for outpt w/u.

Treatment

- Carbamazepine 100 mg BID, increase by 200 mg/d up to 1200 mg/d

Pearl

- Most common cause is compression of the nerve root by an aberrant vessel

---

ACUTE SINUSITIS

Overview

- Definition: Inflammation of the paranasal sinuses, usually viral or allergic, though sometimes bacterial superinfxn (*S. pneumo*, nontypeable *H. influenzae*, *M. catarrhalis*)
- Dangerous pathogens: Pseudomonas (esp HIV, CF, s/p instrumentation), invasive fungal sinusitis (Rhizopus) or mucormycosis (DM, immunosupp); require special tx

History, Physical Exam, & Evaluation

- **HX:** Consider with positional HA, worse bending forward or head movement; pts often have mucopurulent d/c, postnasal drip, sinus pressure, ± tap tenderness; may be afebrile (if +fever, more likely bacterial); progresses over 7–10 d
  - If no resolution w/i 7 d, suggests bacterial dz
- **EXAM:** May have pharyngeal erythema from postnasal drip, ± tap tenderness
- **DX:** Clinical. Imaging not routinely indicated; CT has high Se but low Sp.

Treatment

- Supportive (analgesics, antipyretics, decongestants, antihistamines if allergic)
- Decongestants: Neo-Synephrine nasal spray TID × 3 d, Afrin nasal spray BID × 3 d
- *Abx not routinely indicated:* Reserve for pts w/ sxs >7 d, worsening sxs, fever, purulent d/c, or high risk for severe infection or cx
  - First-line: Amoxicillin 500 mg PO TID × 10 d, TMP-SMX, or azithromycin
  - If no improvement: Amoxicillin–clavulanate, fluoroquinolone, clindamycin

Disposition

- Discharge w/ PCP follow-up; Consider admx if high fever, immunosupp, poor f/u

Pearl

- Sphenoid/ethmoid sinusitis is less common than maxillary sinusitis but has significant potential cx (eg, orbital cellulitis, cavernous sinus thrombosis)

HYPERTENSIVE HEADACHE

History, Physical Exam, & Evaluation

- **HX:** Untreated HTN or other precipitants (pregnancy, drug use, serotonin syndrome)
- **EXAM:** BP often >240/140 (unlikely w/ DBP <120); May have papilledema, encephalopathy, ± focal neuro abnormalities or sz
- **DX:** Assess for e/o end-organ damage (HTN emergency): Head CT (r/o ICH, edema), ECG, e/o aortic injury, pulm edema, renal failure

Treatment

- IV Anti-HTN (↓ MAP by 25% over 1 h (Caution: ↓ BP too quickly could lead to ischemia)
- Common agents: Nitroprusside gtt (CI in pregnancy) or Labetalol gtt

---

CEREBRAL VENOUS SINUS THROMBOSIS

Overview *(NEJM 2005;352(17):1791–1798)*

- **Pathophysiology:** Thrombosis of the sinuses of the brain (eg, sagittal, straight, occipital, transverse) with or without thrombosis of the cortical veins of the brain
- Sinus thrombosis impairs CSF absorption causing ↑ ICP (eg, HA, AMS)
- Cortical vein thrombosis causes venous infarction & localized injury (eg, focal deficits)
- Because of cerebral injury, secondary hemorrhage may develop (40% cases)
- Prothrombotic RF (trauma, hypercoagulable state [esp preg]) present in 85%; other causes include post-LP (2/2 downward traction on cortical veins from pressure chg), sinusitis (cavernous thrombosis) otitis/mastoiditis

History, Physical Exam, & Evaluation

- **HX:** HA present >90%, often gradual over days but can be sudden; ± N/V, vision chgs, focal neuro deficits (see above); Assess PMH for prothrombotic RFs
- **EXAM:** Assess for papilledema, focal neuro deficits; cavernous sinus thrombosis will have CN III/IV/VI compromise, periorbital chemosis/edema, & ↓ vision ipsilaterally
- **DX:** CBC, PT/INR, PTT, Upreg, ± D-dimer; MRI/MRV more Se than CTV but balance accuracy with urgency & desire to r/o other diagnoses (eg, SAH, IPH)
  - D-dimer may help r/o CVST if low pre-TP (weighted Se 94%, Sp 90%) (*J Thromb Haemost* 2012;10(4):582–589)

Treatment

- Anticoagulation (heparin) preferred, often even in presence of hemorrhagic infarcts
- Endovascular thrombolysis can be used, but often reserved for those w/ worst prognosis

Disposition

- Admission to neurology; may warrant ICU care if e/o hemorrhagic conversion or AMS

TEMPORAL ARTERITIS (GIANT CELL ARTERITIS)

Overview

- **Definition:** Granulomatous inflammatory vasculitis of medium/large arteries occurring in pts > 50 y (peak incidence 70–80 y); largely affecting branches of ECA, vertebral, distal subclavian, axillary, arteries, & thoracic aorta; causes ischemic sx by vessel occlusion

History, Physical Exam, & Evaluation

- **HX:** Unilateral HA, jaw/tongue claudication, malaise, low-grade fevers, visual impairment
  - RFs: Age >50 y/o (90% >60 y/o), F > M, h/o PMR (50% of pts)
- **EXAM:** May have tenderness over temporal art. (↓ Se) or ↓ visual acuity (↓ Se)

Evaluation (NEJM 2014;371:50–57)

- ↑ ESR (Se ~84%), ↑ CRP (Se ~86%), combined Se of ESR & CRP may be >95%, but poorly specific in pts w/ other causes for elevation
- Temporal art. bx: high Se for even low-levels of inflammation *if present at site of bx* (requires 1.5–2.0 cm segment); given focality of dz, may need repeat bx or imaging if high pre-TP & first-bx neg
- CTA &/or MRA: Not used to make dx, but may serve as adjunct if -bx &/or assess extent of dz if +bx

Treatment

- Prednisone 1 mg/kg/d (if vision sx, do not wait for bx results) ~2–4 wk, then prolonged taper
- Consult neurology, ophthalmology, rheumatology if concern for dx & to arrange f/u

Disposition

- Admit for visual deficits; Can be discharged on steroids w/ follow-up

---

PSEUDOTUMOR CEREBRI (IDIOPATHIC INTRACRANIAL HTN)

Overview

- **Pathophysiology:** Set of sxs of unclear etiology; due to obstructed venous/CSF outflow rather than ↑ CSF production

History, Physical Exam, & Evaluation (Cephalgia 2015;35(3):248–261)

- **HX:** Gradual onset, global, daily/constant HA (>90%) or retrobulbar pain, ±, N/V, ↓ vision (~70%; may be transient), intracranial noises (~60%); sx can be worst in morning
  - RFs: Young obese females, recent weight gain; some meds (tetracyclines, retinoids)
- **EXAM:** Nl neuro exam (except possible CN VI palsy), check vision & for papilledema
- **DX:** Can be clinical dx (sx, papilledema); LP for opening pressure (>25 cm H_2O in lateral decubitus) confirms dx; Neuroimaging may be normal (or show swelling of optic discs)

Treatment

- Neuro consult (± ophthalmology) if new dx or refractory to tx
- Weight loss remains most effective treatment
- Diuretics to decrease ICP: Acetazolamide 1 mg PO QD
  - May need repeated high-volume LPs; refractory cases may need VP shunt
- Use of steroids controversial & may worsen weight gain

DURAL LEAK/POST-LP HEADACHE

Overview

- **Definition:** HA caused by ICP caused by loss of CSF from recent dural injury (eg, due to LP, myelogram, spinal anesthesia, vigorous coughing)

History, Physical Exam & Evaluation

- **HX:** Occipital HA radiating to shoulders/neck, worse with sitting/standing (± alleviated w/ supine); Worsened by activities that ↑ ICP (eg, coughing, sneezing, Valsalva); Usually present 48–72 h postdural injury (but can be >1 wk); ± N/V, LH, photophobia, tinnitus
- **EXAM:** Nonfocal neuro exam; HA improved w/ lying flat, worse w/ sitting up
- **DX:** None spec; evaluate for other causes of HA, if indicated

Treatment

- As much as 8% will resolve w/o tx; tx indicated for severe or prolonged (>72 h) sx
- Epidural blood patch (clot forms to seal dural defect): 70–98% success
- Methylxanthine derivatives (caffeine IV, aminophylline) may be helpful, limited data
- Surgical closure of dural gap is last-resort effort if blood patch &/or other options fail

Pearls

- Minimize risk of post-LP HA w/ small caliber spinal needle (24–27G), bevel alignment w/ dural fibers, atraumatic needles, minimized number of attempts
- Severe cases can precipitate Sz & SDH (2/2 ↓ ICP → brain pulled → bridging vein strain)

INTRACRANIAL NEOPLASM

Overview (Lancet 2012;379:1984–96)

- **Definition:** Any of a spectrum of neoplasms, each with distinct biology, epidemiology, natural history, & management, & prognosis; often cause acute sx due to mass effect of tumor, vasogenic edema, or secondary hemorrhage on neural tissue, or sz
- Tumors either extraparenchymal (meningioma, pituitary neoplasm) or intraparenchymal
  - Intraparenchymal most commonly glioma (eg, oligodendroglioma, mixed glioma, astrocytoma), primary CNS lymphoma, or metastatic non-CNS primary cancer

History, Physical Exam, & Evaluation

- **HX:** Subacute onset, often daily morning HAs (2/2 ↑ ICP), ± N/V, focal deficits, chgs in personality or speech; sz; alleviation w/ NSAIDs/APAP does not help r/o dx
- **EXAM:** Look for signs of herniation:
  - Uncal (most common): ↓ mental status, blown unilateral pupil, decerebrate posturing
  - Central: AMS, yawning, Cheyne–Stokes breathing, miosis. Decorticate → decerebrate.
  - Tonsillar (posterior): Bradycardia, coma, respiratory arrest
  - Cushing reflex (due to ↑ ICP): HTN, bradycardia, irregular breathing
- **DX:** Neuroimaging w/ CT, usually followed by MRI (w/ contrast); In those suspected w/ pituitary tumors, check lytes, cortisol, TSH
  - Treatment & prognosis depend on tumor phenotype & grade

Treatment (glioma)

- Dexamethasone 4 mg TID for mass effect/minimize edema
- Antiepileptic treatment
- Consult NSGY (consideration of resection), Neuro-oncology

Disposition

- Admit all patients w/ new dx of intracranial neoplasm; or transfer to facility w/ NSGY
- Prognosis heavily dependent on phenotype & grade (mos to yrs)

CNS INFECTIONS

Meningitis

Overview

- **Definition:** Inflammation of the meninges overlying the brain due to either infectious (bacterial, fungal, viral) or noninfectious etiology; sx & tx differ widely based on etiology
- Bacterial meningitis rare in developed nations; common bacteria include S. pneumoniae, N. meningitidis, H. influenzae type b, L. monocytogenes (infants, elderly, pregnant); staph (VPS, trauma, NSGY); seeding of subarachnoid space 2/2 hematogenous spread (eg, from resp tract) or direct spread (eg, sinusitis, acute OM)
- Causes of noninfectious "aseptic" meningitis include drugs (eg, antimicrobials, vaccines, NSAIDs), inflammatory dz (SLE, Behcet); rarely malignancy can p/w leptomeningeal dz

History

- Bacterial: Typically acute (<1 d), high-grade fever, HA, nuchal rigidity, ill appearing, AMS
  - RFs: Extremes of age, immunosupp (esp HIV, steroids, MM/blood ca), crowded living environment (dorms, shelters), splenectomy, ETOH abuse / cirrhosis, IVDU, recent illness (esp sinusitis/OM), dural defect (recent trauma, surgery; congenital, VPS)
  - Classic triad for bacterial etiology: Neck stiffness, fever, AMS (3 of 3 present <50%, 2 of 3 present >95%) (Lancet 2016;388(10063):3036–3047)
- Viral: Typically subacute (1–7 d), also w/ HA, fever, photophobia; unless HSV, usually normal mental status; HSV usually w/ AMS
- Fungal/TB: Subacute (>1 wk), HA, low-grade fever, weight loss, night sweats, ± AMS

Physical Exam
- May have nuchal rigidity, disorientation/AMS, photophobia
  - Brudzinski sign (hip flexion elicited by passive neck flexion) & Kernig sign (inability or reluctance to extend knee when hip is flexed to 90): High Sp, but Se only 5%
- Petechial/purpuric rash suggests meningococcus (N. meningitidis)
- Expect subtle presentation in elderly or immunocompromised pts; may be AMS only

Evaluation
- LP is gold standard for dx but should not delay abx if high pre-TP for bacterial/HSV
  - See table below for indications for CT prior to LP
  - LP tubes: (1 & 4) cell count & diff, (2) gluc & protein, (3) Gram stain, cx ± HSV PCR
  - Gram stain Se depends on etiology: S. pneumoniae (Se >90%), H. influenzae (75%), N. meningitidis (50%), L. monocytogenes (33%); GS & Cx yield may ↓ by 40% if performed after abx, improved by PCR *(Clin Infect Dis 2004;39(9):1267; Lancet 388:3036–3047)*
- BCx, full infectious w/u (CBC, CXR, UA); thrombocytopenia suggests meningococcus

Treatment *(Clin Infect Dis 2004;39(9):1267)*
- Respiratory precautions if suspect meningococcus
- Empiric abx based on suspected etiology (see table); acyclovir 10 mg/kg q8h if c/f HSV
- Early steroids may ↓ inflammatory cascade in bacterial meningitis; therefore, if proven or high pre-TP bacterial etiology, give dexamethasone 0.15 mg/kg w/i 20 min of 1st abx (↑ favorable neuro outcomes & ↓ mortality)
- Consult NSGY in all pts w/indwelling hardware (eg, VPS): removal improves tx success
- Postexposure ppx (if +N. meningitidis): Ciprofloxacin 500 mg PO × 1. Ceftriaxone 250 mg IM (peds), or Ceftriaxone 250 mg IM (pregnancy).
- If viral (non-HSV): Supportive care only, prophylaxis not needed

Disposition
- Admit bacterial, HSV, fungal; Non-HSV viral: D/C vs. Observation based on sx severity

Indications for CT before LP	*(IDSA Guidelines. Clin Infect Dis 2004;39(9):1267)*
Age >60	Any neurologic abnormalities: ↓ GCS*, CN abnlty, abnl visual fields, pronator drift, abnl language (eg, aphasia)
Immunocompromised	
History of CNS/neurologic dz	
Recent seizure w/i 1 wk of presentation	Inability to follow two consecutive commands
Papilledema	Inability to answer two consecutive questions

*No clear data on precise GCS cut-off; some studies suggest CT for any GCS <13, while others suggest CT only if GCS <8. Others simply use "alert" or "not alert" (NEJM 2001;345:1727–1733).

Interpretation of LP Results		
CSF Test	Normal	Implications of Abnormal Results
WBC	<5 WBC <1 PMN	Bacterial: Marked ↑ WBC (usually >1000), ↑ PMN Viral: Usually ↑ WBC but <500, mononuclear *Traumatic tap: if serum WBC nl, expect 1 WBC for every 700 RBC (limited data)**
RBC	None	↑↑ RBC: traumatic LP (if T1 > T4) or SAH (T1–T4) ↑ RBC (& ↑ WBC): Consider HSV Xanthochromia indicates RBCs present 4 h prior
CSF:Serum Gluc	0.6:1	↓ in bacterial/fungal meningitis or hyperglycemia
Protein	15–45 mg/dL	↑ in bacterial/fungal meningitis, syphilis, neoplasm, demyelination, bleed (SAH)
Opening pres.**	<20 mmH₂O	↑ in bacterial, fungal or TB
Gram stain	Negative	Positive in 80% of bacterial meningitis (see above)

*Limited data from adult population. In infants 0–60 d, may be safe to use ratio of 1 WBC: 877 RBCs (Ann Emerg Med 2016:pii:S0196-064(16)31223–31229).
**Can be elevated 2/2 noninfectious etiologies as well.

Common Bacterial Pathogens in Meningitis by Age with Empiric Antibiotics		
Age	Common Pathogens	Empiric Antibiotic Regimen
<1 mo	Group B strep, E. coli, L. monocytogenes, Klebsiella	Ampicillin AND (Cefotaxime OR Gentamicin)
1–24 mo	Group B strep, S. pneumo, H. influenzae, N. meningitidis	Vancomycin AND Ceftriaxone
2–50 yr	S. pneumo, N. meningitidis	Vancomycin 1 g AND Ceftriaxone 2 g
>50 yr	S. pneumo, N. meningitidis, P. aeruginosa, L. monocytogenes	Vancomycin 1 g AND Ceftriaxone 2 g AND Ampicillin 150 mg/kg/d div q4h
Surgery/Trauma	S. aureus, S. epidermidis, P. aeruginosa	Vancomycin 1 g AND Cefepime 2 g

Encephalitis

Overview

- **Definition:** Inflammation of brain parenchyma usually due to infection (often viral); rarely autoimmune/paraneoplastic (*Lancet Neurol* 2016;15(4):391–404)
- HSV (5–10% encephalitis) life-threatening (>70% mortality w/o tx) (*BMJ* 2012;344:e3166)

History & Physical Exam

- **HX:** Acute onset fever (>90% w/ HSV), HA (>80% w/ HSV), behavior chgs (>70% w/ HSV), hallucinations/altered awareness (>60% w/ HSV), confusion/impaired memory (25% w/ HSV); ± diffuse or focal neuro sx (weakness, ataxia, speech disturbance), seizure, or e/o meningeal involvement (+photophobia, +neck stiffness) (*BMJ* 2012;344:e3166)
  - Absence of fever or HA strongly suggests against the dx of HSV encephalitis
  - HSV encephalitis often preceded by nonspecific viral prodrome (fever, malaise, N/V)
  - Assess for immunosupp, recent travel, tick/mosquito bites
- **EXAM:** AMS (may progress to coma), more likely to have focal neuro deficits than isolated meningitis (may progress to diffuse paralysis &/or ataxia); may have e/o concurrent meningeal involvement

Evaluation (*BMJ* 2012;344:e3166)

- LP: CSF ↑ WBC, ± ↑ RBC/xanthochromia, ± ↑ protein levels, nl glucose
  - Important to send HSV PCR, but should not defer tx
- MRI: Imaging modality of choice & helps r/o CI to LP; Se 90% in HSV encephalitis
- EEG: Se 84%, Sp 32% for HSV encephalitis (may help guide need for AEDs)

Treatment

- If concern for HSV encephalitis: Acyclovir 10 mg/kg q8h IV, AEDs
- If low concern for HSV: Supportive ± anticonvulsants, steroids

Disposition

- Admit if confirmed/suspected HSV, not at baseline (eg, AMS), immunosupp

Abscess

Overview

- **Definition:** Purulent collections w/i the CNS (intraparenchymal, epidural, subdural, spinal); form by contiguous spread (sinus, dental) or hematogenous seeding (PNA, endocarditis)
  - RFs: Immunosupp, IVDU, trauma/surgery, local infxn (mastoiditis, sinusitis, dental), & RFs for systemic infxn (eg, endocarditis, line infxn, bacteremia)
  - Certain medical conditions predispose to certain pathogens: HIV (*Toxoplasma gondii, M. tuberculosis*), solid-organ tpx (aspergillus, candida), post-surgical (staph, gram-neg)

History, Physical Exam, Evaluation (*NEJM* 2014;371(5):447–456)

- **HX:** HA (most common), ± low-grade fever; neuro sx only late in dz; AMS often absent
  - Up to 25% of pts may p/w seizures
  - Assess for RFs & ROS suggesting possible source infxn
- **EXAM:** May have nl neuro exam depending on site of abscess & timing of presentation
- **DX:** ↑ WBC, ↑ ESR, blood cultures. CT w/ contrast ("ring-enhancing" lesion)
  - Owing to risk of brain herniation & low Se (25%), LP not routinely performed
  - NSGY consultation for diagnostic stereotactic aspiration for cx & decompression
  - Antitoxoplasma IgG can confirm toxoplasma dx in HIV pts (no need for aspiration)

Treatment

- Although diagnostic NSGY aspiration aims to decompress maximally, therapeutic NSGY aspiration (eg, if pathogen already known) indicated only for large abscesses or those w/ e/o IV abx failure (*NEJM* 2014;371(5):447–456)
- Early abx (before diagnostic aspiration, esp if acute or severe)
- Low threshold to intubate (may progress rapidly)

Disposition

- Admit all pts; may require ICU

Empiric Antibiotics for Brain Abscess (*NEJM* 2014;371(5):447–456)	
Standard	Ceftriaxone* 2 g AND Metronidazole 500 mg ± Vancomycin 1 g
Transplant patients	Ceftriaxone* 2 g AND Metronidazole 500 mg ± Vancomycin 1 g AND Voriconazole AND Trimethoprim-Sulfamethoxazole
HIV-positive patients	Ceftriaxone* 2 g AND Metronidazole 500 mg ± Vancomycin 1 g AND Pyrimethamine AND Sulfadiazine Consider TB tx (INH, Rifampin, Pyrazinamide, Ethambutol)

*Meropenem can be substituted for cephalosporin if allergies present

SEIZURE

Overview

- **Definition:** Spontaneous or provoked abnl synchronous cortical electrical activity; recurrent unprovoked seizures referred to as "epilepsy" (Ann Emerg Med 2014;63(4):437–447)
  - **Simple vs. Complex:** Refers to degree of change of mental status; simple sz cause no chg in mental status, while complex can cause AMS or complete LOC
  - **Partial vs. Generalized:** Refers to location(s) of brain involved & corresponding sx; partial sz are limited to one area of one hemisphere, while generalized are bilateral
  - **Status epilepticus:** >20 min continuous generalized sz activity or continued intermittent sz w/o return to baseline mental status (Ann Emerg Med 2014;63(4):437–447)
- Lifetime risk of nonfebrile seizure is 2–5% (Ann Emerg Med 2004;43(5):605–625)
- May be provoked by numerous etiologies (see below)

Common Etiologies Provoking Seizure	
CNS	Ischemia (eg, CVA), ICH, Vascular malformations (aneurysm, AVM), Neoplasm (primary, met), Sinus thrombosis, Trauma, PRES, HTN enceph, inherited conditions (NF, Tub. sclerosis, Sturge–Weber, etc.)
Infection	Febrile sz (peds), meningitis, encephalitis, brain abscess, HIV OIs, HIV enceph, neurocysticercosis, neurosyphilis, malaria
Toxic	W/D (ETOH, benzo, barb), OD (sympathomimetic, TCA, anticholinergic, SSRI/NSRI, lidocaine, INH), Caffeine
Metabolic	↑↓ glucose, ↑↓ Na, ↓ Ca, ↓ Mg, ↓ O₂, uremia, liver failure, thyrotoxicosis
Obstetric	Eclampsia
Environmental	Heat stroke, Stress, Lack of sleep
Neonatal	CMV, congenital syphilis, rubella, inborn errors of metabolism (eg, PKU)

Common Types of Seizures		
Location	**Type**	**Description**
Generalized	Tonic, Clonic, Tonic–clonic	Abrupt LOC, often apneic; Rigid (tonic), rhythmic jerking (clonic), or tonic phase followed by clonic phase (tonic–clonic); Often a/w incontinence, tongue biting, trauma (eg, shoulder dislocation)
		Followed by post-ictal state of depressed mental status lasting minutes to hours; patients unable to recall event
		Affects all ages; In older adults, more likely 2/2 focal lesion that rapidly generalizes
	Absence	Abrupt LOC; Staring spells or rhythmic blinking; no incontinence
		Minimal post-ictal state but patients unable to recall event
		School-aged children (usually resolves by adulthood)
Partial (focal)	Simple	Isolated unilateral motor (eg, convulsions, automatisms) or sensory (eg, loss or change) or autonomic activity
		No LOC, change in behavior or mental status, or post-ictal state; patients can recall event
	Complex	Isolated unilateral motor (eg, convulsions, automatisms), or sensory (eg, hallucinations), or autonomic activity
		No LOC, but does have behavior change ± postictal confusion

Approach

- If actively seizing: Immediate IV access, roll patient into decubitus (avoid aspiration), suction airway, supplemental O₂, fingerstick glucose, magnesium (if pregnant), antiepileptic agents (IV, IO, IM, IN)
- If not actively seizing: Assess return to baseline mental status, focal deficits

History

- Description of events before, during, & after sz: prodrome, associated sxs (fever, vomiting, HA, trauma, photophobia, visual chg), any focal neuro sxs, AEDs given, type of sz (partial vs. generalized; if partial: simple vs. complex) & duration, post-ictal state
  - **First-time Sz:** Assess possible causal etiologies (see above)
  - **Breakthrough Sz:** Assess similarities &/or differences from prior sz, typical sz frequency, last sz prior to presentation, any changes in AEDs, outpt provider, factors that may lower sz threshold (stress, sleep, noncompliance, new meds, toxins, alcohol, infxn)

- Differentiate from syncope (may have myoclonic jerks, no incontinence or tongue-biting, quick return to baseline mental status)
- Assess for sx of traumatic injury

Physical Exam
- Assess GCS, orientation, & memory (compare with baseline), neuro deficits
- Evaluate for e/o trauma (inc tongue biting) or ingestion; if persistent AMS & unwitnessed sz w/ e/o head trauma or fall, may need temporary C-spine immobilization until cleared

Evaluation (Guidelines: ACEP, Ann Emerg Med 2004;43(5):605–625; AAN, Neurology 2007;69(21):1996–2007)
- **If active seizing:** Defer evaluation until cessation of sz (see Approach)
- **First-time Sz & back to baseline:**
  - Labs: CBC, BMP (glucose, Na), HCG; ± lactate, CPK (↑ lactate & ↑ CPK can help differentiate b/w unwitnessed convulsive sz & syncope w/ myoclonus), LP if immunosupp (even if afebrile); PRN based on hx: Tox screen, LFTs, LP
  - Neuroimaging: Obtain noncontrast CT in ED if feasible
    - May defer neuroimaging to o/p if: Age <40 y, normal neuro exam, no concern for intracranial path (no trauma, no hx malignancy or immunosupp, no fever, no HA, no A/C use), & good o/p f/u; preferred o/p study is MRI w/contrast
    - MRI w/contrast > CT for evaluation of tumors (esp in elderly, hx cancer), but can be done as o/p in most pts if CT negative
  - EEG: May be performed as outpt; indicated only for persistent AMS, SE, dx of viral encephalitis, intubated/paralyzed, r/o nonconvulsive SE
- **Breakthrough sz:**
  - Labs: Electrolytes, UA, AED levels, ± CXR; ± lactate, CPK (↑ lactate & ↑ CPK can help differentiate b/w unwitnessed convulsive sz & syncope w/ myoclonus)
  - Neuroimaging: Consider if different from prior sz, prolonged duration since recent sz, trauma, or other c/f intracranial pathology
  - Keep differential broad even if known sz d/o, esp if therapeutic med levels

Treatment
- Airway: Nasal trumpet, supplemental O_2, suction, positioning, may need to intubate if SE
- **Abortive meds:** Benzodiazepines 1st line (available IV, IM, IN, buccal, PR); ongoing investigations to establish optimal second-line agent
  - IV lorazepam vs. IM midazolam: IM midazolam is noninferior & may be superior to IV lorazepam w/ regard to sz termination/need for rescue tx, & is quicker if no IV access (Epilepsia 2015;56(2):254–262; NEJM 2012;366(7):591–600)
  - IV lorazepam vs. IV diazepam: IV lorazepam superior to IV diazepam w/ regard to sz termination / need for rescue tx (Cochrane 2014;(9):CD003723)
  - Special cases w/ alternative 1st-line tx: Pregnant (Mg 4g IV), INH tox (pyridoxine 1g)
- If not seizing, tx w/AED depends on risk of recurrence: (Ann Emerg Med 2014;63(4):437–447)
  - First-time sz (provoked or unprovoked): No AED indicated if back to baseline mental status, no current or known h/o structural brain disease/injury
  - If h/o sz d/o & ↓ AED levels, load w/ AED (PO or IV; home agent preferred)
  - If h/o sz d/o & nl AED levels (& no clear provoking trigger): Contact o/p prescriber to discuss ↑ o/p AED dose

IV Treatment of Status Epilepticus		
Step	Antiepileptic	Dose
1	Lorazepam OR	2–4 mg (0.1 mg/kg), repeat q5–10min if sz persists
	Diazepam OR	5–10 mg (0.2 mg/kg), repeat q5–10min if sz persists
	Midazolam	5–10 mg (0.2 mg/kg), repeat q5–10min if sz persists
2	Phenytoin OR	1–1.5 g (10–15 mg/kg)* over 20 min
	Fosphenytoin OR	1–1.5 g (15–20 mg/kg) over 5–10 min
	Valproic acid	25–45 mg/kg (absence sz)
	Levetiracetam	1–1.5 g (under study; not included in AAN/ACEP guidelines)
3	Phenobarbital	200–600 mg slow push, then 10–20 mg/kg if no resolution
4	General anesthesia w/ propofol, midazolam, or pentobarbital ± paralytics		

Disposition
- Provoked sz: Disposition depends on underlying cause; if underlying cause cannot be rapidly reversed & pt remains at risk for recurrent provoked sz, admx vs. observation
- Unprovoked sz: Most can be safely discharged w/ close neuro f/u if nl mental status, exam, & w/u (above)
- If on long-term meds or 2nd sz, discuss w/ neurology regarding dose adjustments or starting a long-term med

- Explicit instructions to not drive, operate hazardous machinery or perform tasks where recurrent sz may cause harm; some states have mandatory reporting to DMV
- Admit all pts with 2+ sz in pre-hospital/ED or SE; may need ICU

Pearl
- Treat alcohol w/d sz w/ BZD, almost never responsive to phenytoin

VERTIGO

Definition
- The sensation of disorientation in space combined w/ sensation of motion/spinning
- May be due to benign (usually peripheral) or life-threatening (usually central) causes
  - Central comprise ~10% of cases; CVA comprises ~4% (Mayo Clin Proc 2008;83:765–777)
  - RFs for central vertigo: Older age, males, HTN, CAD, DM, AF, h/o CVA/TIA

Differential Diagnosis for Vertigo	
Peripheral	FB, cerumen impaction, acute otitis media, labyrinthitis, benign paroxysmal positional vertigo, Ménière's dz, vestibular neuronitis, perilymphatic fistula, trauma, motion sickness, acoustic neuroma, ototoxic medications (eg, gentamicin, furosemide)
Central	Infection (encephalitis, meningitis, cerebritis), vertebrobasilar art. insufficiency, subclavian steal syndrome, cerebellar or brainstem hemorrhage or infarction, vertebrobasilar migraine, trauma (temporal bone fracture, postconcussive syndrome), tumor (brainstem or cerebellum), MS, temporal lobe epilepsy

History & Physical Exam
- **HX:** Onset & duration of sxs; changes with position & direction; associated sxs (HA, neuro sx, dysarthria, chg in hearing, CP/LH, palpitations); circumstances surrounding onset (trauma, torsional neck inj, neck manipulation, new meds); PMH including meds
  - Distinguish b/w vertigo & pre-syncope or light-headedness
- **EXAM:** Assess for neuro deficits, nystagmus, cerebellar exam, gait, ± Dix Hallpike; listen for carotid bruits, otoscopy, cardiac murmurs

Historical & Exam Features of Central vs. Peripheral Vertigo		
	Peripheral	Central
Timing	Acute-onset (seconds) Can be intermittent or constant Often self-resolves (sec–hrs) Present early in course	Gradual-onset (min–hr) Progressive & constant Present later in course
Intensity	Severe	Mild–moderate
Nystagmus	Always present: Unidirectional, fatigable horizontal or rotatory (never vertical)	May be absent, can be bidirectional. Vertical nystagmus almost always central in origin.
Associated sxs	Intense N/V Provoked by movement/position ± hearing loss or tinnitus Nl brainstem/cerebellar exam	Mild nausea, often HA Not affected by movement Usually no auditory sxs May have abnl neuro exam

Evaluation
- ECG (r/o arrhythmia), glucose & electrolytes, UA, HCG (if child-bearing age)
- Neuroimaging: Preferred modality is MRI; head CT PRN to r/o hemorrhage (eg, HA, trauma, A/C), limited utility for cerebellum/brainstem
  - Consider CTA or MRA to evaluate for vascular dz (carotid, vertebrobasilar)

Treatment
- **Central:** Symptomatic relief (antiemetics, benzodiazepines); Neurology consult, ASA (if ischemic CVA); NSGY (if hemorrhagic CVA) & anticoagulation reversal
- **Peripheral:** usually supportive care w/ antivertigo medications (Diazepam 2–4 mg IV/5–10 mg PO, meclizine 25 mg PO, diphenhydramine, promethazine)
  - For BPPV, consider trying Epley maneuver (or modified self-Epley maneuver at home)
  - For acute bacterial labyrinthitis: ENT consult, IV abx, usually need admission
  - For Ménière's: Supportive medications, encourage decreased salt intake, close ENT f/u

Disposition
- Home once sxs improve w/ PCP/ENT f/u
- Admit if (a) central/CVA, (b) peripheral w/ refractory sx, (c) acute bacterial labyrinthitis

Pearl

- More than half of pts presenting to ED with a chief complaint of "dizziness" or "vertigo" may have nonneurologic processes *(Mayo Clin Proc 2008;83:765–777)*

Common Causes of Peripheral Vertigo	
Etiology	**Findings**
Benign paroxysmal positional vertigo	• Due to otolith disruption w/i semicircular canals (often posterior) • Most common cause of peripheral vertigo (lifetime prev 2.4%; annual rate of recurrence 15%) *(NEJM 2014;370:1138–1147)* • **HX:** Brief (sec/min) spinning sensation, episodic (<1 min each), precipitated by chg in head position (eg, rolling over in bed), severe, a/w N/V • **DX:** Dix-Hallpike causes sx & unidirectional nystagmus in >70% pts, depending on canal involved: start in seated position, rapidly lie flat on back, extend pt's head back 45°, then immediately to left or right 45°, keep pt's eyes open, monitor nystagmus & sxs, repeat on other side. • **TX:** Usually resolves w/o tx (median duration 7 d w/ horizontal canal, 17 d w/ posterior canal); Epley's maneuver may cure sx in >80% w/ one cycle & >92% w/ four cycles
Labyrinthitis - Viral - Acute bacterial - Toxic	• Inflammatory d/o of inner ear 2/2 infection or external toxin • Distinguished from vestibular neuronitis by hearing involvement • **Viral/Serous:** Usually coexisting or recent URI/OM, may have hearing loss; usually nontoxic, may have mild fever; r/o VZV (Ramsay Hunt) requiring IV acyclovir & admx; usual tx is supportive care (antiemetics, hydration) • **Acute bacterial:** Coexisting OM ± cholesteatoma (esp if s/p abx); severe sxs, hearing loss; toxic; tx w/ IV abx, ± ENT consult for myringotomy; admit (only cause of peripheral vertigo that usually needs admx) • **Toxic:** Due to medication ototoxicity; progressive sxs, often w/ hearing loss, tinnitus, NO nystagmus.
Vestibular neuronitis	• Noninflammatory d/o of vestibular system (unclear etiology) • **HX:** Sudden onset, severe, isolated vertigo (no auditory sx); progressive over hours & then gradually subsides, but may have persistent mild sxs for wks/mos; May have h/o prior infxn/toxin; ± nystagmus.
Ménière's Dz	• Increased pressure w/i inner ear endolymphatic system, either due to known cause (metabolic, endocrine, trauma, meds, etc.) or idiopathic • **HX:** Classic tetrad: Episodic severe vertigo (a/w N/V, lasting min to hrs, often wo/se severe sx), unilateral chgs in hearing, tinnitus, & sensation of ear fullness or pressure; sx followed nonspecific fatigue & nausea × days, then prolonged sx-free remission • **TX:** Supportive care, trigger avoidance, if severe may warrant trial of diuretics or steroids (limited supporting data)
Acoustic neuroma	• Intracranial benign neoplasm arising from Schwann cells encasing vestibular or cochlear nerve; cause sx both by affecting signal transmission on affected nerve or by mass effect • **HX:** Gradual onset, progressive unilateral sensorineural hearing loss (most common sx), ± tinnitus, HA, imbalance (rarely frank vertigo), facial weakness/numbness • **DX:** Unlike other causes of peripheral vertigo, dx requires neuroimaging (MRI w/ contrast) • **TX:** Observation (if few sx), surgical excision, stereotactic XRT

FACIAL DROOP

Approach

- **Definition:** Unilateral weakness of the facial muscles, w/ or w/o other neuro deficits; either due to central (upper motor neuron) or peripheral (lower motor neuron) etiologies
- Strength of eye closure & eyebrow elevation helps differentiate central vs. peripheral:
  - Central etiology *spares* forehead due to bilateral innervation → w/u for stroke
- Bedside fingerstick blood glucose early b/c hypoglycemia can cause this

Differential Diagnosis for Facial Droop	
Location	**Differential**
Peripheral	Bell's palsy (idiopathic), facial nerve injury, postsurgical (parotidectomy), infectious (Lyme dz, HSV, mastoiditis), acoustic neuroma, parotid malignancy, botulism
Central	CVA/TIA, intracranial bleed, Todd's paralysis, Guillain–Barré syndrome, cerebral vasculitis/arteritis, multiple sclerosis, myasthenia gravis, progressive supranuclear palsy, infection (meningitis, encephalitis, brain abscess), mass lesion, sarcoidosis, Lyme

Localizing the Lesion in Facial Droop					
Location	**Upper Face**	**Lacrim***	**Saliva** Taste***	**± Associated sx**	**Common Causes**
Cortex****	Intact	Intact	Intact	UE weak	Infarct
Subcortical****	Intact	Intact	Intact	UE weak	Infarct
Pons	Weak	Intact	Intact	UE weak/numb, ataxia, nystagmus, CN VI palsy	Infarct, glioma, MS
CPA	Weak	Intact	Intact	Tinnitus, face numb ataxia, nystagmus	Neoplasm, AVM, sarcoid
IAC proximal to geniculate gang	Weak	Change	Change	Tinnitus, hearing loss, nystagmus	Bell's palsy, acoustic neur.
IAC/FC distal to geniculate gang	Weak	Change	Change	Tinnitus, hearing loss, nystagmus	Bell's palsy, acoustic neur., AOM
FN distal to SMF	Weak	Intact	Intact	None (except if trauma, parotid)	Head injury, parotid path

*Lacrimation innervated from nucleus superior salivatory nerve in pons, via nervus intermedius (traverses w/ CN VII in internal auditory canal).

**Salivation innervated from nucleus superior salivatory nerve in pons, via nervus intermedius (traverses w/ CN VII in IAC) & chorda tympani (traverses w/ CN VII in FC).

***Taste innervated from nucleus of fascia solitarius in pons, via nervus intermedius (traverses w/ CN VII in IAC) & chorda tympani (traverses w/ CN VII in FC).

****Cortical and subcortical lesions contralateral to sx (all others ipsilateral).

IAC, internal auditory canal; FC, facial canal; FN, facial nerve; SMF, stylomastoid foramen. *NEJM* 2004;351(13):1323–1331.

BELL'S PALSY

History
- Acute onset (over hours) painless unilateral facial droop not sparing the forehead, ± aching of ear (60%), taste disturbances (60%), hyperacusis (30%), dry eye, ± cheek/mouth paresthesias (but true sensory loss suggests central lesion)
  - RFs: Adult, diabetics, pregnancy, tick exposure
- Evaluate risk for more concerning pathology: RFs for TIA/CVA, sx of neoplasm, etc.
- Accounts for ~50% of all facial palsies. Can be bilateral, but this requires further w/u.
- Unclear etiology (proposed: ischemic mononeuropathy, HSV reactivation in geniculate g.)

Physical Exam
- Paralysis *must include forehead;* inability to smile or close eye, drooling, hyperacusis
  - Assess for changes in lacrimation, salivation, & taste (see above)
- Look for findings of spec etiology; eg, erythema migrans (Lyme), vesicles (HSV)

Evaluation
- Labs & imaging not routinely indicated if typical presentation
- If atypical presentation, other signs, systemic sxs: Neuroimaging & neuro consult

Treatment (*Neurology* 2012;79(22):2209)
- Artificial tears, tape eyelid before sleeping to prevent corneal injury (cannot close lids)
- Prednisone 60 mg QD × 5, then slow taper (NNT 11) (*Cochrane* 2010;3:CD001942)
- *No empiric abx*, but consider if concerned or severe: Acyclovir (HSV), doxycycline (Lyme)
  - No clear benefit of antiviral tx in Bell's (*Cochrane* 2009;4:CD001869)

Disposition
- Home w/ reassurance, neuro f/u if paralysis persists for months
- Prognosis: 80–90% complete recovery in 2–3 mo, 10% permanent, 14% recurrence.

INTRACRANIAL HEMORRHAGE

Overview

Approach

- Immediate IV access; low threshold for intubation if GCS <8 or declining; assess for e/o herniation (give empiric hyperosmolar tx); emergent neuroimaging, NSGY/neurology c/s
  - Attend to concurrent life-threatening pathology (eg, ATLS, ACLS)
- Pts w/ ICH can decompensate rapidly 2/2 ↑ ICP

History & Physical Exam

- **HX:** Acuity/timing of onset, position, severity, duration, circumstances surrounding onset (trauma, exertion, Valsalva, cocaine), associated sx (HA, N/V, vision chgs, focal neuro sx, speech or behavior chg, fatigue, neck pain), PMH (HTN, cancer, connective tissue d/o), FHx (ICH, aneurysm/AVM, PCKD), Meds (A/C, anti-plt agents)
- **EXAM:** VS; Assess GCS, motor/sensory & coordination, meningeal signs, e/o trauma
  - Signs of impending herniation: Asymmetric nonreactive pupil, decorticate/decerebrate posturing, Cushing's reflex (↑ BP, ↓ HR)

Evaluation

- CBC, BMP, PT/INR, PTT, Type & Screen
- STAT Noncontrast CT head to evaluate location & extent of bleeding; based on type of ICH, CTA may help clarify vascular etiology (eg, AVM, aneurysm)
- NSGY consultation: if ↑ ICP & ↓ GCS, may need bolt, drain, craniotomy vs. craniectomy

Treatment

- Reverse anticoagulation: See section on Anticoagulation Reversal (Ch. 11)
- Optimize BP (SBP 90–140 mmHg): Nicardipine, Labetalol, Esmolol gtt first-line; Consider IV enalaprilat if unable to take PO but no need for continuous gtt
- Cerebral protection: HOB elevation to 30 degrees, minimize ↑↓ glucose, hyperthermia, ↓ BP, ↓ O_2, ↓ CO_2, seizures

Subarachnoid Hemorrhage

Overview

- **Definition:** Acute bleed into subarachnoid space between pial & arachnoid mater; can be traumatic (often focal) or atraumatic (eg, ruptured aneurysm, AVM; often generalized)
  - 80% of atraumatic SAH from ruptured aneurysm, but 30–50% of these may have had prior sentinel bleed (eg, leak); important to consider sentinel bleed in ddx of HA

Clinical Grading Scale for SAH (World Federation of Neurologic Surgeons)		
Grade	GCS	Clinical Appearance
1	15	No motor deficit
2	13–14	No motor deficit
3	13–14	Motor deficit
4	7–12	With or without motor deficit
5	3–6	With or without motor deficit

History & Physical Exam

- **HX:** Classically sudden "thunderclap" HA, max pain w/i 1 h, "worst HA of life", ± neck pain, N/V, photophobia, syncope or AMS, focal neuro deficits, sz
  - Red flags: Exertional/Valsalva, neck pain, arrival by ambulance, LOC, N/V
  - RFs: Age >60, FH (4× risk), HTN, smoking, alcohol, cocaine, amphetamine use, PCKD, collagen/connective tissue d/o
- **EXAM:** Ranges based on severity; if sentinel bleed with low-grade, may have nl neuro exam, or if high-grade with low GCS, may be obtunded; Assess for photophobia & nuchal rigidity; May have ocular motor palsy 2/2 aneurysm compression.

Evaluation

- Noncontrast head CT: In pts with low pre-TP (low risk by hx & nl neuro exam): Se 100% (–LR 0.01) if performed w/i 6 h & read by neuroradiologist, 89% after 6 h (*BMJ* 2011;343:d4277; *Acad Emerg Med* 2016;23(9):963–1003).
- LP (gold standard): ↑ opening pressure (>20 cm H_2O), Xanthochromia (100% Se if >12 h)
  - No established "lower limit" for RBCs: Multiple "test thresholds" have been studied, including visible xanthochromia (Se 31%, Sp 98%), RBC <1 K × 10^6/L in Tube 4 (pooled Se 76%, Sp 88%; +LR 5.7, –LR 0.21); Spectrophotometric bilirubin (Se 100%, Sp 95%; +LR 28.8, –LR 0.22) (*Acad Emerg Med* 2016;23(9):963–1003)
- CTA: Reaches sens of 98% for bleed, but is improving & will likely play greater role; obtain CTA if SAH is diagnosed in order to localize aneurysm/AVM
- Conventional angiography: gold standard for localizing aneurysm/AVM if CTA neg

Treatment
- See Approach above; early consultation to NSGY critical
- 70% of SAH will have vasospasm (usually 3–21d, peak 7–10d), causing delayed cerebral ischemia; nimodipine (60 mg q4h PO) should be started w/i 96h of SAH

Disposition
- Admit, may need ICU; prognosis dependent on WFNS Grade/GCS

Subdural & Epidural Hematoma
Overview
- **Definition:** Bleeding into the subdural or epidural spaces due either to trauma (EDH, SDH) or tearing of the bridging veins from rapid acceleration/deceleration injury (SDH), occasionally, no h/o trauma present (SDH)
- Both cause sx as a result of mass effect on brain parenchyma & are NSGY emergencies

History, Physical Exam, Evaluation, Treatment
- See section on EDH & SDH in Trauma chapter as well as General Approach above to ICH

Nontraumatic Intraparenchymal Hemorrhage
Overview
- **Definition:** Hemorrhage often within the subcortical white matter or (less likely) brainstem, causing sx due to mass effect, vasogenic edema & localized inflammation
- Classified as either primary (HTN, amyloid angiopathy) or secondary (coagulopathy, AVM, neoplasm, cerebral venous sinus thrombosis, hemorrhagic conversion of ischemic infarct)

Characteristic Appearance & Location of Common Nontraumatic Etiologies		
Cause	**Typical Location**	**Typical Appearance**
HTN	Int capsule, thalamus, cerebellum/pons	Round, homogenous
CAA	Lobar (cortical/subcortical)	Round, homogenous
Coagulopathy	Lobar	Irregularly shaped
*Neoplasm	Variable; may be multiple	Surrounding edema

*Common neoplasms: Primary CNS tumors, melanoma, lung, breast (Semin Roentgenol 2014:49(1):112–126)

History, Physical Exam, Evaluation, Treatment
- See Approach above to ICH

Disposition
- Admit to neurology if no e/o aneurysm/AVM; often require ICU

ISCHEMIC STROKE

Overview
Approach
- Requires immediate & rapid assessment; utility of thrombolysis is time-limited
- Immediate IV access, telemetry, supplemental O_2 if hypoxic, neuro c/s if tPA candidate
- Quick assessment of ABCs: if GCS < 8 but RR & O_2 nl, weigh risk-benefits of sending pt to CT scan w/o intubation, intubate if concern for imminent deterioration
  - If possible, obtain patient advanced directive (goals of care) to guide resuscitation
- All patients need STAT fingerstick glucose to r/o hypoglycemia as cause of sx
- Goal to R/O TIA, Sz, & ICH ASAP & provide lytics if w/i eligible time frame

History
- Establish time of onset (if unwitnessed, establish time "last seen nl"), sx progression (stable vs. improving), circumstances surrounding onset (recent health, trauma, sz, toxins)
  - Complaints may be vague (AMS, numb, weak, vision Δ, dysarthria)
- Assess RFs for ischemic CVA (HTN/HLD, DM, AF, CAD/PVD, CHF, Valve dz, hypercoagulable states, PFO [5–10% of pop w/ clinically significant PFO])
- Assess for other causes (see table), inc. recrudescence ("unmasking") of old CVA

Differential Diagnosis for Ischemic Stroke	
CNS	TIA, ICH, Neoplasm, Seizure (Todd's paralysis), Recrudescence of prior CVA (eg, 2/2 infxn, metabolic, GIB; may not have known CVA hx), Complex migraine, Cerebral venous sinus thrombosis
Vascular	Aortic dissection, Cervical arterial dissection (carotid, vertebral), Endocarditis, HTN encephalopathy
Tox/Metabolic	↓ glucose, ↑↓ Na, Wernicke's encephalopathy, Drug toxicity
Hematologic	TTP
Other	Bell's palsy, Conversion d/o, Cryptogenic (no known cause; 25%)

Physical
- Quick but detailed neuro exam using NIH Stroke Scale (see below)
- Check for arrhythmia, murmur, bruits, & rectal for occult blood if considering lytics

NIH Stroke Scale		
Variable	Finding	Points
Consciousness	Alert, keenly responsive	0
	Arouses w/ minor stimulation	1
	Arouses w/ repeat or painful stimulation	2
	Coma	3
Orientation (month, age)	Answers both correctly	0
	Answers one correctly	1
	Answers none correctly	2
Commands (close eyes, grip)	Performs both correctly	0
	Performs one correctly	1
	Performs none correctly	2
Best gaze	nl	0
	Partial palsy (no forced deviation)	1
	Total gaze paresis or forced deviation	2
Visual fields	No visual loss	0
	Partial hemianopsia	1
	Complete hemianopsia	2
	Bilateral hemianopsia (blind)	3
Facial palsy	None	0
	Minor paralysis (eg, flattened nasolabial fold)	1
	Partial paralysis (near total in lower face)	2
	Complete paralysis (total lower/upper face)	3
Motor arm (10 s drift)	No drift	0
	Drift but does not hit bed	1
	Some effort but drifts to bed	2
	No effort against gravity	3
	No movement	4
Motor leg (5 s drift)	No drift	0
	Drift but does not hit bed	1
	Some effort but drifts to bed	2
	No effort against gravity	3
	No movement	4
Ataxia (finger/nose, heel/shin)	Absent	0
	Present in 1 limb	1
	Present in 2 limbs	2
Sensory	nl	0
	Mild–Moderate loss ("pinprick feels less sharp")	1
	Severe–total loss	2
Language (writing if intubated) (Naming objects, pictures)	nl, no aphasia	0
	Some loss of fluency or comprehension	1
	Severe aphasia; fragmented	2
	Mute, global aphasia	3
Dysarthria (Have pt read list of words)	nl	0
	Slurs some words but understandable	1
	Severe, unintelligible	2
Extinction/Inattention (Bilateral stimulation)	No abnlty	0
	Inattention or extinction to bilateral stimulation	1
	Profound hemi-inattention	2
Score <5 = minor, Score >20 = severe neurologic deficit		

Evaluation:
- CBC, BMP, PT/INR, Troponin, UA, T & S
- ECG: May reveal AF; cerebral T waves (deep symmetric precordial) suggest ↑ ICP (rare)
- Noncontrast CT: r/o hemorrhage & exclude other etiologies; eval for early e/o infarction (hyperdense vessel segment; loss of grey-white differentiation, gyral effacement)

- CT Angiography: r/o arterial dissection; localize thrombus & map vasculature limitations (eg, stenosis, tortuosity) to help guide potential IA tx
- MRI: Highest Se & Sp for CVA in acute setting (initially ↑ DWI & ↓ ADC signal; after 6 h ↑ T2 FLAIR; after 16 h ↓ T1 signal), but often not immediately available
- Echocardiography: Eval for atrial/LV thrombus, mitral valve pathology, myxoma, PFO; diagnostic yield 4–10% (TTE) & 11–41% (TEE), but +findings often chg long-term mgmt; most useful in pts w/ abnl ECG or c/f embolic source *(Postgrad Med)* 2014;90(1066):434–438).
- Once CVA dx'ed: addx tests to evaluate RF (HgbA1c, Lipid panel) & guide 2° prevention

Transient Ischemic Attack

Overview:
- **Definition:** Acute focal neurologic dysfxn 2/2 ischemia from arterial occlusion (thrombotic or embolic) but completely resolving within 24 h (usually <1 h) & not a/w residual tissue infarction; signals ↑ CVA risk 2/2 shared underlying pathophysiology w/ CVA
- Etiologies: Often thromboembolic event (AF, PFO, Atherosclerosis), small vessel dz, or fixed large-vessel stenosis w/ transient ↓ BP
- Risk of CVA after TIA: 3% w/i 2 d, 5% w/i 7 d; ABCD² Score may predict individual risk, but should not supplant clinical judgment (see footnotes in table) or dictate f/u urgency

ABCD² Score: Stroke Risk after TIA				
Factor	**Criteria**	**Pts**	**7-d CVA Risk***	**7-d CVA Risk****
Age	Age >60	1	0 pts 0%	<4 pts 2.3%
BP	First BP >140/90	1	1 pt 0%	≥4 pts 10.2%
Clinical signs	Motor weakness ± speech	2	2 pts 0%	
	Isolated speech disturbance	1	3 pts 0%	**90-d CVA Risk²**
Duration	>60 min	2	4 pts 2.2%	<4 pts 2.4%
	10–59 min	1	5 pts 16.3%	≥4 pts 7.2%
Diabetes	Requiring meds/insulin	1	6 pts 35.5%	

*Original study (single-community, UK) *(Lancet 2005;366(9479):29–36.*

**Pooled meta-analysis of 29 cohorts *(Neurology 2015;85(4):304–305)*. Up to 1/3 of pts w/ TIA-mimics may have ABCD² ≥4, and 1/3 of pts w/ true TIA have ABCD² <4.Additionally, 1/5 pts w/ ABCD² <4 have >50% carotid stenosis, needing urgent f/u. Thus, score should accompany clinical judgement, eval of other CVA RFs (cervical arterial stenosis), and strong consideration should be given to ED neurology c/s to guide mgmt & urgency of f/u.

History & Physical Exam
- See Approach; If acute, emphasis should be placed on assessing degree of resolution

Evaluation
- If sx not fully resolved (NIHSS > 0): W/U as acute CVA (Noncontrast CT & CTA)
- If sx fully resolved (NIHSS = 0): May defer CT & obtain MRI/MRA w/i 24 h, unless c/f other etiologies (eg, partial sz 2/2 underlying neoplasm)
- Need to find etiology of TIA (echo, carotid imaging, Holter, MRI/MRA), usually as inpt

Treatment *(Stroke 2013;44(3):870–947; Stroke 2014;45(7):2160–236)*
- Tx focuses on short- & long-term risk reduction
- ASA (325 mg QD) ± clopidogrel (75 mg QD) based on severity of intracranial stenosis
- BP control: In acute setting, may be reasonable to avoid active BP control for >24 h unless markedly elevated (>220/120) or concurrent medical condition requiring ↓ BP; if BP remains elevated after first several days, tx w/ goal BP < 140/90
- Statin therapy if LDL-C >100 mg/dL
- Anti-coagulation if e/o Afib/Aflutter (VKA or NOAC); if CI to A/C, ASA ± clopidogrel
- Carotid revascularization: Recommended for high-grade (>70%) & moderate (50–69%, NNT 15; if not otw high surgical risk) stenosis no risk reduction if stenosis <50%; if able to undergo CEA, CEA preferred over CAS *(Cochrane 2012;9:10:662–668)*
- Lifestyle modifications: Weight loss, diet/low-salt, exercise, ↓ ETOH, ↓ tobacco

Disposition
- Admit if 1st TIA, mx TIAs in short time, cardiogenic, or posterior circulation
  - In some stroke centers, select cases can be managed outpt (eg, recent full w/u)
- ABCD² is a useful data point but not well validated as a disposition tool

Pearl
- Recurrent TIAs w/ different sxs are likely cardiac emboli; if same sxs, likely cerebral

Ischemic Stroke

Overview
- **Definition:** Acute focal neurologic dysfxn 2/2 ischemia causing tissue infarction, often due to acute arterial occlusion (embolic >25% thrombotic > vascular dissection, etc) or fixed stenosis w/ hypotension

History, Physical Exam, & Evaluation

- See Approach; If acute, initial assessment should not delay imaging & decision to provide lytic tx (apart from reviewing CIs)
- Sxs & exam findings will depend on arterial distribution affected (see table)
  - Anterior circulation: Unilateral motor/sensory deficit (eg, numbness, weakness, facial droop, monocular blindness [amaurosis fugax], aphasia)
  - Posterior circulation: Nonlateralizing sxs (eg, diplopia, dysarthria, dysphagia, ataxia)

Common Ischemic Stroke Patterns	
Stroke Location	**Presentation**
Ophthalmic Art.	Transient painless monocular vision loss (often embolic from ICA)
Internal Carotid Art.	See ACA & MCA: profound motor & sensory deficits
Ant. Cerebral Art.	C/L hemiparesis & sensory loss (leg, perineum > arm, face) ± impaired judgment/confusion, ± incontinence (pelvic floor weakness), ± disconnection syndrome (↓ awareness of I/L body, 2/2 corpus callosum infarction)
Mid. Cerebral Art.	C/L hemiparesis & sensory loss (face, arm > leg, perineum) ± aphasia (if dominant hemisphere; Broca/receptive [frontal] or Wernicke/expressive [temporal]) or neglect (if nondominant)
Post. Cerebral Art.	Homonymous hemianopia ± cortical blindness ± Agnosia (object recognition), alexia (word recognition), prosopagnosia (face recognition), memory deficits ± Prominent contralateral sensory chgs w/o paralysis (thalamus)
Lacunar Art.	Pure hemiplegia (pons/internal capsule), pure sensory (thalamus), clumsy hand & dysarthria syndrome (pons), unilateral leg paresis & ataxia (pons/internal capsule)
Common Posterior Fossa Syndromes (QJM 2013;106(7):607–615)	
Post. Inf. Cerebellar Art. (Lateral Medullary Synd, Wallenberg)	NO motor deficits Sensory: *Crossed* sensory loss on I/L face, C/L arm/leg Ataxia: I/L limb & truncal (veer/lean) ataxia Oculobulbar: Ocular (diplopia, nystagmus, ocular torsion), bulbar (dysarthria, dysphagia, hiccups, uvular deviation) Autonomic sx: Horner syndrome
Ant. Inf. Cerebellar Art. (Lat Pontine Synd.)	I/L facial weakness & sensory loss I/L sensorineural hearing loss (labyrinthine art.) Ataxia, nystagmus
Basilar Art. (pontine)	Impaired or alternating responsiveness (may present w/ coma) Various B/L motor sxs, including bulbar ± Visual impairment/cortical blindness • "Locked-in syndrome": Only ocular muscles remain intact

Treatment (Stroke 2013;44(3):870–947; Stroke 2014;45(7):2160–236)

- Early Neurology C/S & imaging: Recommended door-to-physician, ≤10 min; door-to-stroke team, ≤15 min; door-to-CT initiation, ≤25 min; door-to-CT interpretation, ≤45 min
- ASA 325 mg PO/PR. May use clopidogrel, ticlopidine, or warfarin per neurology.
- BP control: Labetalol (IV) & Nicardipine (gtt) first-line, use short-acting IV agents
  - If TPA candidate: BP goal <185/110 (lysis contraindicated if >185/110 after 2 doses)
  - If not TPA candidate: Treat only if persistently >220/120, s/sx other end-organ damage (eg, AMI), or alternative med condition needing BP control; lower ≤10–20%
- Fibrinolytic therapy (rtPA 0.9 mg/kg): In selected pts w/i appropriate timeframe & w/o CIs
  - Odds of favorable recovery decrease with time after sx onset (see table)
  - Risks of tPA: ICH (6% risk, clinically significant 1–2%), angioedema (1-5), systemic bleeding; ↑ 7 d mortality, but no ↑ mortality at final f/u (Lancet 2012;379(9834):2364–2372)
  - See table below for inclusion criteria, absolute & relative CIs
  - Intra-arterial tPA (available at some stroke centers) may be preferred (w/ or w/o prior IV tPA) for proximal lesions (distal ICA, MCA, basilar), severe sx, CI to systemic tPA, or delayed presentation after sx onset (4.5–6 h, investigations ongoing 6–12 h)
  - Thrombectomy (typically w/ tPA) (eg, Merci retrieval system): Recanalization w/ Merci retrieval 57%, in combo w/ IA tPA 70%; ICH risk 7–10% (Stroke 2008;39(4):1205–1212)
- If arterial dissection or suspected cardioembolic stroke, may consider heparin

Pooled Odds of Favorable Outcome After TPA			
Time of TPA administration after sx	0–1.5 h	1.5–3.0 h	3.0–4.5 h
Odds of favorable neuro recovery at 3 mo	2.81	1.55	1.40

Data pooled from 6 RCTs (Lancet 2004;363(9411):768–774); no change in mortality w/ different timing of tx.

Criteria for Thrombolysis in Acute Stroke

Inclusion Criteria

- Age >18
- Clinical Dx of acute ischemic stroke w/ measurable neuro deficit
- Time of onset <3 h (well established), or <4.5 h in some centers

Absolute CIs to Lysis

- CTH shows ICH or very large stroke (>33% of hemisphere)
- High clinical suspicion for SAH (even w/ nl CTH)
- Active internal bleeding (eg, GIB)
- Bleeding diathesis (PLT <100000, heparin in past 48 h, anticoagulation w/ INR >1.7)
- Stroke, intracranial surgery, or head trauma in past 3 mo
- LP in past 1 wk
- Recent arterial puncture at noncompressible site
- Prior ICH, AVM, or aneurysm
- Refractory HTN (SBP >185 mmHg & DBP ≥110 mmHg despite tx)

Relative CIs (weigh risk–benefit)

- Minor or rapidly resolving sxs
- Witnessed sz at time of stroke onset
- Acute MI in past 3 mo
- Recent GI/GU hemorrhage in past 3 wk
- Major surgery or serious trauma in past 2 wk
- Pregnancy

Additional Relative CIs (for use after 3 h & before 4.5 h)

- Age >80
- NIHSS >25 (suggests large stroke)
- Oral anticoagulant use (regardless of INR)
- Combination of prior ischemic strokes & diabetes mellitus

Disposition
- Admit all patients; Large strokes may need ICU (risk of edema, hemorrhagic conversion)

Pearls
- Inpt w/u includes carotid imaging, echo, Holter monitor, advanced serology (hypercoagulability, lipids, bleeding diathesis, ESR, ANA)
- NIHSS correlates w/ neurologic outcome at 3 mo but poor predictor for posterior CVAs

NEUROMUSCULAR SYNDROMES

MYASTHENIA GRAVIS

Overview
- **Definition:** Autoimmune d/o (Abs against *post*synaptic ACh nicotinic receptors) causing progressive weakness of incremental muscle groups, with intermittent crises marked my potential need for ventilatory support
- Epidemiology: Most commonly affects women in 20s–30s, men in 60s–70s (peak)
- DDx includes Lambert–Eaton syndrome (similar pathophysiology, paraneoplastic)

History
- Gradual onset, symmetric, fluctuating proximal & ocular muscle weakness
  - Common: Extraocular/ptosis (present in 50% initially), bulbar, limb (prox > distal); however, w/i 1 y most pts have generalized involvement
  - Sx least severe in morning; worsen w/ repetitive activity & throughout day
- Assess for triggers of crisis: Stress, infection, pregnancy, surgery, meds (abx, steroids)
- If advanced dz: Obtain clear goals of care in case need for intubation

Physical Exam
- Proximal weakness & fatigability worse w/ repetitive activity, relieved by rest
- CN affected early (ocular: Ptosis, diplopia; bulbar: Dysarthria, dysphagia)

Evaluation
- Neuro C/S: if new onset, poor o/p f/u, or probable need for admx
- If new dx: AChR Ab test has high Sp, but poor Se, esp in localized dz; Tensilon (edrophonium) test (2 mg IV over 15 s; binds to AChE, blocking ACh hydrolysis)
  - Tensilon test may precipitate bradycardia or heart block – have atropine at bedside
- If known dx: Differentiate MG crisis from cholinergic crisis (most pts on cholinergic meds)
  - Cholinergic tox: lacrimation, salivation, perspiration, bronchorrhea, N/V, diarrhea, brady

- Measuring NIF (negative inspiratory force) can identify pts at risk of respiratory failure; NIF <20 cm H_2O suggests severe resp weakness

Treatment
- Ventilatory support as indicated (NIPPV, intubation)
- Long term txs include AChE-inh (pyridostigmine) & immunomod (steroids, etc.)
- Corticosteroids given in crisis but can worsen sx initially; minimal short-term effect
- Plasmapheresis & IVIG: mainstays of tx for acute crisis

Disposition
- Admit all pts w/myasthenia crisis
- If no e/o crisis & good o/p f/u, can d/c with close o/p f/u

GUILLAIN–BARRÉ SYNDROME

Overview
- **Definition:** Acute autoimmune demyelinating peripheral neuropathy, often in response to external infectious exposure & characterized by loss of peripheral nerve reflexes
- Common associated pathogens: *Campylobacter* (~30%), EBV, HSV, HIV, *Mycoplasma*
- Slow recovery (can take mo in worst affected); 5% die from cx (sepsis, PE, dysautonomia)

History, Physical Exam, & Evaluation
- **HX:** Progressive ascending weakness; can start w/ numbness/paresthesias or pain in LE's, f/b symmetric b/l weakness over hrs to wks
  - Usually (2/3) heralded by recent URI or diarrheal illness days – wks prior to sx
- **EXAM:** Acute ascending symmetric weakness, sensory chgs, ↓ DTRs (however, 10% of early cases will have DTRs), 20% will have autonomic dysfxn & potentially-fatal arrhythmias (*NEJM 2012;366: 2294–2304*); ± CNS (hallucinations, psychosis, vivid dreams) (*NEJM 2012;366: 2294–2304*)
  - Miller-Fisher variant = ataxia, areflexia, ophthalmoplegia.
- **DX:** Clinical dx; w/u generally to r/o other dx
  - CPK nl (acute myopathy may present similarly but nl sensation & ↑ CPK)
  - LP (can r/o lyme, lymphoma): Albuminocytologic dissociation (↑ protein, no WBCs or bacteria) only present 50% of cases in 1st wk, 75% by 3rd wk (*NEJM 2012;366:2294–2304*)

Treatment (*NEJM 2012;366:2294–2304*)
- Consult neurology
- Hemodynamic stabilization: telemetry (risk for arrhythmia; some pts may need PPM), rapidly titratable vasoactive agents as needed for dysautonomia
- Respiratory support as indicated (25% pts need intubation): avoid succinylcholine for RSI
- Plasmapheresis & IVIG equally effective; combo not superior
- Steroids have limited effectiveness in speeding recovery

Disposition:
- Admit until no e/o progression; ICU if respiratory compromise
- Prognosis: Full recovery can take mo & can be c/b mx dz (PNA, sepsis, PE, etc)

AMYOTROPHIC LATERAL SCLEROSIS (ALS)

Overview
- **Definition:** Degenerative dz of UMNs & LMNs
- Epidemiology: Age >40, M = F

History, Physical Exam, & Evaluation
- **HX:** Progressive motor weakness & atrophy, fasciculations, spasm; NO sensory loss.
  - Assess pt goals of care regarding life-support interventions including airway
- **EXAM:** UMN & LMN findings, initially distal; fasciculations 2/2 denervation; may have bulbar findings (dysphagia, dysarthria) in advanced dz, spasticity, ↑ DTRs, +Babinski
  - Bladder & bowel sphincters & ocular muscles often spared
- **DX:** If new onset, neuro consult & consider MRI brain & spinal cord

Treatment
- Supportive care (Respiratory support, antispasmodics)
- In pts w/ known dx, treat cx (DVT from immobility, asp PNA, UTI, decubitus ulcers)

Disposition
- Depends on respiratory status, acuity

MULTIPLE SCLEROSIS (MS)

Overview
- **Definition:** Progressive chronic immune-mediated demyelinating dz of the CNS
  - Generally follows relapsing-remitting (85–90%; may not have complete recovery b/w relapses) or primary progressive course (usually w/o relapses)
- Epidemiology: Relapsing-remitting presents young (30 y) & F>M (3:1); primary-progressive presents older (40 y) & F=M; ↑↑ risk if 1st-degree relative also affected
- Dx requires 2+ distinct episodes w/ differential neurologic sxs (ie, diff anatomic lesion)

History
- Acute episodes develop over hours–days (also remit over same time course)
  - Look for precipitating factors for exacerbation (eg, infection, hyperthermia)
- Sx can be highly variable: vision, sensation, mobility/balance, cognition, sphincter control
  - See table for typical presentations, ocular sx common
  - Uhthoff phenomenon: Sxs worsen w/ ↑ body temp (exercise, hot bath, fever)

Typical Multiple Sclerosis Presentations (Lancet 2017;389(10076):1336–1346)	
Acute unilateral optic neuritis*	Sensory sx in a CNS pattern
Diplopia (2/2 INO or CN VI palsy)*	Lhermitte's sign
Facial sensory loss or trigeminal neuralgia	Asymmetric limb weakness
Cerebellar ataxia, nystagmus	Urge incontinence, erectile dysfxn
Partial myelopathy	

*Optic Neuritis: Painful EOM, afferent pupillary defect, decreased visual acuity, ± papilledema.
**INO: Inter-nuclear ophthalmoplegia (affected eye is able to abduct but not adduct; unaffected eye EOM nl) due to MLF lesion; Lhermitte's sign: Electric-shock sensation travelling down spine with neck flexion.

Evaluation (Lancet 2017;389(10076):1336–1346)
- Neuro consult indicated due to clinical benefit of early dx
- MRI Brain (Se 80% in pts w/ isolated syndrome): multifocal T2 hyperint white matter lesions
- MRI Spine (Se 50% in pts w/ isolated syndrome; mostly c-spine): indicated if sx localize to spinal cord or MRI Brain nondiagnostic
- LP: Indicated only if uncertainty based on MRI findings; may show pleocytosis (50%) & IgG oligoclonal bands (85–95%)

Treatment
- Treat any reversible underlying triggers (eg, infxn, dehydration, fevers)
- High-dose corticosteroids are 1st line for acute relapses; may consider addition of 2nd-line plasmapheresis in fulminant cases (Neurology 2011;76(3):294–300)
- Supportive: spasticity (baclofen, benzo), pain (carbamazepine/TCA), fatigue (amantadine)

Disposition
- Admit all new-dx for further w/u
- Most pts are admitted for relapses; can D/C if mild sx, nonprogressive, & close neuro f/u

Pearl
- Due to complexity of dx, rates of mis-dx pts (ie, w/o dz) may be as high as 10% (Lancet 2017;389(10076):1336–1346)

TRANSVERSE MYELITIS

Overview (NEJM 2010;363:564–572)
- **Definition:** Acute or subacute inflammation & varying demyelination of a limited length of spinal cord causing motor, sensory, & autonomic dysfxn w/ sx correlating to level affected
- Often >2 vertebral seg involved; MS-associated TM can be <2 seg & partial cord
- Epidemiology: All ages affected; bimodal peak (10–19y & 30–39y); M = F; unrelated to FHx
- Etiologies: Postvaccination (60% in children), postinfection, systemic autoimmune dz, or acquired demyelination dz (eg, MS), neuromyelitis optica, idiopathic (15–30%)

History, Physical Exam, & Evaluation
- **HX:** Acute or subacute paraplegia, sensory changes (with definitive spinal cord level), & sphincter loss (below level); onset over hours to days; bilateral but often asymmetric, often w/ neuropathic back/midline pain
  - Ask about recent viral illness, immunization, FHx of MS, vision sx (NMO)

- **EXAM:** Symmetric or asymmetric weakness & sensory loss referable to a spinal cord level, hyperreflexia, +Babinski, +Lhermitte's sign (+electric radiating back pain w/ neck flexion)
- **DX:** MRI entire spine w/ contrast; Neurology consult; If confirmed by imaging, may need LP (+pleocytosis) to help differentiate etiology & prognosticate

Treatment
- Ventilatory support as indicated by level of cord involvement & sx
- Supportive care: Analgesia (TCA, carbamazepine), Spasticity (baclofen, benzos), fatigue
- High-dose steroids (1-g methylprednisolone QD IV) are 1st-line, esp for postinfectious or demyelinating etiology (NEJM 2010;363:564–572)
- May consider plasmapheresis if fulminant or refractory to steroids; limited data

Disposition
- Admit to neurology
- Prognosis depends on etiology: Most recovery takes mo to yr
  - MS-associated TM: Quicker & complete recovery; but ↑ risk of relapse c/w idiopathic, post-viral, or post-immunization

DYSURIA

(Am Fam Phys. 2015;92:778)

Definition
- Sensation of pain, burning, or discomfort on urination; generally indicates infection or inflammation of the bladder &/or urethra

Approach to the Patient
History
- Onset/frequency/severity/location? Hematuria? Urinary frequency/hesitancy/urgency? Abnl penile or vaginal d/c? Lesions? Perineal pain? Pain on intercourse?
- ROS (fever, trauma, flank pain, abdominal or suprapubic pain, joint/back pain)
- PMH (STDs or PID, DM or immunocompromised)
- MEDS (topical irritants)
- SOCIAL (recent intercourse, multiple sexual partners)

Physical Exam
- Most pts should have at least an assessment of costovertebral angle tenderness & an abdominal exam
- Women: Consider pelvic exam if at risk for STDs, w/ vaginal sxs, postmenopausal
- Men: Should perform penile exam, testicular exam & prostate exam given risk of complicated dz

Evaluation
- Urine studies (clean catch UA, hCG ± culture, NAAT for GC/Chlamydia); CBC/Chemistries rarely indicated, unless suspected complicated dz (see below)
- Consider vaginal/urethral studies (smear w/ wet mount, cx), renal u/s, IV pyelography, CT abdomen/pelvis if warranted
- Further studies may include urine cytology, voiding cystourethrography, cystoscopy, urodynamic testing, but not routinely performed in ED

Dysuria Differential	
Pathophysiology	Differential
Structural	Urolithiasis, BPH, urethral stricture/diverticula, atrophic vaginitis
Infectious	Vulvovaginitis, urethritis, cervicitis, prostatitis, epididymo-orchitis, cystitis, pyelonephritis, STDs
Meds	PCN, Cytoxan, topical hygiene products (vaginal spray/douche/lubricant)
Neoplastic/autoimmune	GU cancer (penile, vulvar/vaginal, prostate, bladder), Behçet, Reiter, SLE
Other	Instrumentation, urethral trauma, interstitial cystitis

URINARY TRACT INFECTIONS

(Emerg Med Clin North Am. 2011;29:539)

Definitions
UTIs are classified according to a spectrum of dz & the predominant clinical sxs: Asymptomatic bacteriuria, uncomplicated lower UTI (cystitis), uncomplicated pyelonephritis, complicated UTI w/ or w/o pyelonephritis, recurrent UTI

Asymptomatic bacteriuria: Absence of urinary sxs w/ Ucx ≥10^5 cfu/mL uropathogen. Screening/ tx not recommended except in pregnant women

Acute uncomplicated UTI: Acute dysuria, urgency, frequency, suprapubic pain w/ UA ≥10 WBC/mm^3 & Ucx ≥10^3 cfu/mL

Acute uncomplicated pyelonephritis: Fever, chills, flank pain in the absence of alternative Dx & urologic abnlty w/ UA ≥10 WBC/mm^3 & Ucx ≥10^4 cfu/mL

Complicated UTI: Features of uncomplicated UTI/pyelonephritis AND 1 or more of the following—pregnancy, diabetes, male gender, immunosuppression (eg, chemo, AIDS), functional GU abnlty (indwelling catheter, neurogenic bladder), structural GU abnlty (renal stone, intestinal fistula, PCKD, kidney transplant pt)

Recurrent UTI: At least 3 episodes of uncomplicated UTI documented by culture in the last 12 mo in the absence of structural/functional abx

Male urogenital tract infections: Urethritis, prostatitis, epididymitis, orchitis

Asymptomatic Bacteriuria

(Guideline: U.S. Preventive Services Task Force. Screening for Asymptomatic Bacteriuria. In Adults: USPSTF Reaffirmation Recommendation Statement. *Ann Intern Med.* 2008;149:43.)

(Nicolle LE, Bradley S, Colgan R, et al. Infectious Disease Society of America Guidelines for the Diagnosis and Treatment of Asymptomatic Bacteriuria in Adults. *Clin Infect Dis.* 2005;40:643.)

Definition

- Absence of urinary sxs w/ UA ≥10 WBC/mm^3 & Ucx ≥10^5 cfu/mL of the same uropathogen in 2 consecutive midstream urine samples ≥24 h apart; however, a single positive midstream urine is generally accepted as adequate & more practical
- USPSTF recommends screening for asymptomatic bacteriuria w/ Ucx for pregnant women at 12–16 wk gestation given increased risk of pyelonephritis, preterm labor & low birth weight
- USPSTF recommends against screening for asymptomatic bacteriuria in men or nonpregnant women
- The IDSA recommends against routine screening for or tx of asymptomatic bacteriuria in diabetic women, older persons >65 y/o residing in the community or institutionalized residents of long-term care facilities, spinal cord injury, & pts w/ indwelling urethral catheters

Treatment (Asymptomatic Bacteriuria in Pregnancy)

- 3–7-d course of nitrofurantoin or cephalosporin (cephalexin, cefpodoxime, cefdinir, cefaclor)

Pearl

- Given the high PPV of leukocyte esterase & nitrites on UA for bacteriuria, a positive test result in an asymptomatic pregnant pt in the ED should be considered for tx pending culture data

Acute Uncomplicated Urinary Tract Infection (Acute Cystitis)

Definition

Acute dysuria, urgency, frequency, suprapubic pain w/ UA ≥10 WBC/mm^3 & Ucx ≥10^3 cfu/mL, but ≥10^5 cfu/mL also used to define UTI; absence of structural/functional UG tract abnormalities

Occurs when uropathogen from bowel or vagina colonize periurethral mucosa & ascend through urethra & bladder

Predominant uropathogens: *E. coli* (75–95%), *K. pneumoniae, P. mirabilis, E. faecalis, S. saprophyticus,* & *S. agalactiae* (group B Strep); rarely *P. aeruginosa, Ureaplasma* species

Probability of dz in pts presenting w/ 1 or more UTI sxs is ~50%

History

- Combination of dysuria, frequency, hematuria, fever, back pain, &/or self-diagnosis all increase the probability of UTI, whereas their absence decreases its probability
- Vaginal d/c or irritation w/o the above sxs decreases probability of UTI
- RFs: Prior UTI, family h/o UTI, sexual intercourse, new sex partner (w/i 1 yr), use of spermicide

Physical Exam

- ±Fever; tenderness w/ suprapubic palpation; CVA tenderness
- GU exam if vaginal d/c or irritation present

Evaluation

- CBC/Chemistries rarely indicated
- Urine hCG, UA (+leukocyte esterase AND +nitrite has best diagnostic utility, where *either* +LE or +nitrite helpful w/ high pretest probability pts)
- Routine Ucx not needed in uncomplicated cases

Treatment

(Gupta K, Hooton TM, Naber KG, et al. International clinical practice guidelines for the treatment of acute uncomplicated cystitis and pyelonephritis in women. *Clin Infect Dis.* 2011;52:e103.)

- Spontaneous resolution observed in 25–42% of untreated women
- Antibiotic regimens:
  1st-line:
  - Nitrofurantoin 100 mg BID × 5 d
  - Trimethoprim–sulfamethoxazole 160/800 mg (1 DS tablet) BID × 3 d (if <20% resistance in community)
  - Fosfomycin 3 g in a single dose
  Alternative regimens:
  - Fluoroquinolones (ofloxacin, ciprofloxacin, levofloxacin) for 3 d
  - β-lactams (amoxicillin–clavulanate, cefdinir, cefaclor, cefpodoxime) for 3–7 d
- Symptomatic tx: NSAIDs, phenazopyridine (variable efficacy)

Disposition
- Home

Pearls
- Probability of cystitis >90% in women w/ sxs of UTI in the absence of vaginal d/c or irritation, thus consider empiric tx w/o UA or w/ nl UA (negative LE & nitrites do not reliably r/o UTI)
- UTI in males is rare thus consider STD, prostatitis
- Increasing *E. coli* resistance to amoxicillin & trimethoprim–sulfamethoxazole

Acute Uncomplicated Pyelonephritis
Definition
- Upper UTI of renal pelvis & kidney secondary to ascending lower UTI (*see Acute Uncomplicated UTI for Pathogenesis & Uropathogens*)
- Fever, chills, flank pain in absence of alternative Dx & urologic abnlty w/ UA ≥10 WBC/mm^3 & Ucx ≥10^4 cfu/mL

History
- Highest incidence 15–29 y/o, followed by infants & elderly
- Combination of constitutional sx (fever, chills, malaise), lower urinary tract sx (dysuria, frequency, hematuria) & upper urinary tract sx (flank pain); N/V
- RFs: Prior UTI, sexual intercourse (esp ≥3/wk in last 30 d), new sex partner (w/ i 1 yr), use of spermicide, stress incontinence in previous 30 d, diabetes mellitus

Physical Exam
- ±Fever, tachycardia, hypotension; CVA tenderness (~25% bilateral)

Evaluation
- CBC may show leukocytosis, but can be nl (rarely guides decision making)
- Chemistries (esp BUN/Cr) if renal impairment suspected
- Urine hCG, UA (+leukocyte esterase AND + nitrite has best diagnostic utility, where *either* + LE or + nitrite helpful w/ high pretest probability pts; WBC casts)
- Ucx & susceptibility should always be performed (usually reveals ≥10^5 cfu/mL of single uropathogen)
- Routine blood cultures not indicated
- Diagnostic imaging usually not indicated; can be considered to r/o alternative Dx, if complicated dz suspected, if sxs do not improve, or if recurrence → CT abdomen/pelvis study of choice over u/s

Treatment
(Gupta K, Hooton TM, Naber KG, et al. International clinical practice guidelines for the treatment of acute uncomplicated cystitis and pyelonephritis in women. *Clin Infect Dis.* 2011;52:e103.)
- Outpt tx:
  - Ciprofloxacin 500 mg PO BID × 7 d
  - levofloxacin 750 mg PO QD × 5 d
  - Trimethoprim–sulfamethoxazole 160/800 mg (1 DS tablet) BID × 14 d
  - Oral β-lactam for 10–14 d

*Above regimens can be given w/ (esp if resistance in community is known to exceed 10% or Bactrim/β-lactam are used) or w/o an initial 400 mg IV dose of ciprofloxacin, 1 g IV dose ceftriaxone, or consolidated 24-h dose of aminoglycoside

- Inpt tx:
  - IV fluoroquinolone, an aminoglycoside (w/ or w/o ampicillin), an extended spectrum cephalosporin or PCN (w/ or w/o an aminoglycoside), or a carbapenem

Disposition
- Home: Most cases in o/w well appearing, healthy women
- ED Obs: Persistent emesis requiring IVFs or antiemetics
- Admit: Inability to take PO/intractable vomiting, age >65 y/o, toxic appearance, suspected sepsis, obstructive uropathy, inadequate f/u, poor social disposition (ie, homeless)

Pearl
- Cx: Emphysematous pyelonephritis, perinephric abscess, urosepsis, ARF, renal scarring

Complicated Urinary Tract Infection
History
(*See Uncomplicated Cystitis & Pyelonephritis*)

Physical Exam
(*See Uncomplicated Cystitis & Pyelonephritis*)

Evaluation
- CBC may show leukocytosis, but can be nl (rarely guides decision making)
- Chemistries (esp BUN/Cr)

- Urine hCG, UA (+leukocyte esterase AND + nitrite has best diagnostic utility, where *either* + LE or + nitrite helpful w/ high pretest probability pts; WBC casts)
- Ucx & susceptibility should always be performed (usually reveals ≥10⁵ cfu/mL of single uropathogen when positive)
- Routine blood cultures not indicated, but should be obtained in suspected sepsis
- Diagnostic imaging should be considered → CT abdomen/pelvis study of choice over u/s
- Urology consultation: Esp w/ known or suspected structural/functional abx, recent urologic procedure, UG tract FB, obstructive uropathy, UTI in male

Treatment
- Empiric parenteral therapy w/ fluoroquinolone, carbapenem (ie, ertapenem, meropenem, or imipenem), or 3rd-generation cephalosporin (ie, ceftriaxone, cefotaxime), or piperacillin/tazobactam
- Duration: 7–10 d for complicated cystitis; 10–14 d for complicated pyelonephritis

Disposition
- Typically admit

Catheter-associated UTI (CA-UTI)
(Hooton TM, Bradley SF, Cardena DD, et al. Diagnosis, prevention, and treatment of catheter-associated urinary tract infection in adults: 2009 international clinical practice guidelines from the IDSA. *Clin Infect Dis.* 2010;50:625)

Definition
- **CA-UTI:** Sxs or signs compatible w/ UTI w/ no other identifiable source of infection w/ ≥10³ cfu/mL uropathogen in pts w/ indwelling urethral, suprapubic, or intermittent straight catheter in urine sample obtained w/i 48 h of removal
- **Catheter-associated asymptomatic bacteriuria (CA-ASB):** Presence of ≥10⁵ cfu/mL uropathogen in a catheter urine specimen in a pt w/o sxs
- Pt scenarios may include pts transferred from long-term care facilities w/ chronic indwelling foley/suprapubic catheters, paraplegic pts w/ chronic indwelling catheters, pts w/ urinary obstruction w/ temporary foley catheter or intermittent straight catheterization, etc.

History
- New onset or worsening fever, rigors, AMS, malaise, or lethargy w/o identifiable cause in pt w/ catheter
- Dysuria, frequency, urgency, suprapubic pain, flank pain, hematuria in those whose catheters were recently removed

Physical Exam
- ±Fever, tachycardia, hypotension; CVA tenderness; suprapubic tenderness
- Cloudy/malodorous urine should not be used to differentiate CA-UTI & CA-ASB

Evaluation
(See *Complicated UTI*)

Treatment
(See *Complicated UTI* for Antimicrobials)
- Screening for & tx of CA-ASB are not recommended except pregnant women
- 3-d regimen may be considered in CA-UTI pts ≤65 y/o w/o upper tract sxs
- 5-d regimen of levofloxacin may be considered in CA-UTI pts not severely ill
- 7-d regimen recommended for CA-UTI pts w/ prompt resolution of sxs
- 10–14-d regimen recommended in those w/ delayed response

Prevention
- Strongly consider indication for catheter insertion, limit catheterization changes, aseptic technique w/ placement, among others

Disposition
- Home in majority of cases
- Admit: Age >65 y/o, toxic appearance, suspected sepsis, immunocompromised (DM, sickle cell, cancer on chemotherapy, organ transplant recipient, immunosuppressives), inadequate f/u, poor social disposition (ie, homeless)

Recurrent Urinary Tract Infection
(Dason S, Dason JT, Kapoor A. Guidelines for the diagnosis and management of recurrent urinary tract infection in women. *Can Urol Assoc J.* 2011;5:316)

Definition
- At least 3 episodes of uncomplicated UTI documented by culture in the last 12 mo in the absence of structural/functional abx
- **Relapse** (5–10% women) occurs w/i 2 wk of completing antimicrobial therapy & is caused by persistence of the same uropathogen, suggesting antibiotic resistance

- **Reinfection** occurs >2 wk after completing antimicrobial therapy & is generally secondary to infection w/ different organism or strain

History
(*See Uncomplicated Cystitis and Pyelonephritis*)

Physical Exam
(*See Uncomplicated Cystitis and Pyelonephritis*)

Evaluation
- CBC/Chemistries rarely indicated
- Urine hCG, UA (+leukocyte esterase AND + nitrite has best diagnostic utility, where *either* + LE or + nitrite helpful w/ high pretest probability pts)
- Ucx should be obtained on representation to assess for antimicrobial resistance
- Postvoid residual if incomplete emptying suspected
- Imaging: Renal u/s, IV pyelography, CT abdomen/pelvis if warranted although not routine needed on emergent basis
- Further studies may include voiding cystourethrography, cystoscopy, urodynamic testing, but not routinely performed in ED

Treatment
(*See Uncomplicated UTI for Antimicrobials*)
- Consider starting prophylactic, continuous low-dose abx for 6-mo duration:
  - Nitrofurantoin 50–100 mg PO QD
  - Fosfomycin 3 g sachet PO q10d
  - Ciprofloxacin 125 mg PO QD
  - Cephalexin 125–250 mg PO QD, cefaclor 250 mg PO QD
  - Trimethoprim–sulfamethoxazole 40/200 mg QD or 3 times weekly
- May alternatively consider postcoital antimicrobial prophylaxis w/ a single dose w/i 2 h after intercourse (esp if UTI temporally a/w coitus):
  - Nitrofurantoin 50–100 mg
  - Trimethoprim–sulfamethoxazole 40/200 mg or 80/400 mg
  - Cephalexin 250 mg
- Self-start antibiotic therapy is an additional option (pt must be instructed to contact a medical provider w/i 48 h if sxs do not resolve)

Disposition
- Home w/ urology f/u to assess for anatomical/functional etiology

Urethritis
(Workowski KA. CDC STD Treatment Guidelines. *Clin Infect Dis*. 2015:61:S759.)

Definition
- Urogenital inflammatory condition characterized by urethral inflammation which can result from infectious & noninfectious etiologies
- Infectious causes include gonococcal (*N. gonorrhoeae*) & nongonococcal (*C. trachomatis*, *M. genitalium*, *T. vaginalis*, HSV, adenovirus)
- Rare causes include syphilis, CMV, & enteric bacteria

History
- Highest prevalence in adolescent, sexually active men
- Dysuria, urethral pruritus, mucopurulent or purulent urethral d/c; however, asymptomatic infections are common
- Urinary frequency & urgency typically absent
- Sexual hx: Current sexual activity, type (oral, vaginal, anal), MSM, number of sex partners, condom use, h/o STDs (esp GC/*Chlamydia*), sex w/ prostitutes
- Systemic sxs? (Fever, sore throat, arthritis, rash, back pain)

Physical Exam
- GU exam: Urethral meatus for skin lesions, erythema, d/c; milk urethra for d/c; testicular/epididymal exam in men, pelvic exam in women

Evaluation
- First-void ("dirty") UA (may reveal + LE & ≥10 WBC/hpf), urine hCG
- Gram stain of urethral secretions w/ ≥5 WBC/hpf (presence of gram-negative intracellular diplococci c/w gonococcal dz) & culture
- Urine NAAT for *N. gonorrhoeae* & *C. trachomatis* most sens

Treatment
- GC & *Chlamydia* coinfection common so therapy should be geared toward both:
  - Azithromycin 1 g orally in a single dose OR doxycycline 100 mg PO BID × 7 d
  - -AND-
  - Ceftriaxone 250 mg in a single IM dose

- Abstain from intercourse for 7 d & until all sex partners (w/i previous 60 d) are evaluated or empirically treated

Disposition
- Home w/ PCP referral for counseling & further STD testing

Pearl
- GC & *Chlamydia* are reportable to state health department
Guideline: Center for Disease Control and Prevention. Sexually transmitted diseases treatment guidelines, 2010. *MMWR Recomm Rep.* 2010;59(RR-12):1–110.

Male Urogenital Tract Infections

Acute Bacterial Prostatitis
(Curr Opin Infect Dis. 2016;29:86)

Definition
- The NIH consensus classification of prostatitis syndromes includes 4 categories:
  - I. Acute bacterial prostatitis
  - II. Chronic bacterial prostatitis (≥3 mo of sxs)
  - III. Chronic bacterial prostatitis/chronic pelvic pain syndrome (CP/CPPS)
    - A. Inflammatory
    - B. Noninflammatory
  - IV. Asymptomatic inflammatory prostatitis
- Acute bacterial prostatitis is an acute bacterial infection of prostate w/ + Ucx, lower urinary tract sxs, obstructive voiding sxs, & systemic sxs
- Bacterial prostatitis can be spontaneous or secondary to urologic intervention
- Bacterial spectrum similar to uropathogens seen in other UTIs (*see Uncomplicated UTI*); however, uropathogens of prostatitis carry greater number of virulence factors. Also, *C. trachomatis, T. vaginalis, U. urealyticum, N. gonorrhoeae,* & viruses rare causes

History
- Typical age 20–45 y/o; most common urologic Dx in men <50 y/o
- Acute onset fevers, chills, malaise, frequency, dysuria, poor urine stream, feeling of incomplete bladder emptying, & lower back/abdominal/pelvic pain
- Sexual Dysfxn (ejaculatory discomfort & hematospermia) may be present
- RFs: Recent urologic intervention/instrumentation, urethral stricture, urethritis

Physical Exam
- ±Fever; suprapubic abdominal discomfort
- Testicular exam should be performed to r/o epididymitis/orchitis
- DRE w/ warm, tender, swollen prostate

Evaluation
- Consider CBC & Bcx, esp if toxic appearing
- UA (+nitrites & LE, PPV 95%, NPV ~70%), Ucx
- Consider post-void residual urine measurement, urinary retention may not be evident
- Consider transrectal u/s if prostate abscess suspected (poor response to abx)
- Prostate biopsy as an outpt

Treatment
- Systemically ill pts should receive parenteral abx: IV ciprofloxacin 400 mg BID, IV levofloxacin 500 mg IV QD OR ceftriaxone 2 g IV QD
- Clinically stable pts may be treated w/ oral therapy (usually fluoroquinolone)
  - Ciprofloxacin 500 mg PO BID or levofloxacin 500–750 mg PO QD × 2–4 weeks
  - Trimethoprim–sulfamethoxazole 160/800 mg (1 DS tablet) BID × 2–4 weeks
  - Sexually transmitted: Ceftriaxone 250 mg IM × 1 AND doxycycline 100 mg BID × 14 d

Disposition
- Home w/ urology f/u
- Admit if systemically ill, known antibiotic resistant pathogen, etc.

Pearls
- 10% men w/ acute bacterial prostatitis go on to suffer chronic prostatitis, & 10% progress to chronic prostatitis/chronic pelvic pain syndrome
- Cx: Chronic prostatitis (10%), acute urinary retention, prostatic abscess (~2%), sepsis

Epididymitis/Orchitis
(Workowski KA. CDC STD Treatment Guidelines. Clin Infect Dis. 2015:61:S759.)

Definition
- Epididymitis & orchitis are inflammation of the epididymis & testes, respectively, w/ or w/o infection

- Can be acute (<6 wk), subacute (6 wk–3 mo), or chronic (>3 mo) based on symptom duration
- Orchitis usually occurs when inflammation spreads from epididymis to adjacent testicle (epididymo-orchitis), but isolated orchitis w/o epididymitis can be seen w/ mumps
- Epididymitis can be sexually transmitted, caused by N. gonorrhoeae or C. trachomatis, or by ascending lower UTI by common uropathogens (see *Uncomplicated UTI*); M. tuberculosis should be considered in high-risk pts, & fungal or viral causes found in pts w/ immunodeficiency
- Noninfectious causes of epididymitis include postinfectious inflammatory rxn to pathogens (ie, M. pneumoniae, adenoviruses), vasculitides, meds (ie, amiodarone)

History
- Primarily affects young men aged 18–35 y/o, bimodal distribution 16–30 y/o & 50–70 y/o
- Testicular pain, swelling usually beginning posteriorly overlying epididymis; lower urinary tract sxs may be present
- RFs: Unprotected intercourse (esp anal), MSM, increased number of sex partners, h/o STDs (esp GC/Chlamydia), sex w/ prostitutes, structural/functional GU abnlty, urinary tract instrumentation

Physical Exam
- ±Fever; assess for CVA tenderness, suprapubic pain as e/o other urinary tract dz
- Testicular exam: Palpation of epididymis, testes, cremasteric reflex; tender, erythematous, swollen spermatic cord & testicular contents c/w epididymitis-orchitis
  - Prehn sign: Relief of pain w/ elevation of testes can be seen w/ epididymitis. Inguinal exam for hernia or swollen, tender nodes.

Evaluation
- First-void ("dirty") UA (+LE & ≥10
- WBC/hpf suggests urethritis, favoring Dx of epididymitis); Ucx
- Gram stain of urethral secretions w/ ≥5 WBC/hpf (presence of gram-negative intra-cellular diplococci c/w gonococcal dz) & culture
- Urine NAAT for N. gonorrhoeae & C. trachomatis most sens
- Imaging: Testicular color Doppler ultrasonography (Findings: Thickened epididymis w/ increased blood flow suggesting hyperemia)

Treatment
- Sexually active men <35 y/o & older men w/ RFs for STDs:
  - Ceftriaxone 250 mg IM × 1
    -AND-
  - Doxycycline 100 mg PO BID × 10 d
- Abstain from intercourse for 7 d & until all sex partners (w/i previous 60 d) are evaluated or empirically treated
- Men >35 y/o or no RFs for STDs (thus likely caused by enteric organisms):
  - Levofloxacin 500 mg PO QD × 10 d
  - Ofloxacin 300 mg PO BID × 10 d

*Note: Above fluoroquinolones have activity against C. trachomatis & favorable UG tissue Penetration

- Supportive: NSAIDs for pain, ice/elevation of testes while at rest

Disposition
- Home

Pearl
- Pts <35 y/o likely to have an STD organism as etiology; >35 y/o more likely enteric pathogen

FLANK PAIN

Approach to the Patient
History
- Onset (sudden vs. progressive)? Location? Dysuria/hematuria/urinary frequency? Prior h/o similar sxs
- ROS (fever, rash, trauma, nausea, vomiting, weakness, abdominal pain), PMH (kidney stones, gout, cancer, AAA, congenital kidney dz, cardiac or vascular dz)

Evaluation
- CBC, Cr; consider renal u/s or noncontrast abdominal CT

Flank Pain Differential	
Pathophysiology	**Differential**
Renal	Nephrolithiasis, urolithiasis, retroperitoneal hematoma, ruptured renal cyst, ureteral stricture
Infectious	Pyelonephritis, perinephric abscess, psoas abscess, pneumonia, discitis, vertebral osteomyelitis, epidural abscess
Vascular	Ruptured AAA, renal infarct, renal vein thrombosis, PE
GI	Biliary dz
Other	PCKD (ruptured cyst), renal malignancy, varicella-zoster
Trauma	Lumbar spasm, radiculopathy

Urolithiasis (Nephrolithiasis and Ureterolithiasis)
(Emerg Med Clin North Am. 2011;29:519)

Definition
- Urolithiasis denotes calculi (of mineral or organic solids) that form anywhere in the urinary tract; nephrolithiasis & ureterolithiasis more specifically denote calculi present in the kidney or ureter, respectively
- Kidney stones form when urine becomes saturated w/ stone-forming salts
- Types of calculi:
  - Calcium oxalate stones (~80%): Predisposing conditions include hypercalciuria (hyperparathyroidism, sarcoidosis, type I RTA, hypercalcemia of malignancy, thiazides) & hyperoxaluria (Crohn's dz other ileal dz)
  - Magnesium ammonium phosphate (struvite) stones (~15): Requires combination of ammonia & alkaline urine. Source of ammonia from splitting of urea by urease-producing bacteria (*Proteus, Klebsiella, Pseudomonas,* & *Staphylococcus*)
  - Uric acid stones (~5–10%): Secondary to hyperuricosuria (gout, DM2, HTN)
  - Cystine stones: Secondary to inherited defects of tubular amino acid reabsorption
  - Drug-induced calculi: 2/2 metabolic abnormalities that favor stone formation or crystallization of drug or metabolites
- Stones lodged in ureter are typically found in 3 locations: Ureteropelvic junction, at the level of the iliac vessels, & ureterovesicular junction

History
- M:F, 2:1; Caucasian > Hispanic > Asian > African; peak incidence 20–50 y/o
- Renal colic (acute, spasmodic, unilateral flank pain radiating to groin/testes/labium) & visceral sxs (N/V/diaphoresis)
- Distal stones may cause lower abdominal pain & lower urinary tract sxs (dysuria, frequency, hematuria)
- PMH: FH nephrolithiasis, hyperparathyroidism, sarcoidosis, RTA, malignancy, Crohn's, jejunoileal bypass, recurrent UTI, gout, DM2, HTN, structural urologic abnormalities
- Meds: Indinavir, loop/thiazide diuretics, laxatives, carbonic anhydrase inhibitors, cipro-floxacin, sulfonamides have been a/w drug-induced calculi

Physical Exam
- Fever? Tachycardic? Generally uncomfortable appearing, diaphoretic, cool/clammy skin
- CVA tenderness; lower abdominal/pelvic tenderness (if stone has migrated)
- Assess for midline spinal TTP, acute abdomen, etc. which suggest alterative dx

Evaluation
- UA (may show +RBCs, though sens 84% spec 48% for stone; proteinuria, crystalluria), Ucx
- Consider BUN/Cr; CBC usually nonspecific & not helpful
- Imaging:
  Renal U/S (sens 45%, spec 94% for stones; sens 85–90% spec 90–100% for hydro):
  - May be initial radiographic exam w/ high pretest probability or if CT not possible (pregnancy); esp useful for detection of hydronephrosis or ureteral dilatation; not sens stones <5 mm; can be done point-of-care
  Nonenhanced helical CT (sens 96–98%, spec 100%)
  - Useful as initial radiographic exam, particularly w/ 1st presentation of suspected stone or low-moderate probability; able to make alternative diagnoses; modality of choice when available

*Indinavir stones not visible on CT

Treatment
- Data suggests IVFs likely not useful for acute renal colic from urolithiasis, but consider if pt appears dehydrated or has AKI

- Pain control: NSAIDs (ibuprofen 600 mg PO TID or ketorolac 15–30 mg IV if unable to take PO [caution in renal insufficiency]) & morphine 0.1 mg/kg × 1 then titrated for further relief
- Medical expulsive therapy: Tamsulosin 0.4 mg PO QD × 14 d or until stone passage; other alpha-antagonists (doxazosin, terazosin, alfuzosin) & nifedipine still used by many. SUSPEND trial (RCT 1167 pts tamsulosin, nifedipine or placebo) showed no increase in stone passage with MET. (Health Tech Assess. 2015;19:1)
- Urology consult: For concomitant infection, renal insufficiency, or low likelihood of stone passage (>10 mm)

Disposition
- Home: Adequate pain control in ED, nl Cr; f/u w/ urology in 24–48 h if stone >5 mm
- Admit: Intractable pain, unable to tolerate POs, renal failure, infection, renal transplant, single kidney, comorbid conditions (DM, baseline CRI), infected stone w/ obstruction

Pearls
- Presence or absence of hematuria alone cannot be used to diagnose or exclude nephrolithiasis
- Most stones ≤5 mm (70–98%) will pass spontaneously. Stones >5 mm have smaller chance (25–51%) of spontaneous passage & are more likely to need urologic intervention. (J Urol. 2015;194:1009)
- Send pts home w/ strainer, esp 1st-time stone formers for stone analysis
- Cx: Obstructed infected kidney (urologic emergency requiring urgent decompression), renal insufficiency, failed expulsion

HEMATURIA

(Davis R, Jones JS, Barocas DA, et al. Diagnosis, evaluation and follow-up of asymptomatic microhematuria (AMH) in adults: AUA guideline. J Urol. 2012;188:2473)
(Adv Chronic Kidney Dis. 2015;22:289)

Definition
- Hematuria is blood in the urine. Gloss hematuria is visible. Microscopic hematuria is ≥3 RBCs/hpf in urine sediment.
- Hematuria must be distinguished from pigmenturia (discoloration of urine). Pigmenturia can be caused endogenously by melanin, porphyrins, bilirubin, myoglobin, or hemoglobin or exogenously by meds (ie, warfarin, rifampin, phenazopyridine, phenytoin, etc.), beets

History
- Onset (sudden vs. chronic)? Dysuria/urinary frequency/renal colic? During entire or part of urine stream? (hematuria at beginning of urination → urethral; throughout urination → upper urinary tract or proximal bladder; end of urination → bladder neck or prostatic urethra)
- Painless hematuria should raise suspicion for genitourinary malignancy
- ROS (fever, weight loss, night sweats, rash, sore throat, abdominal pain, N/V, recent viral infection or UTI; trauma; excessive exercises; pelvic radiation)
- PMH (kidney stones, HTN, cancer, congenital kidney dz, vascular dz, bleeding diathesis, SCD, hereditary spherocytosis)
- MEDS:
  - Drugs that cause pigmenturia: Warfarin, rifampin, phenazopyridine, phenytoin, azathioprine, deferoxamine, doxorubicin, riboflavin
  - Drugs that cause myoglobinuria: Amphotericin B, barbiturates, cocaine, diazepam, ethanol, heroin, methadone, statins
  - Drugs that cause hematuria: NSAIDs, anticoagulations, busulfan, cyclophosphamide, OCPs, quinine, vincristine
- Social (smoking, benzene or aromatic amine exposure)

Physical
- Evaluate for HTN, petechiae, arthritis, rash
- Assess for suprapubic & CVA tenderness; thorough GU exam including prostate exam
- Postvoid residual if concern for urinary retention

Evaluation
Key question: Is this truly hematuria?
- Urine dipstick + blood (can be seen w/ hematuria, hemoglobinuria, myoglobinuria, or other pigmenturias); urine sediment necessary to confirm >5 RBCs/hpf as well as identify protein, RBC casts (suggests glomerulonephritis), & crystalluria (suggests urolithiasis)
- Other urine studies: Urine cytology
- CBC, BUN/Cr, coags (if isolated hematuria—erythrocytes in sediment, but no protein—suggests bleeding diathesis)
- Outpt imaging: CT urography (1st line), renal u/s, MRI. Cystoscopy if ≥35 y/o.

Disposition
- Large, gross hematuria may warrant continuous monitoring of HCT & urology eval. If microscopic, can obtain further outpt eval by nephrology or urology.

Hematuria Differential	
Pathophysiology	**Differential**
Structural	Urolithiasis, BPH, PKD, analgesic nephropathy, papillary necrosis, menstruation
Infectious	UTI, STDs, renal TB, malaria
Vascular	AVM, renal artery dz (thrombosis, dissection, malignant HTN), renal vein thrombosis, sickle cell crisis
Meds	Cyclophosphamide, anticoagulants
Inflammatory	Glomerulonephritides (poststrep, postinfectious, IgA nephropathy, lupus nephritis, Alport's syndrome, thin basement membrane dz, etc.), vasculitis (HSP, granulomatosis w/ polyangiitis, etc.), transfusion rxn
Trauma/Other	Renal trauma, urethral or ureteral trauma, recent instrumentation, paroxysmal nocturnal hemoglobinuria, vigorous exercise
Neoplastic	Renal Ca, urethral Ca, bladder Ca, prostate Ca

ACUTE KIDNEY INJURY

(Lancet. 2012;380:756)
(Kidney Disease: Improving Global Outcomes (KDIGO) Acute Kidney Injury Work Group. KDIGO Clinical Practice Guideline for Acute Kidney Injury. Kidney Int Suppl. 2012;2:1)

Approach to the Patient
Definition & Staging
- AKI is defined as any of the following:
  - Increase in serum Cr by ≥0.3 mg/dL (≥26.5 µmol/l) w/i 48 h; or
  - Increase in serum Cr by ≥1.5 times baseline, which is known or presumed to have occurred w/i prior 7 d; or
  - Urine volume <0.5 mL/kg/h for 6 h
- AKI is staged for severity according to the following criteria:

Staging of Acute Kidney Injury				
Stage	**RIFLE Criteria**	**Serum Cr**	**Urine Output**	**Management**
1	**R**isk	1.5–1.9 times baseline -OR- GFR decrease >25%	<0.5 mL/kg/h for 6–12 h	• D/c nephrotoxins • Ensure volume status/ perfusion pressure • Monitor Cr & UOP • Avoid hyperglycemia • Consider alternative to using radiocontrast • Noninvasive w/u • Consider invasive w/u
2	**I**njury	2–2.9 times baseline -OR- GFR decrease >50%	<0.5 mL/kg/h for ≥12 h	-AND- • Check for changes in drug dosing • Consider RRT • Consider ICU admit

3	**F**ailure	3 times baseline -OR- ↑ in serum Cr to ≥4 mg/dL -OR- GFR decrease >75%	<0.3 mL/kg/h for ≥24 h -OR- Anuria for ≥12 h	-AND- • Avoid subclavian catheters if possible
	Loss	Persistent ARF = complete loss of kidney function for >4 wk		
	ESKD	End-stage kidney disease (>3 mo)		

History

- ARF is usually asymptomatic & diagnosed when labs reveal renal abnormalities
- Sxs may include decreased urine output, weight gain, fluid retention (peripheral edema, anasarca, ascites), fatigue, anorexia, N/V, pruritus, altered sensorium, thirst/ orthostasis (prerenal)
- ROS (fever, rash, flank pain, hematuria)
- PMH: Baseline renal impairment, CHF, liver dz, SLE, multiple myeloma
- MEDS (ACEI/ARB, NSAIDs, aminoglycosides, other abx, cisplatin, amphotericin B, diuretics)

Physical

- Assess volume status; myoclonus, pericardial or pl rub, rash, mental status, edema
- Stigmata of CHF, liver dz, collagen vascular dzs

Evaluation

- CBC, Chem 10 (BUN/Cr ratio), serum osmolality; consider VBG w/ STAT potassium
- Urinalysis/sediment, urine lytes (urine Na, urine K, urine Cr, urine osmolality)
  - $FE_{Na}\% = (Urine\ Na \times Plasma\ Cr)/(Plasma\ Na \times Urine\ Cr) \times 100$
- Consider LFTs, BNP if indicated
- EKG for cardiac electrical instability from potential electrolyte abx
- Consider point-of-care cardiac, IVC, renal u/s
- Imaging: Renal u/s (r/o obstruction, assess flow); consider CT abdomen if c/f pelvic mass, Doppler u/s of renal vasculature
- Other studies: Renal biopsy

Differential Diagnosis of AKI/ARF	
Pathophysiology	**Differential**
Prerenal	**Hypovolemia:** Dehydration, hypotension/shock, hemorrhage, vomiting/diarrhea, diuresis, burns, pancreatitis, severe hypoalbuminemia **Altered Renal Hemodynamics:** Low cardiac output states (CHF, severe valvular heart dz, tamponade, massive PE, abdominal compartment syndrome), sepsis, anaphylaxis, Meds (NSAIDs, ACEI/ARBs), hepatorenal syndrome
Intrinsic renal	**Renovascular Obstruction:** Renal artery atherosclerosis/thrombosis/embolism/dissection/vasculitis Renal vein thrombosis/external compression **Glomerular Dz:** Glomerulonephritis, vasculitis, malignant HTN, preeclampsia, DIC, collagen vascular dzs (SLE, scleroderma) **Intratubular Obstruction:** Multiple myeloma, uric acid, acyclovir, MTX, indinavir **Acute Tubular Necrosis:** Profound ischemia, infection, radiocontrast, calcineurin inhibitors, abx (ie, aminoglycosides), antifungals (amphotericin B), chemo (ie, cisplatin), ethylene glycol, rhabdomyolysis, HUS/TTP **Interstitial Nephritis:** Allergic nephritis (β-lactams, fluoroquinolones, sulfa, NSAIDs), pyelonephritis, leukemia/lymphoma, sarcoid
Postrenal	**Ureter:** Calculi, clot, cancer (pelvic mass), external compression **Bladder Neck:** Calculi, clot, cancer (pancreatic), BPH, neurogenic bladder **Urethra:** Stricture, valves

Interpreting Laboratory Data in AKI/ARF						
	BUN/Cr	FE_{Na}	Urine$_{Na}$	SpGrav	Urine$_{osm}$	Other
Prerenal	≥20	<1%	<10 mmol/L	>1.018	>500	Hyaline casts
Intrinsic renal	10–20	>1%	>20 mmol/L	<1.015	300–500	• Muddy brown casts (ATN) • RBC casts (glomerular injury, tubulointerstitial nephritis) • WBC casts (interstitial nephritis) • Broad granular casts (CKD) • Eosinophiluria (allergic nephritis) • Uric acid crystals (urate nephropathy) • Oxalate/Hippurate crystals (ethylene glycol tox)
Postrenal	<10	>1%	—	—	<350	

Treatment
- *Prerenal:* Correct volume status/perfusion pressure (IVFs, pressors, PRBCs if indicated, diuresis/inotropes if cardiorenal)
- *Intrinsic:* Eliminate nephrotoxins, treat underlying cause, consider glucocorticoids
- *Postrenal:* Transurethral or suprapubic catheter placement; may require ureteric stents or percutaneous nephrostomy tube placement
- Consider sodium bicarbonate if pH <7.2 or HCO_3 <15 mmol/L as bridge to dialysis

Indications for Emergent Dialysis and Renal Replacement Therapy "A, E, I, O, U"
- Acidosis (pH < 7.1)
- Electrolyte imbalance (hyperkalemia, hypocalcemia, hyperphosphatemia)
- Intoxication (lithium, salicylates, ethylene glycol, methanol, among others)
- Overload (volume overload)
- Uremia (pericarditis, encephalopathy, neuropathy, bleeding)

Disposition
- Home: Mild prerenal azotemia may be adequately treated w/ hydration; pts w/ postobstructive ARF can be sent home if obstruction is relieved (ie, w/ bladder catheter) & no significant comorbidities
- Admit: Pts w/ uremia, significant electrolyte abnormalities, volume overload, severe metabolic acidosis, unexplained ARF

Pearl
- Cx: Intravascular volume overload, hyponatremia, hyperkalemia, hyperphosphatemia, hypocalcemia, hypermagnesemia, metabolic acidosis, uremia, anemia, arrhythmias

TESTICULAR TORSION/TORSION OF TESTICULAR APPENDIX

(*Emerg Med Clin North Am.* 2011;29:469)

History
Testicular Torsion
- Sudden onset pain (± swelling) in scrotum w/ radiation into abdomen; pain may be intermittent; N/V; most commonly in puberty

Torsion of Appendix
- Similar presentation to testicular torsion but pain can be localized to superior pole of testicle; benign condition

Physical Exam
Testicular Torsion
- Ill appearing, very tender/swollen/elevated testicle that may lie horizontally or anteriorly rotated; presence of cremasteric reflex does not r/o dz

Torsion of Appendix
- Normal-appearing testes; tenderness localized to superior pole of testicle; may have nodular "blue dot" at superior pole of testicle

Evaluation
- Labs: Preop labs if surgery anticipated
- Imaging: Scrotal duplex u/s to assess flow to testicle, but imaging should not delay time to OR; HRUS if duplex equivocal

Treatment
- Consult urology immediately if concern for testicular torsion as time to OR is critical for survival of testicle; if delay to OR, may attempt manual detorsion in medial to lateral direction ("open book" technique)
- Analgesia
- Antiemetics

Pearls
- >90% salvage rate if detorsion occurs <6 h
- Continuous pain >24 h is a/w an infarcted testicle

PHIMOSIS AND PARAPHIMOSIS

(Emerg Med Clin North Am. 2011;29:485)

History
Phimosis
- Inability to retract the distal foreskin over the glans penis; "ballooning" of the prepuce during urination; painful erection, preputial pain, weak urinary stream

Paraphimosis
- Inability to completely reduce foreskin distally back to natural position over glans penis. Entrapped foreskin forms constricting band, leads to pain & swelling.
- A/w vigorous sexual activity & chronic balanoposthitis
- Occurs exclusively in uncircumcised males & is a urologic emergency
- Pediatric: Often seen w/ forceful retraction or forgetting to reduce foreskin after bathing/voiding; irritability may be the only sign in nonverbal children

Physical Exam
Phimosis
- Inability to retract foreskin proximally over glans penis

Paraphimosis
- Foreskin retracted behind the glans & cannot be replaced to nl position; proximal shaft is soft (unless there is accompanying infection) w/ glans appearing erythematous/edematous & eventually blue/black & firm

Treatment
- If significant manipulation is expected, you may perform a penile block. On the dorsal aspect of the penis in the 2- & 10-o'clock positions, deposit 1% lidocaine; subsequently complete a ring block by depositing anesthetic circumferentially around the proximal shaft.

Phimosis
- No acute intervention needed unless infection suspected. Consider topical steroids (0.05–0.1% betamethasone) × 4–6 wk for mild–moderate cases.

Paraphimosis
- Compress the foreskin & glans by snugly grasping it w/ the palm of the hand & apply pressure for several minutes. Other methods to reduce edema include:
  - *Dundee micropuncture technique:* Make ~20 puncture holes in edematous foreskin tissue w/ a small needle (27 gauge) & express the fluid
  - *Hyaluronidase technique:* Inject 1 cc of hyaluronidase (150 U/mL) using a tuberculin syringe into the site of edematous foreskin
  - *Sugar technique:* Soak a swab of 50 mL of 50% dextrose solution & leave it wrapped around the foreskin for 1 h
- Attempt manual reduction by placing index fingers on dorsal border of glans behind retracted prepuce & thumbs on glans; may facilitate w/ ice, elastic bandage over glans or spreading hyperosmolar agents (such as sugar/dextrose) over glans to reduce swelling
- Consult urology if manual reduction unsuccessful

Disposition
- Home: Phimosis ± abx for accompanying infection; paraphimosis if skin is in the nl position. Urology f/u for all paraphimoses.
- Admit: Paraphimosis not reduced by conservative methods

Pearls
- Educate parents/caretakers of children on importance of avoiding forcible retractions & of gentle reduction of foreskin after bathing & voiding
- Paraphimoses that are not immediately treated are at risk for necrosis & autoamputation

PRIAPISM

(Emerg Med Clin North Am. 2011;29:485)

Definitions
- Priapism is defined as a prolonged erection lasting generally >4 h in the absence of sexual stimulation
- Ischemic (low-flow) priapism is the most common subtype & is due to painful engorgement of the corpora cavernosa. This can lead to intracavernosal acidosis, sludging of blood, thrombosis of cavernal arteries, & impotence
- Nonischemia (high-flow) priapism is rare, painless, & is caused by increased arterial inflow to the penis as a result of traumatic arterial–cavernosal fistulas

History
- Painful, persistent erection lasting >4 h, not relieved by ejaculation
- RFs: impotence agents (sildenafil), SCD, leukemia, urogenital malignancies (prostate, bladder), CVA, spinal cord injury antihypertensives (hydralazine, prazosin, doxazosin), antidepressants (trazodone, fluoxetine, sertraline), antipsychotics (phenothiazines & atypicals), phosphodiesterase inhibitors, cocaine, toxins (scorpion, black widow, CO)

Physical Exam
- Obvious erection, generally involving only the corporal cavernosa & flaccid corpora spongiosum

Evaluation
- Labs: Preoperative labs if contemplating OR
- May send a blood gas from penile aspirate

Treatment
- Pain control
- To reduce flow/vasoconstriction:
  - Oral/IM: Terbutaline 5 mg PO × 1; terbutaline 0.25–0.5 mg IM × 1 (unclear benefit)
  - Intracavernosal phenylephrine injection: Using a 25- or 27-gauge needle (or tuber-culin syringe), inject 0.2–0.5 mg of phenylephrine into corporus q10–15min (maximum 4–5 doses) 2 cm distal to origin of shaft on dorsal penis at 2- or 10-o'clock position
  Note: Must dilute phenylephrine solution. Take phenylephrine 1% solution (10 mg/mL) & extract 1 mL (10 mg) from solution. Add this 1 mL to 9 mL of saline, which will give you 1 mg/mL of phenylephrine solution. You can then extract 0.2–0.5 mL (0.2–0.5 mg) of this for intracavernosal injection.
- If unsuccessful, aspiration/irrigation technique:
  - Perform penile nerve block: On the dorsal aspect of the penis in the 2- & 10-o'clock positions, deposit 1% lidocaine; subsequently complete a ring block by depositing anesthetic circumferentially around the proximal shaft
  - Prep & drape penis in sterile fashion
  - At 2- or 10-o'clock position insert a 16–18 g needle (also consider 18-gauge dialysis butterfly access needle), & using a 10–30 mL syringe, slowly aspirate while milking corporus w/ other hand until return if bright red blood & detumescence occurs
  - If this fails, you can attempt to irrigate by injecting 20–30 mL of phenylephrine & NS solution (10 mg phenylephrine in 500 mL NS) as exchange for 20–30 mL aspirate
- W/ sickle cell crisis: IVFs, O_2, pain control, consider exchange transfusion
- Consult urology for refractory priapism (may necessitate surgical decompression)

Disposition
- Recommended to observe for at least 2 h to assess for recurrence
- Home: Once detumescence achieved. Recommended to d/c w/ 3-d course of oral α-adrenergic agent (pseudoephedrine)
- Admit: If priapism not responsive to ED tx

Pearls
- >12 h of priapism a/w onset of tissue demise w/ >24 h a/w permanent impotence
- Cx: Hematoma, infection, systemic absorption of vasoactive agents (severe HTN), recurrence, impotence (this risk should be discussed w/ pt & is a possibility despite efforts & timeliness of therapy)

EMERGENCIES IN DIALYSIS PATIENTS

(Am J Emerg Med. 2006;24:847)

Definition
- Any complication involving dialysis catheters or fistulas as well as infection, electrolyte imbalances, cardiac complaints, or signs of fluid overload among others
- Common complaints & special considerations include:

Common Chief Complaints and Special Considerations in Dialysis Patients	
Chief Complaint	**Differential/*Special Considerations**
Fever	PNA (healthcare associated), UTI, bacteremia, *peritonitis (particularly w/ peritoneal dialysis), *Access-related infection (hematogenous spread can lead to endocarditis, septic pulmonary emboli, septic arthritis, vertebral osteomyelitis, epidural abscess)
Dyspnea	*Fluid overload/pulmonary edema, *high-output cardiac failure (AV fistula), *pl effusion (uremic, chronic fluid overload), *anemia (decreased EPO production), PTX (after subclavian or IJ HC access), *pericardial effusion (uremic), PE
Chest pain	ACS, PE, AD, *uremic pericarditis, *uremic pleuritis
Syncope	*Intradialytic hypotension, *uremic autonomic neuropathy, *dysrhythmias, other frequent causes of syncope
Hypotension	*Intradialytic hypotension, dysautonomia, antihypertensives, pericardial effusion/tamponade, sepsis, *anaphylaxis (oversulfated chondroitin sulfate contaminants in heparin)
Abdominal pain	Consider common causes of abdominal pain, *uremic gastritis/colitis, *peritonitis (particularly w/ peritoneal dialysis), *abdominal wall hernias (from increased abdominal pressures w/ ascites)
Headache/ AMS	*Dialysis dysequilibrium syndrome, *uremic/HTN encephalopathy, *hypertensive emergency, ICH, CVA, *medication effects from altered pharmacodynamics (benzodiazepines, morphine, meperidine, etc.), hyponatremia
Skin changes	*Uremic pruritus, *prurigo nodularis, *calciphylaxis (cutaneous uremic artiolopathy)
HD access sx	AV access "steal syndrome," AV fistula/catheter access vein thrombosis, AV fistula hemorrhage
Other	Electrolyte abnormalities (hyperkalemia, hyperphosphatemia, hypermagnesemia, hypocalcemia, hyponatremia), metabolic acidosis, uremic polyneuropathy (restless leg syndrome, paresthesias)

Approach to the Patient
History
- Should focus on assessing for common causes of respective chief complaints, w/ attention to special considerations unique to ESRD pt

Physical
- Attention to abnl vital signs
- Pulmonary & cardiac exam including assessment of friction rub, rhonchi, & rales
- Abdominal exam, esp in pts w/ PD catheters
- Extremity exam & JVP for signs of fluid overload
- Skin exam for e/o calciphylaxis
- Assess graft site for thrill & signs of bleeding, infection, edema, & bruising; assess tunneled catheter site for e/o cellulitis or underlying abscess formation

Diagnostics
- CBC, Chem 10; consider ABG w/ STAT potassium & to assess acid–base status
- Consider LFTs, BNP, cardiac markers if indicated
- Consider contacting PD access nurse for sample of PD dialysate fluid (cell count [WBC >50–100 cell/mm^3 suggest peritonitis], Gram stain, culture)
- EKG for cardiac electrical instability from potential electrolyte abx, ischemia

- Consider point-of-care cardiac & lung u/s & FAST exam to assess for effusion & ascites, respectively
- Imaging: Appropriate imaging for respective complaints; Doppler imaging of AF fistula site if concern for thrombosis

Treatment
- Refer to appropriate sections for tx of conditions noted above
- Special considerations:
  - **Peritonitis:** Vancomycin 2 g AND cefepime/ceftazidime 1 g each added to 1 bag of dialysate infused into & allowed to dwell in the peritoneal cavity for 6 h
  - **Dialysis disequilibrium syndrome:** Reduce ICP (HOB elevation >30°, hyperosmolar therapy [mannitol, hypertonic saline], euglycemia, euthermia, eunatremia, MAP > 65, CO_2 40 mmHg, CPP 50–70 mmHg); renal consult
  - **Clotted AV graft/fistula:** Immediate vascular surgery consultation for consideration of catheter-directed thrombolysis, pharmacomechanical thrombolysis, surgical thrombectomy
  - **Clotted Vascular Access Catheters:** Consult institutional policies; if feasible, attempt catheter-directed tPA via infusion of 2 mg tPA into occluded lumen & fill remainder w/ saline. After 15 min, inject 0.3 mL saline to move the active enzyme toward the tip of the catheter. After another 15 min, inject another 0.3 mL to move the active enzyme toward the tip of the catheter. After another 15 min, try to aspirate catheter. If unsuccessful, send pt for catheter exchange.
  - **Vascular Access Hemorrhage:** Apply direct pressure for 10–15 min; if occurs w/ hours of dialysis, consider protamine 1 mg per 100 U heparin received (or 10–20 mg if dose unknown) to reverse heparin anticoagulation; consider application of gelfoam, surgical, or other hemostatic agent; immediate vascular surgery consultation for uncontrolled hemorrhage

Disposition
- Depends upon presenting complaint, but most will invariably require admission

Pearls
- BP measurement over & use of AV fistula sites for blood draw/administering therapy is contraindicated
- BNP levels are not reliable in diagnosing fluid overload/HF in dialysis pts as basal BNP levels are typically elevated & increased BNP levels from baseline may not correlate w/ clinical HF
- Chronically elevated troponin common & a/w increased mortality; makes assessment of ACS challenging; however, the National Academy of Clinical Biochemistry (NACB) recommends a 20% change in troponin concentration from baseline for Dx of AMI

VAGINAL BLEEDING

(Emerg Med Clin North Am. 2012;30:991)

History
- Onset? Painful? Quality (dark vs. clots vs. bright red)? Quantity (number of pads/h)? Pregnant or postpartum? LMP? Last intercourse? Use of protection? Gravida & parity? Trauma? ROS: Dizziness or light-headedness? Presyncopal? Other bleeding? Fever? PMH (clotting disorder, hypo- or hyperthyroid, liver dz) MEDS (anticoagulants or antiplatelet tx, contraceptives, hormonal therapy), SOCIAL (domestic violence)

Diagnostics
- CBC, type & screen (Rh), urine hCG; quantitative hCG if pt is pregnant; crossmatch (if heavily bleeding); consider pelvic u/s

Pearls
- Average pad holds 5–15 cc of blood
- Average tampon holds 5 cc of blood

Vaginal Bleeding Differential	
Pathophysiology	**Differential**
Nonpregnant	Abnl uterine bleeding, PCOS, IUD or oral contraceptives, endometritis, cervicitis, fibroids, uterine polyps, adenomyosis, endometrial hyperplasia or cancer, coagulopathies, postcoital bleeding
1st trimester	Implantation bleeding, miscarriage, ectopic pregnancy, hydatidiform mole
2nd/3rd trimester	Placenta previa, vasa previa, placental abruption, uterine rupture
Other	Postpartum hemorrhage, retained products of conception

Miscarriage
(Emerg Med Clin North Am. 2012;30:837)

History
- Vaginal bleeding ± passage of clots or tissue at <20 wk; abd pain/cramps

Physical Exam
- Speculum & bimanual exam to assess for passage of blood/POC & whether os is open or closed. (If copious bleeding, remove POC w/ gentle traction to allow uterus to clamp.)

Evaluation
- Labs: UA, quant hCG, HCT, type & screen (crossmatch if HD unstable). If products expelled, send to pathology.
- Imaging: Pelvic u/s to determine location of pregnancy

Classification of Miscarriage
- Threatened: Os closed, no passage of POC, viable fetus w/ heart tones, mild cramping/ bleeding (~20% will eventually abort)
- Inevitable: Os dilated & effaced; POC not passed; cramps, moderate bleeding
- Complete: POC expelled, cervical os closed; little cramping or bleeding
- Incomplete: Some, but not all products have passed. Retained fetal or placental tissue
- Missed: Pregnancy loss after development of embryo/fetus, os closed

Treatment
- ED:
  - Supportive management: IVFs, O_2, monitoring, position on L side
  - Blood products: Transfuse if HD unstable
- Medication therapy:
  - Rh immunoglobulin: 50 mcg <12 wk, 300 mcg >12 wk if Rh-negative
  - Consult: Gyn service if HD unstable or if need for D&C anticipated (inevitable, incomplete or missed abortion)
- Home management:
  - Hormonal therapy: Methotrexate may be indicated under guidance of OB/Gyn
  - Consider prophylaxis w/ doxycycline or testing for STD if discharging home w/ open os

Disposition
- Home: Stable pts w/ complete or threatened abortion; f/u w/ OB/Gyn w/i 72 h to monitor hCG levels
- Admit: Uncontrolled bleeding or pts requiring immediate D&C

Pearl
- Threatened & missed abortions can only be distinguished by pelvic u/s

Ectopic Pregnancy
(Emerg Med Clin North Am. 2012;30:837)

History
- Unruptured: abd pain, cramping, amenorrhea or abd pain.
- Ruptured: hypotension, tachycardia, abd pain
- RFs: H/o PID, IUD, fertility tx, recent abortion or prior ectopic

Physical Exam
- Assess for HD stability. Signs of peritonitis if rupture has occurred. Speculum & bimanual exam may reveal pelvic tenderness &/or adnexal mass.

Evaluation
- Labs: Quant hCG, HCT, Rh screen, PT/PTT & type & crossmatch 4 U (if HD unstable)
- Imaging: Pelvic US (TVUS should identify IUP at 5.5 wk); if HD unstable, FAST exam to assess for free fluid

Treatment
- Supportive: 2 large-bore IVs, IVF resuscitation, monitor
- Transfusion: If HD unstable
- Rh immunoglobulin: 50 mcg <12 wk, 300 mcg >12 wk if Rh-negative
- Consult: Urgent Gyn eval for consideration of medical (MTX) vs. surgical (laparoscopy/laparotomy) tx options

Pearl
- Heterotopic pregnancies (co-occurrence of IUP & ectopic) have incidence of 1/30,000 in spontaneous pregnancies but 1/100 in assisted pregnancies.

Placenta Previa and Abruptio Placentae
(Emerg Med Clin North Am. 2012;30:919)

History
- Placenta previa: Placental implantation adjacent to or over os. Presents as painless, bright red, vaginal bleeding usually after 28 wk. RFs: Multiple gestation, multiparity, advanced maternal age, previous placenta previa/C-section, maternal smoking, HTN
- Abruptio placentae: Separation of implanted placenta b/w 20 wk & delivery. Presents as painful, dark red bleeding (80%); may also present w/ signs/sxs of DIC. RFs: Eclampsia, DM, HTN, abdominal trauma, cocaine, cigarette smoking

Physical Exam
- Check fundal height, contractions, & uterine tenderness:
  - Firm/tender uterus = placental abruption until proven o/w
- AVOID SPECULUM & VAGINAL EXAM

Evaluation
- Labs: CBC, Chem 7, LFTs, PT/PTT, fibrinogen (r/o DIC), UA, type/crossmatch 2 U
- Imaging: Doppler u/s (fetal heart tones); bedside abdominal u/s to assess placenta & signs of fetal movement, though may not always detect abruption

Treatment
- Supportive: Place on L side, 2 large-bore IVs, IVF resuscitation, monitor pt & fetus
- Transfusion: Blood products ± FFP (HD unstable or signs of DIC)
- Medications: Rh immunoglobulin 300 mcg if Rh-negative, magnesium for fetal neuroprotection if emergent delivery under 32 wk
- Consult: Urgent Gyn eval for possible STAT C-section

Disposition
- Admit: All pts to the OB service even if HD stable for close monitoring

Retained Products of Conception and Postabortion Sepsis
(Ob Gyn. 2015;125:1042)

History
- Infection of placenta &/or POC which can spread to the uterus → systemic
- Retained POC: Cramping, heavy bleeding
- Postabortion sepsis: Cramping, bloody or purulent d/c, fever

Physical Exam
- Fever, vaginal bleeding or purulent/bloody d/c, uterine tenderness

Evaluation
- Labs: Quant hCG, type & cross, preop labs
- Imaging: Pelvic u/s

Treatment
- Supportive: Stabilize (see Sepsis chapter), correct coagulopathy/anemia

- Abx: If suspected infection, clindamycin 900 mg IV q8h PLUS gentamicin 5 mg/kg/d OR ampicillin 2 g q4h PLUS gentamycin PLUS metronidazole 500 mg q8h OR levofloxacin 500 mg QD PLU metronidazole OR piperacillin–tazobactam 4.5 g q8h.
- Consult: Gyn service for D&C

Disposition
- Admit: All pts to OB/Gyn for D&C

Postcoital Bleeding

History
- Trauma during intercourse? Vaginal d/c, assess domestic violence or abuse.
- RFs: Cervical abnormalities, STDs, postmenopausal

Physical Exam
- Ongoing bleeding; vaginal lacerations, abrasions

Evaluation
- Labs: Urine hCG, GC/*Chlamydia* testing; HCT

Treatment
- ED:
  - Abx: Treat STI appropriately (see *Vaginal Discharge* below)
  - Consult: Gyn service for laceration requiring extensive repair; social services if concern for domestic violence

PREECLAMPSIA AND ECLAMPSIA

(*Emerg Med Clin North Am.* 2012;30:903)

Definition
- Chronic HTN: Systolic BP >140/90 before 20 wk gestation or longer than 12 wk postpartum
- Gestational HTN: BP >140/90 on 2 occasions after 20 wk gestation.
- Preeclampsia: Gestational HTN & proteinuria, can be classified as mild to severe based on end-organ damage
- Eclampsia: Preeclampsia w/ szs or coma; generally 3rd trimester or postpartum

Approach to the Patient

History
- HA, visual disturbances, mental status changes, abd pain, edema. ROS plural gestation? PMH (prior preeclampsia, nulliparity, extremes of age, HTN, obesity, antiphospholipid antibody syndrome, DM, chronic renal dz, connective tissue disorder)

Physical Exam
- HTN, abdominal tenderness, hyperreflexia/clonus, peripheral edema, papilledema, AMS

Evaluation
- UA, CBC, Chem 7, LFTs, LDH, uric acid, coags, type & cross, fetal/maternal monitoring

Treatment
- BP: Hydralazine, labetalol, or nifedipine (goal BP <140/90)
- Sz prophylaxis: Magnesium 2–6 g IV load + 1–2 g/h
- Szs: Magnesium (2–4 g IV q5–10min); refractory szs: Diazepam (5 mg IV q5min up to 20 mg) OR phenobarbital (200 mg IV)
- Consult: Gyn for all pts; delivery = only definitive tx for eclampsia

Disposition
- Home: Mild preeclampsia; schedule OB f/u in 24 h
- Admit: Eclamptic & most severe preeclamptic pts need urgent delivery (pending BP & sz control) & ICU admission

HYPEREMESIS GRAVIDARUM

(*JAMA.* 2016;316:1392)

Definition: Nausea & vomiting that result in weight loss or failure to gain weight
History: Pregnancy (1st trimester, usually week 8–12), nausea/vomiting, inability to PO
Physical Findings: Tachycardia, dehydration
Evaluation: Labs: Electrolytes, UA; often have ketosis & electrolyte derangements

Treatment: IV fluids (w/ dextrose), antiemetics (metoclopramide, doxylamine, pyridoxine). Ondansetron in 1st trimester may ↑risk of cardiac malformations. (*Reprod Toxicol.* 2014;50:134)

Disposition: Home if tolerating PO, admit if severe dehydration

EMERGENCY DELIVERY

(*Emerg Med Clin North Am.* 2012;30:961)

Definition
- True labor: Regular uterine contractions of increasing intensity at decreasing intervals
- 1st stage: Cervical dilatation & effacement (up to 12 h)
- 2nd stage: Complete cervical dilatation, culminating in delivery (up to 2 h)

Approach to the Patient
History
- Frequency & intensity of contractions, rupture of membranes, fetal movement, has pt had prenatal care for eval of cx of pregnancy, screening tests, etc.

Physical Exam
- External exam: Assess for crowning or active bleeding (if so, defer speculum/bimanual exam)
- Sterile speculum exam: Confirm ROM by checking for ferning &/or Nitrazine test
- Bimanual exam: Assess cervical effacement & dilatation (10 cm = complete), position, presentation (fetal part in canal), lie (relation of long axis to mother → longitudinal or transverse), & station (−3 to +3; 0 is at level of ischial spines); cord prolapse?

Diagnostics
- Abdominal u/s if placenta previa of concern

Treatment
- Basics of Delivery
  - Cord prolapse: Manually place hand in vaginal vault, lift presenting part away from cord; place pt in knee–chest position or deep Trendelenburg. Administer tocolytics (magnesium 4–6 g IV, terbutaline 0.25 mg SQ).
  - Vaginal delivery: Place mother in lithotomy position; cleanse/drape perineum if possible; w/ contractions, ask mother to "bear down"
    - Head: One hand on occipital area & other on perineum, maintain fetal head in flexed position; if cord wrapped at neck reduce over head or bring cord caudally over shoulders & deliver baby through cord. In extreme circumstances can cut cord first.
    - Shoulders: Rotate head & exert gentle pressure until anterior shoulder delivered; lift head upward to deliver posterior shoulders, attempt to guide posterior shoulder over perineum.
    - Body: Support head & catch body w/ the other hand. Suction mouth & nose.
    - Cord: Clamp cord twice & cut, send cord blood for serology & Rh. Clamp cord 1–3 cm distal to navel.
    - Placenta: Apply pressure above symphysis w/ minimal traction on cord (too much traction will cause uterine inversion); sudden gush of blood & lengthening cord will signify imminent placental delivery.
    - Aftercare: Massage uterus ± oxytocin 20 U IV (can be given as 10 U IM if no IV access for ongoing hemorrhage); inspect & repair lacerations of cervix, vagina
    - Infant care: Suction mouth & nose, stimulate with warm blanket. BVM if no spontaneous respirations. If pulse <60 start CPR, neonatal resusc per PALS. Obtain Apgar scores at 1 & 5 min.
- Shoulder Dystocia:
  - McRoberts: Hyperflexion of hips to abdomen w/ external rotation & slight abduction
  - Rubin I maneuver: Downward pressure just proximal to symphysis pubis
  - Woods screw maneuver: Insert hand into vagina & apply pressure to anterior aspect of posterior shoulder to abduct/extend shoulder & free it
  - Delivery of the posterior arm: Insert hand into vagina, flex posterior arm of the fetus, bringing it across the chest. Deliver posterior arm & then rotate fetus out
  - Gaskin position: Place Mom in hands-and-knees position, allows gravity to help open space
- Breech: Ideally OB present, or delivery in OR for c/s. If imminent, touch fetus as little as possible & let delivery happen spontaneously, do not pull on fetus which can entrap fetal head. If head becomes entrapped, uterine relaxant like terbutaline can be given.

- Perimortem delivery: >23 wk gestational age (obvious gravid uterus), should initiate w/i 5 min of maternal arrest. (Emerg Med Clin North Am. 2012;30:937)
  - Vertical incision from epigastrium to pubic symphysis & extend through all layers to the peritoneal cavity.
  - Uterus is exposed & incised at bladder reflection, retract bladder caudally
  - Incision extended to uterine fundus, with operator's hand used to palpate fetal parts & prevent damage. Infant extracted, clamp & cut umbilical cord.

FEMALE PELVIC PAIN

(Emerg Med Clin North Am. 2011;29:621)

History
- Dyspareunia, vaginal bleeding or d/c? Urinary sxs, ROS PMH (STDs, recent procedure) MEDS (contraceptive devices, hormonal therapy), social (domestic violence)

Physical Exam
- Abdominal exam; Gyn exam (d/c or bleeding, masses or tenderness)

Diagnostics
- Labs: UA, GC/Chlamydia, Wet mount
- Imaging: Pelvic US (assess flow, torsion, mass, fluid)

Ovarian Cyst
History
- Dull, vague, unilateral sensation of pelvic pain or dyspareunia
- Rupture: Sudden, unilateral, sharp pelvic pain; can also present as diffuse peritonitis

Physical Exam
- Lower quadrant abdominal tenderness, adnexal tenderness/mass, vaginal bleeding

Evaluation
- Labs: CBC, type & screen (crossmatch if HD unstable)
- Imaging: Pelvic u/s to assess for size, complexity, torsion, presence of free fluid. Bedside FAST if HD unstable.

Treatment
- Supportive: IVFs, transfuse if HD unstable
- Analgesia: NSAIDs, Narcotics prn
- Consult: Gyn Service for persistent pain, large-volume hemorrhage

Disposition
- Home: Stable, pain well controlled; f/u w/ Gyn or PCP in 1–2 mo for repeat u/s to reassess size
- Admit: HD unstable

Ovarian Torsion
History
- Acutely worsening unilateral lower abd/pelvic pain, N/V
- Can present as intermittent torsion w/ intermittent sxs
- RFs: Ovarian cysts, dermoid & other tumors, pregnancy

Physical Exam
- Nonspecific & variable; Gyn exam reveals unilateral, adnexal mass in majority of cases ± tenderness (though tenderness absent ~30% of the time)

Evaluation
- Labs: Urine hCG, pre-op labs
- Imaging: Pelvic US to assess for ovarian edema, cyst/mass, blood flow

Treatment
- Analgesia/antiemetics
- Consult: Gyn service for urgent laparoscopy

VAGINAL DISCHARGE (SEXUALLY TRANSMITTED INFECTION)

(Workowski KA. CDC STD Treatment Guidelines. Clin Infect Dis. 2015;61:S759.)

History
- Purulent or malodorous d/c? Dyspareunia? Pruritus? Postcoital bleeding? Dysuria, urinary frequency or urgency? Vaginal hygiene, self-tx? Menses?
- RFs: Multiple sexual partners & unprotected intercourse

Physical Exam
- External: Inspect for lesions, ulcerations; adenopathy
- Speculum: Vaginal wall inflammation/d/c; cervical inflammation/d/c
- Bimanual: If cervical motion tenderness or adnexal tenderness, think PID (see below)

Evaluation
- Labs: GC/Chlamydia testing; wet mount

Treatment
- N. gonorrhoeae: Ceftriaxone 125 mg IM × 1
- C. trachomatis: Azithromycin 1 g PO × 1 OR doxycycline 100 mg PO BID × 7 d OR levofloxacin 500 mg PO QD × 7 d
- T. vaginalis: Metronidazole 2 g PO ×1 OR 500 mg PO BID × 7 d
- Bacterial vaginosis: metronidazole 500 mg PO BID ×7d OR metronidazole 0.75% gel intravaginally 5 g/d × 5 d OR clindamycin 2% cream intravaginally 5 g × 7 d
- Candidiasis: Topical azoles (over the counter) × 7 d OR fluconazole 150 mg PO × 1

Pearls
- Educate pts on safe sex practices & advise pts to tell their partners to get tested/ treated
- Encourage HIV testing outpt if not offered in ED
- Drinking alcohol on metronidazole can cause disulfiram-like reaction (flushing, ↑ HR, ↓ BP)

PELVIC INFLAMMATORY DISEASE AND TUBO-OVARIAN ABSCESS

(Workowski KA. CDC STD Treatment Guidelines. *Clin Infect Dis*. 2015:61:S759.)

Definition
- Spectrum of inflammatory disorders, any combination of endometritis, salpingitis, tubo-ovarian abscess & pelvic peritonitis.
- Commonly a/w gonorrhea, chlamydia but <50% of pts with PID test positive for these organisms. Involves other bacteria (eg, GNR, anaerobes) & viruses (eg, M. genitalium)
- Cx include abscess, perihepatitis (Fitz-Hugh-Curtis), sepsis, chronic pain, increased risk of ectopic pregnancy, infertility

History
- Lower abd pain, vaginal d/c, dysuria, dyspareunia, nausea ± fevers
- RFs: Age <25, multiple sexual partners, unprotected sex, h/o PID, IUD placement in the last month, recent instrumentation of the cervix, douching, smoking

Physical Exam
- Lower abdominal tenderness, cervical discharge, cervical friability, cervical motion tenderness, adnexal tenderness/fullness
- Clinical exam has poor sensitivity; presentation is often atypical

Evaluation
- Labs: Always check pregnancy test; cervical cultures, UA, CBC (not sens)
- Abdominal CT or pelvic US only required if TOA is suspected (unilateral tenderness or palpable mass, systemically ill)

Treatment
- Low threshold for empiric tx: Minimum criteria in sexually active young women or others at risk are pelvic pain & cervical, uterine or adnexal tenderness
- Outpt: Ceftriaxone 250 mg IM × 1 + doxycycline for 14 d
- Consider adding metronidazole for anaerobes
- Azithromycin is considered insufficient for PID; may be used in isolated cervicitis or 2nd line
- If severe PCN allergy, options are hospitalization or azithromycin &/or levofloxacin depending on regional antibiogram
- Inpt: (Cefotetan or cefoxitin) + doxycycline OR clindamycin + gentamicin
- Consult: Gyn service if concern for TOA

Disposition
- Admit if toxic appearing, severe vomiting, TOA, failure of outpt therapy, pregnancy, immunocompromised, young age, poor f/u w/i 72 h
- Discharged pts need f/u in 3 d to ensure sx resolving. Partners should be tested.

Pearls
- Given ↑ resistance to antibiotic regimens, CDC updates recommendations frequently
- PID in pregnancy is rare but does happen; alternative diagnoses should be considered

RASH

Definition
- One or more skin lesions originating from a common cause (often over a short prd) & having a spec distribution & morphology

Approach
- HPI: Onset (timing, location); evolution (distribution, morphology); periodicity (constant vs waxing & waning, temporal associations); sxs (pain, pruritus, burning, fever, bleeding); new exposures or inciting events (topical or systemic exposures, recent travel, occupational exposures, sick contacts, animals, sexual hx)
- PMH & Meds (including immunizations, new formulations or doses, supplements, illicits)
- Ensure a good ROS (rashes can be first sign of an occult internal process)
- PE: Determine distribution, shape (if applicable), morphology, & secondary changes
  - Distribution: Localized/grouped/regional/generalized, central/peripheral, flexor/extensor surface, dermatomal, acral, intertriginous, follicular, mucosal, sun-exposed areas
  - Shape (if applicable): Annular (ring), round/nummular/discoid (coin), targetoid, arcuate (arc), linear, serpiginous, reticular (net-like/lacey), whorled (marble-like), polycyclic (coalescing circular/ring-shaped lesions)
  - Morphology & secondary changes: See tables

Common Dermatologic Morphologies		
Flat	Macule	Flat circumscribed area of discoloration (compared to surrounding skin) <1.0 cm diam
	Patch	Flat circumscribed area of discoloration (compared to surrounding skin) >1.0 cm diam, or similarly sized confluence of macules
Raised	Papule	Raised solid lesion <1.0 cm diam; compared to nodule, papule is superficial; can be any color
	Plaque	Raised plate-like solid area >1.0 cm diam, or similarly-sized confluence of papules; can be any color
	Nodule	Raised often-round solid lump; compared to papule, nodule is larger & deeper (epidermal, epidermal-dermal, dermal, dermal-subdermal, subcut); can be any color
	Wheal	Raised variously-shaped, often-erythematous, edematous, pruritic area often >1.0 cm diam; compared to plaque, wheal is often w/ irregular & sharp borders
Fluid-filled	Vesicle	Raised fluid-filled lesion <0.5 cm diam; compared to pustule, vesicle fluid is clear; compared to cyst, vesicle is superficial, thin-walled, & smaller
	Pustule	Raised fluid-filled lesion <0.5 cm diam; compared to vesicle, pustule fluid is purulent; coalescing groups of pustules are referred to as "lakes"
	Bulla	Raised fluid-filled lesion >0.5 cm diam; fluid can be clear or hemorrhagic
	Cyst	Firmly encapsulated cavity/sac filled w/ fluid or semi-solid material; compared to vesicle, cyst is deeper & firmer
Vascular	Petechia	Numerous, uniform, small (pinpoint), nonblanching, red/purple, asx macules; 2/2 thrombocytopenia
	Purpura	Irregularly shaped, circumscribed, nonblanching, macules or patches; occasionally painful; 2/2 blood extravasation, often a/w small-vessel thrombosis
Depressed	Eschar	Circumscribed depressed lesion covered by dry, adherent black necrotic tissue
	Erosion	Circumscribed minimally-depressed lesion w/ open/exposed moist dermal tissue
	Ulcer	Circumscribed depressed lesion w/ open/exposed moist dermal or subcutaneous tissue

Common Secondary Changes	
Scaling	Thickened outer epidermis (stratum corneum), usually white
Crusting	Dried liquid debris (eg, serum, blood, exudates), usually yellow–brown
Lichenification	Thickening of epidermis w/ accentuated skin lines/markings
Excoriation	Superficial abrasions, usually due to scratching

Typical Manifestations of Common or Critical Acute Disseminated Rashes

Viral Etiologies

Acute HIV	Pink **maculopapular** 2–3 wk after initial infxn; a/w const sx
Dengue fever	Pink **maculopapular/confluent macules** w/ islands of sparing a/w high fever, HA, retro-orbital & severe body pain; lasts 2–3 d
Measles	Pink **maculopapular**, starts behind ears & face/neck, spreads to trunk & extremities (w/ palms/soles), ± confluence; a/w fever, cough, coryza, conjunctivitis; lasts 3–7 d, leaves as arrived
Mononucleosis	Pink **maculopapular**; no palms/soles; a/w const sx
Parvovirus B19	Red ("slapped") cheeks w/ circumoral pallor (lasts 1–4 d), then generalized **reticular/lacey** rash, esp extensor surfaces (spares palms/soles) w/ progression to trunk/buttocks (can last 3 wk)
Pityriasis rosea	Pink/salmon small oval **plaques** distributed on lines of cleavage on trunk/prox extremities (spares face, palms, soles); often 1–3 wk after herald patch (single 2–4 cm pink plaque w/ fine scaling borders & depressed pale center); rash lasts 5 wk – 5 mo
Roseola	**Pink macules**; starts neck/trunk after defervescence & spreads to face/extremities; lasts 1–2 d
Rubella	Pink **maculopapular**, starts on face/forehead then to trunk/ extremities, ± coalesce; a/w fever, HA, arthralgias; lasts ~3 d
Varicella (Chicken pox)	Pruritic **macules**, progress to **papules & vesicles**, crusting w/i 48 h; trunk/face > extremities; ± mucous membranes; crusts fall off after 1–2 wk; may leave hypopigmented scars long-term

Bacterial Etiologies

Gonococcemia	Few scattered **hemorrhagic pustules** (often over joints) occurring after mucosal infxn; a/w arthralgias & low-grade fever; tx w/ CTX (1 g IV QD × 7d) & azithromycin (1 g PO ×1); admx
Leptospirosis	Initially warm & flushed, can develop **transient petechia**, later **purpura**; a/w fever, HA, myalgias, GI sx, subconjunctival hem; sx can be bimodal; severe dz (Weil syndrome) a/w liver failure
Lyme	Mx **erythema migrans** in 20% of primary lyme; Secondary lyme (3–10 wk after infxn) small pink oval **macules/patches**, a/w neuro (CN), visual, cardiac (get ECG), msk complications
Meningococcemia	Rapidly progressive **petechia & purpura**; pt toxic-appearing; ±2–3 d prodrome of HA, URI sx (but 20% pts present w/ sepsis); tx w/ CTX × 7d; mortality 10–15% w/ tx (Intern Med 2016;55(6):567–572)
RMSF	Numerous red **macules** w/ **central petechia** start on wrists/ ankles, then palms/soles, then arms/legs/trunk; 10–15% may not have rash; a/w abrupt fever, severe HA, N/V, abd pain, myalgias
Scarlet fever	Diffuse fine erythematous **coalescent "sandpaper" eruption**; starts on neck & spreads to trunk/extremities, becomes **macules coalescing into patches**; flushed face w/ circumoral pallor; a/w recent strep infxn; lasts 7 d then fine desquamation
Staph scalded skin syndrome	Diffuse painful **light erythema** w/ **widespread exfoliation** of thin sheets of skin; no mucous membranes; a/w malaise, fever
Secondary syphilis	Diffuse **macules, papules** (± pustules), including on palms/soles & mucous membranes
Toxic shock syndrome	Diffuse erythematous **coalescent "sandpaper" macules & patches**, ± hemorrhagic bullae; mucous membranes involved; a/w fever, GI sx, confusion, multiorgan failure

Arthropod Bites

Bed bugs	Painless pruritic red **papules** on exposed areas; occasionally wheals, hemorrhagic nodules, vesicles 2/2 bug proteases
Lice	Painless pruritic red **papules & wheals**, often concentrated in covered areas (axilla/groin/trunk) & sparing extremities
Scabies	Painless pruritic red **papules**, often clustered, starts on hand/foot, spreads to trunk; look for intertriginous burrows

Vascular/Hematologic

HSP	Erythematous **macules & papules** becoming **purpuric** (palpable purpura) symmetrically on lower extremities; spares soles; a/w abd pain & joint pain

ITP	**Petechia**, esp in lower extremities & palette; can be asx
TTP	**Petechia**, a/w fever, AMS/neuro deficits, ± jaundice
DIC	**Petechia, purpura, hemorrhagic bullae**, acral cyanosis, localized necrosis/gangrene (inc. extremities); a/w multiorgan failure

Hypersensitivity Reactions

Acute generalized pustular psoriasis	Diffuse small sterile pruritic **pustules** on erythematous base, a/w fever; trunk & intertriginous areas common (no mucous membranes); may have multiorgan dysfxn
Allergic contact dermatitis	*Poison Ivy/Oak:* Wheals & vesicles (± malaise) on exposed areas *Topical (eg, hair dye):* **Vesicles & papules** w/ crusting, edema
Bullous pemphigoid	Acute or subacute pruritic, diffuse, tense **bullae** on nl, erythematous, or urticarial base; many causal associations (diuretics, NSAIDs, captopril); bx dx
DRESS Syndrome	**Maculopapular, papulosquamous, pustular, bullous,** or **urticarial** exanthem; a/w fever, LAN, systemic sx; 2/2 drug
Erythema multiforme	Diffuse erythematous **macules/papules** w/ evolving morphology (become targetoid, then polycyclic & annular configuration); trunk, extremities (inc palms/soles), face (mucous memb ~70%)
Erythema nodosum	Painful pink/purple, round, oval **nodules** (1–6 cm diam), can coalesce; symmetric & usually anterior tibia (also knees, ankles, thighs, forearms); self-resolves after 1–6 wk
Erythroderma	**Generalized erythema** (>90% TBSA; spares palms/soles), progresses to scaling & desquamation; pruritic; often w/ edema; LAN ± e/o high-output HF, hepatomegaly, splenomegaly
Morbilliform drug eruption	Diffuse erythematous morbilliform **macules/papules** (less commonly erythroderma, pustules, targetoid lesions), can coalesce & become edematous; trunk, extremities, face
Pemphigus vulgaris	Diffuse small or confluent painful **flaccid blisters & erosions** on erythematous base (+Nikolsky); inc on mucous membranes
SJS/TEN	Diffuse erythematous dusky confluent purpuric **macules** or **patches**, rapidly evolve to coalesce & blister (+Nikolsky); often starts on trunk & spreads to extremities (inc palms/soles) & face (inc mucous membranes); eventually epidermal sloughing
Scromboid	Diffuse **macular** or **papular** erythema w/ urticaria <30 min after ingesting scombroid fish; a/w HA, N/V, palpitations
Serum-sickness & serum sickness-like rxn	Diffuse **urticarial** or serpiginous **macules & patches**, well-demarcated w/ intense red border & central clearing; trunk, face, extremities (no palms/soles), a/w arthralgias
Sweet syndrome	Tender, violaceous, well-demarcated painful **papules & plaques** (± central pustules, bullae, or ulcers), can evolve to coalesce; common esp on upper body (inc face, mucous memb), a/w fever
Urticaria	Pruritic, pink-erythematous **wheals**, ranging in size from a few mm to several cm in size; may be round or irregular in shape

Miscellaneous

Guttate psoriasis	Diffuse dewdrop-like 1–10 mm salmon-colored **papules** w/ fine scaling; can coalesce; may be preceded by URI or grp A strep infxn
Photosensitive rash	**Erythema** or bulla (inc hemorrhagic) at area of UV exposure
Pityriasis versicolor	Subacute hypo- or hyperpigmented **macules & patches**, often neck/trunk/UEs; 2/2 *malassezia* fungus, not contagious; RFs are humidity, immunosupp, OCPs, poor nutrition; tx topically for localized dz (azole, terbinafine), systemic for extensive dz (azoles)

VIRAL EXANTHEMS

Measles (Rubeola; "First Disease")
Definition (*Lancet* 2012;379(9811):153–164)
- Highly contagious dz caused by the measles virus, spread by droplet contact
- Epidemiology: Usually nonimmunized or immunosupp (1° vaccine failure <0.2%); can occur in immunized adults (2° vaccine failure 5% >15 yr after vaccination) esp if no herd immunity (though often milder); winter/spring common; incubation prd ~1 wk

History & Physical Exam
- Assess vaccination status
- Prodrome (lasts 3 d): Acute febrile illness, cough, coryza (nasal mucosal inflammation), conjunctivitis, Koplik spots (small irreg-shaped blue-white macules on buccal mucosa)
- Exanthem (lasts 3–7 d): Starts behind ears, on face/neck as discrete purple-red macules & papules; spreads to trunk & extremities (inc palms/soles), becoming confluent; disappears in same order as arrived

Evaluation
- Routine labs rarely indicated (CBC may show leukopenia)
- Lab confirmation: Measles serologies (enzyme immunoassay for measles IgG & IgM), throat or nasopharyngeal swab for viral isolation/RT-PCR. Contact lab specialist.

Treatment
- Supportive, consult ID
- Two-dose Vit A may reduce mortality in children <2 yr (Cochrane 2005;(4):CD001479)

Complications
- During/post-infxn: Otitis media (most common) & mastoiditis, keratitis, corneal ulcerations & blindness, croup, PNA (most common severe complication), myopericarditis, TTP, febrile sz, encephalomyelitis (1:1000 incidence ~2 wk after infxn; 2/3 autoimm demyelination; fever/sz / various neuro sx) (Lancet 2012;379(9811):153–164)
- Late complications (rare): Inclusion body encephalitis (mo after infxn; fatal), subacute sclerosing panencephalitis (yrs after infxn; fatal)

Disposition
- Home if absence if cx
- Notifiable infectious dz at national level by CDC; requires notification w/i 24 h

Rubella (German Measles; Three-day Measles; "Third Disease")
Definition
- Contagious dz of childhood caused by rubella virus, spread by droplet contact
- Epidemiology: Usually children, but adults can get too (long-term vaccine failure <10%); winter/spring common; incubation prd 2–3 wk (Lancet 2004;363(9415):1127–1137)
- Rubella infxn in children/adults is distinct from congenital rubella syndrome (CRS), a severe teratogenic congenital infxn (not discussed here)

History & Physical Exam
- Assess vaccination status
- Prodrome: Malaise, low-grade fever, HA, sore throat, adenopathy, arthralgias
- Exanthem: Erythematous macules & papules begin on face/forehead, spread to trunk/extremities, may coalesce; typically lasts 3 d then resolves

Evaluation
- Routine labs rarely indicated (CBC may show leukopenia, thrombocytopenia)
- Lab confirmation: Rubella serologies (enzyme immunoassay, latex agglutination, IFA), throat or nasopharyngeal swab for viral isolation/RT-PCR. Contact lab specialist.
- Confirmation important in pregnant patients

Treatment
- Supportive

Complications
(Lancet 2004;363(9415):1127–1137)
- During/post-infxn: Inflammatory arthritis (most common), encephalopathy (1:5000–1:30,000), transient thrombocytopenia, hemolytic anemia (rare), GBS
- If pt is pregnant: Congenital rubella syndrome (highest risk in first trimester)

Disposition
- Home, avoid contact w/ pregnant women (severe congenital defects)
- Notifiable infectious dz at national level by CDC; requires notification w/i 24 h

Erythema Infectiosum ("Fifth Disease")
Definition
- Highly contagious dz caused by Parvovirus B19, spread by respiratory droplets
- Epidemiology: Mainly school-age children (2–14 y/o); winter/spring common; incubation prd 1–2 wk; transmission via blood products rare (virus lives in RBC precursor)

History & Physical Exam
- Prodrome: Malaise, low-grade fever, HA, arthralgias
- Exanthem: Intensely red face ("slapped cheek") w/ circumoral pallor (lasts 1–4 d), then generalized reticular/lacey rash, esp extensor surfaces (spares palms/soles) w/ progression to trunk/buttocks (can last 3 wk); rash uncommon in adults

Evaluation
- Routine labs rarely indicated; consider CBC, reticulocyte count, & haptoglobin in pts w/ hx hemolytic anemia (eg, hereditary spherocytosis) or hemoglobinopathies (ie, SCD)
- Lab confirmation: Serologic testing, DNA assays (direct hybridization)

Treatment
- Supportive
- If complicated (see below), can consider course of IVIG in consultation w/ hematology

Complications
- During infxn: Inflammatory arthritis (most common, esp adults), transient aplastic crisis (esp in pts w/ hemolytic anemias & hemoglobinopathies), pure red cell aplasia
  - Parvovirus temporarily shuts down RBC production during infxn
- In pregnant pts, risk of fetal loss 5–10%; greatest in 2nd trimester (CMAJ 2005;172(6):743)

Disposition
- Home; CDC does not recommend avoidance of school or workplace

Roseola Infantum (Exanthema Subitum; "Sixth Disease")
Definition
- Dz of children 6–36 mo (95%) caused by HHV-6 & HHV-7, spread by salivary secretions
- Three stages of infxn: acute, latent, reactivation
- Epidemiology: Acute dz is most common viral exanthem in children <3 yr (10–20% of all acute febrile illnesses in this age), no seasonality, incubation prd 1–2 wk; Reactivation can be severe in immunosupp (esp recent HSCT) (Clin Microbiol Rev 2015;28(2):313–335).

History & Physical Exam
- Prodrome: Abrupt high fevers (± febrile sz), HA, coryza, periorbital edema
- Exanthem: Begins after defervescence; erythematous macules; starts neck/trunk & spreads to face/extremities; clears in 1–2 d

Evaluation
- Routine labs rarely indicated (CBC may show leukopenia)
- Primary infxn w/ HHV-6 is difficult to confirm diagnostically

Treatment
- Supportive for primary infxn
- Reactivation in immunosuppressed: May tx w/ ganciclovir or foscarnet

Complications
- Primary infxn: febrile sz (most common complication)
- Reactivation infxn (most severe in transplant pts, esp recent HSCT): encephalitis, bone marrow suppression, pneumonitis, hepatitis, transplant failure, GVHD

Disposition
- Home

Herpes Simplex 1 and 2 (HHV-1 and HHV-2)
Definition
- Historically, HSV-1 a/w orofacial dz & HSV-2 a/w genital dz; now both can cause both dz; transmission by contact w/ active lesions, but also by resp droplets & infected secretions
- Three stages: primary, latent (asx), reactivation; reactivation triggers include illness or fever, menstruation, sun exposure, psychological stress (but usually spontaneous)
- **Herpes gingivostomatitis:** Affects oral/perioral mucous membranes, usually 1° infxn
- **Herpes labialis:** Affects perioral skin & mucous membranes; difficult to distinguish 1° & 2° dz; latent virus lives in trigeminal ganglion; reactivation in >1/3 pts
- **Herpes genitalis:** Affects genitals (inc suprapubic, perineum, thighs, perianal) & mucous membranes; difficult to distinguish 1° & 2° dz; 60–70% of primary infxn can be asx; reactivation is common & can be sx (1-yr reactivation 20–50% [HSV-1], 70–90% [HSV-2]) or asx (80–90% of HSV-2 pts have transient asx shedding); up to 25% of infected pts unaware they have dz (NEJM 2016;375(7):666–674)

History & Physical Exam
- Herpes gingivostomatitis & labialis:
  - Prodrome: Malaise, fever, localized pruritus/tingling/burning, dysphagia if intraoral
  - Rash (gingivostomatitis): Oral/perioral vesicles, oral ulcers, gingivitis (lasts 1–2 wk)
  - Rash (labialis): Clustered vesicles on erythematous base, often outside of mouth at vermillion border (but can be on nose); ± LAN & sore throat; distinguish from aphthous stomatitis (canker sore), which are discrete painful intraoral lesions
- Herpes genitalis:
  - Prodrome: Malaise, fever, HA, tender LAN; localized burning/pain in genital region
  - Rash: Clustered vesicles on erythematous base, crusted ulcers if on dry skin
  - Risk factors: Number lifetime sexual partners, mx partners, h/o STI/HIV

Evaluation

- Generally not needed in ED; if recurrent, determining HSV-1 vs HSV-2 guides prog & tx
- PCR (best), Tzanck smear (can't differentiate HSV-1 vs HSV-2), viral cx (slow), biopsy

Treatment

- Pain control, hydration
- Herpes labialis: Topical therapy (docosanol 10% cream, penciclovir 1% cream, acyclovir 5% ointment, cidofovir 0.3 or 1% gel) & oral therapy (Acyclovir, Famciclovir, Valacyclovir) may decrease sxs & time to healing; sunscreen may decrease relapses.
- Herpes genitalis: Tx differs for first infxn, recurrent infxn, & suppressive tx
  - First infxn: Acyclovir 400 mg TID, Famciclovir 250 mg TID, Valacyclovir 1 g BID (7–10 d)
  - Recurrent: Acyclovir 400 mg TID, Famciclovir 125 mg BID, Valacyclovir 1g QD (5 d)
- Severe or disseminated dz: IV acyclovir 5–10 mg/kg q8h

Complications

- Bacterial superinfxn (eg, impetigo), keratitis (2/2 autoinoculation), disseminated dz (eg, meningoencephalitis, hepatitis, pneumonitis) esp in neonates & immunosupp

Disposition

- Home unless severe/disseminated (requires IV antivirals) or unable to tolerate PO
- Herpes genitalis pts should be counseled on safe sex & prevention (MMWR 2010;59:1–110)

Varicella ("Chickenpox," HHV-3)

Definition

- Primary infxn w/ VZV; highly contagious (~90% transmission among household contacts; 10–35% w/ limited exposure); transmission by resp droplets or vesicle secretion
- Epidemiology: Mostly children (5–10 y/o), but can affect infants & adults (esp if from tropical regions, 2/2 childhood dz less common); mortality low, but ~4× higher in infants & ~25× higher in adults, including most among immunocompetent; winter/spring common; incubation prd ~14 d (Lancet 2006;368(9544):1365–1376)

History & Physical Exam

- Prodrome (24–48 h before rash): Fever, malaise, HA, abd pain usually lasting 24–48 h before skin lesions. Rash & new lesion formation over 1–7-d prd.
- Exanthem: Pruritic macules, progress to papules & vesicles, crusting w/i 48 h; trunk/face > extremities; crusts fall off after 1–2 wk; may leave hypopigmented scars long-term
- Mucous membranes can be involved: conjunctiva, genitals, oropharynx
- "Breakthrough varicella" in immunized pts is similar but mild (ie, <50 lesions)

Evaluation

- Routine labs rarely indicated (CBC may show lymphopenia & transaminitis)

Treatment

- Healthy children: Supportive (calamine lotion, colloidal oatmeal baths; AVOID salicylates 2/2 Reye syndrome); oral acyclovir w/i 24 h of dz onset may reduce fever by 1 d & sx severity by 15–30%, but not recommended by CDC (Lancet 2006;368(9544):1365–1376)
- High-risk groups (infants, age >12, pregnant, steroids (inc inhaled) or any immunosupp, chronic skin or pulm dz, long-term ASA use, pregnant) or complicated dz: IV acyclovir
- Precautions: put pts on airborne (neg pressure) & contact precautions until crusted
  - Pts should not be managed by providers w/o immunity or those who are pregnant

Complications

- Bacterial superinfxn (impetigo, cellulitis; most common); invasive bacterial infxns (PNA, arthritis, osteomyelitis, necrotizing fasciitis, sepsis) & varicella PNA; neuro cx (cerebellar ataxia [1:4000], encephalitis, myelitis); heme cx (thrombocytopenia, purpura fulminans); vasculitis (inc intracranial); hepatitis (Lancet 2006;368(9544):1365–1376)
- In rare cases, maternal varicella in early gestation can result in a congenital varicella syndrome (microcephaly, mental retardation limb hypoplasias, cutaneous defects, etc.); later in pregnancy, varicella can cause preterm delivery & neonatal varicella

Postexposure Prophylaxis

- Antivirals not recommended for PEP
- If eligible for VZV vaccine: give vaccine w/i 3–5 d of exposure, if no e/o prior immunity
- If not eligible for VZV vaccine (allergy, immunosupp, pregnancy, infant): Varicella zoster immune globulin can prevent varicella or lessen severity, give w/i 96 h of exposure

Disposition

- Home for uncomplicated cases
- Admission for high-risk groups or those w/ complications

Herpes Zoster ("Shingles," HHV-3)

Definitions (NEJM 2013;369(3):255–263; Cochrane 2008;1:CD005582)
- Reactivation of VZV from sensory ganglia; 20–50% lifetime risk (if nonvaccinated)
- **Herpes zoster ophthalmicus:** (V1 branch of CN V) Rash on forehead, periocular, nose
- **Herpes zoster oticus (Ramsay Hunt syndrome):** (CN VII/geniculate ganglion) Rash on ear, hard palate, anterior 2/3 of tongue; can get ipsilateral facial nerve palsy; a/w variable other CN findings (tinnitus, hearing loss, N/V, vertigo, nystagmus, etc.)
- Zoster sine herpete: Clinical features similar to VZV but w/o rash

History & Physical Exam
- Risk factors: Previous VZV infxn, age, immunosupp, neoplastic disease (esp hematologic)
- Prodrome (may be absent): 2–3 d of localized skin sensations (tingling, hot/cold sensation, pruritus, burning pain) prior to rash; can be a/w HA, photophobia, malaise,
- Exanthem: Grouped vesicles on erythematous base, eventually crusting; pain; distributed in dermatomal pattern, not crossing midline; overlap adjacent dermatomes in 20% cases
- Sensory changes vary: Paresthesias (tingling), dysesthesia (altered), allodynia (pain), hyperesthesia (exaggerated), pruritus

Evaluation
- Clinical dx; testing may be indicated if rash is atypical or pt has comorbidities
- DFA for VZV Ag (~80% Se), PCR (lesion base) (95–100% Se) (NEJM 2013;369(3):255–263)

Treatment
- Antivirals indicated if w/i 72 h of rash onset, but recommended even >72 h if new vesicles forming, complications present (inc eye), or pt risk factors (immunosupp, elderly)
- Antivirals (valacyclovir, acyclovir, famciclovir) decrease course & neuralgic pain
  - Acyclovir 800 mg PO q4h 5 times daily × 7–10 d
  - Valacyclovir 1000 mg PO q8h × 7 d (may have better bioavailability than acyclovir)
  - Famciclovir 500 mg PO q8h × 7 d (may have better bioavailability than acyclovir)
- Corticosteroids: Data equivocal; may accelerate healing & possibly reduce pain; may not help prevent postherpetic neuralgia (NEJM 2013;369(3):255–263; Cochrane 2008;1:CD005582)
- Herpes zoster ophthalmicus: Consult ophthalmology
- Supportive care (NSAIDs/acetaminophen; may need opiates during acute rash)
- Postherpetic neuralgia: tx disappointing (<50% pts have >50% reduction in pain); topical agents (lidocaine patch [NNT 2.0], capsaicin cream [NNT 3.3]); systemic tx (gabapentin [NNT 4.4], pregabalin [NNT 4.2], TCAs [NNT 2.6]); combo tx better than mono-tx (if tolerated); pain specialist c/s if considering opiates (NEJM 2014;371(16):1526–1533)

Complications (NEJM 2013;369(3):255–263; NEJM 2014;371(16):1526–1533)
- Postherpetic neuralgia (pain >90 d after rash, can be long-term; ~20% incidence after VZV, risk inc w/ age); bell's palsy; transverse myelitis, cerebrovascular disease; disseminated dz (pneumonitis, hepatitis, pancreatitis, CNS) esp in immunosupp
- Herpes zoster ophthalmicus: ~50% can have ocular comp (eg, iritis, episcleritis, keratitis)

Disposition
- Home unless disseminated

Pityriasis Rosea (associated HHV-6 and HHV-7)
Definition
- Acute, self-healing exanthema of unclear etiology: may be viral (a/w HHV-6 & HHV-7), but can also be a/w drugs (esp if no herald patch & longer duration) (BMJ 2015;351:h5233)
- Epidemiology: Mainly adolescents/young adults (age 10–35); a/w asthma, eczema, URIs

History & Physical Exam
- Const sx in only ~50%: Fever, HA, arthralgia, cough, N/V, LAN (BMJ 2015;351:h5233)
- Herald patch present in 40–75%: Single pink/salmon-colored oval plaque 2–4 cm diam w/ fine scaling borders & pale depressed center; precedes rash by up to 3 wk
- Exanthem: Numerous lesions similar in appearance to herald patch on trunk & prox. extremities but in characteristic lines of cleavage ("Christmas tree pattern"); spares face, scalp, palms, & soles typically; lasts 5 wk but can last up to 5 mo

Treatment
- Supportive (oatmeal baths & emollients may help): No recommended role for steroids, abx, or antivirals including acyclovir. In severe cases, topical agents may be tried locally, & if improvement can then use widely. (BMJ 2015;351:h5233)

Disposition
- Home; can f/u w/ dermatology esp if >3 mo duration

Molluscum Contagiosum (associated Poxvirus)
Definition
- Benign, self-limiting but long-lasting eruption 2/2 poxvirus; spread by fomite, skin-to-skin, & sexual contact & auto-inoculation
- Can serve as marker or opportunistic infxn in pts w/ HIV

History & Physical Exam
- Exanthem: Nonpainful smooth tan dome-shaped papules (2–5 mm diam) w/ umbilicated center on face, trunk, extremities (but can see in axilla, groin, a/c fossa, etc.); can last up to 12–18 mo

Treatment
- Self-limited & asx: no tx needed; can refer to dermatology for lesion eradication to dec risk of spread (cryotherapy, laser, curettage, imiquimod cream, trichloroacetic acid, or tretinoin), esp if numerous prd or HIV+ (Curr Opin Pediatr 2016;28(2):250–257)

Disposition
- Home ± dermatology f/u

BACTERIAL EXANTHEMS

Refer to Chapter 4 ("Soft Tissue Infections") for the following: Cellulitis, Erysipelas, Staph Scalded Skin Syndrome, Toxic Shock Syndrome, & Necrotizing Fasciitis

Scarlet Fever (Scarlatina, "Second Disease")
Definition
- Rash in children (3–12 yr) 2/2 erythrogenic toxin-producing strains of gpr A β-hemolytic streptococci; transmitted via airborne droplets & fomites from ppl w/ dz & asx carriers; incubation 1–4 d; winter/spring common

History, Physical Exam, & Evaluation
- PRODROME: Acute onset sore throat, fever, HA, vomiting, ± abd pain (can be severe)
- EXAM: Diffuse fine erythematous coalescent "sandpaper" eruption ("goosebump" appearance); starts on neck/axilla/groin & spreads to trunk/extremities (w/o palms/soles), becomes macules coalescing into patches; lasts 7d then fine desquamation
- Characteristic features: Flushed face w/ circumoral pallor; inc intensity at flexor folds (Pastia lines are transverse red streaks in skin folds); strawberry tongue; beefy red pharynx & tonsils w/ or w/o exudate
- DX: Rapid strep test (Se 60–90%, Sp 90%), throat cx; CBC rarely indicated but usually leukocytosis w/ PMN predominance present

Treatment
- PCN VK QID × 10 d, benzathine PCN 1.2 million U IM × 1, or macrolide in PCN-allergic

Disposition
- Home

Impetigo
Definition
- Highly contagious superficial infxn 2/2 S. aureus & group A β-hemolytic streptococci; transmitted via direct contact (inc autoinoculation) & fomites; summer common
- Two types: Nonbullous (majority of cases; represents host response to infxn), Bullous (caused by bacterial toxins, esp staph exfoliative toxins)
- Epidemiology: Affects mainly children (2–5 yr; most common pediatric bacterial skin infxn)

History & Physical Exam
- Nonbullous impetigo: Begins as red macule or papule that becomes a vesicle; vesicle ruptures to form an erosion, & its contents dry to form honey-colored crusts; usually on face (cheeks or under lips) or extremities; self-limited over 2 wk
- Bullous impetigo: Begins as rapidly enlarging vesicles that form sharply demarcated bullae w/ little to no surrounding erythema; these rupture, forming yellow oozing crusts; usually moist intertriginous areas involved (neck fold, axilla, groin, perineum); self-limited

Evaluation
- Dx is clinical; gram stain & culture rarely indicated

Complications
- Cellulitis, lymphangitis, poststreptococcal GMN, TSS, SSSS; invasive bact infxns

Treatment (Cochrane 2012;1:CD003261)
- Most will resolve spontaneously, but abx recommended
- Topical abx equally if not more effective than oral abx (mupirocin 2% ointment TID 3–5 d)

- Oral abx may be indicated in those who cannot tolerate topical tx or w/ extensive dz: Amoxicillin/clavulanate, dicloxacillin, cephalexin, macrolide for PCN-allergic pts

Disposition
- Home w/ instruction to prevent spreading

FUNGAL EXANTHEMS

Dermatophytoses
Definitions
- Superficial fungal infxns involving the stratum corneum, hair, or nails:
  - Tinea capitis: infxn of hair & scalp
  - Tinea corporis: infxn of smooth, hairless skin (except palms, soles, & groin)
  - Tinea cruris: infxn of groin, genitals, pubic area, or perineum
  - Tinea pedis: infxn of feet, commonly interdigital regions
  - Tinea manuum: infxn of hand, commonly interdigital regions
  - Tinea unguium/Onychomycosis: infxn of the nail

Clinical Features and Treatment of Dermatophytoses		
Dermatophytosis	**Historical & Physical Exam**	***Treatment**
Tinea capitis	Hx: Often children 3–14 yr; RFs - poor hygiene, overcrowding, ↓ SES PE: Scalp w/ hair loss, scaling, pruritus Dx: Clinical; wood's lamp may reveal green fluorescence	• Topical tx ineffective but selenium shampoo can reduce transmission • Systemic tx preferred: -Terbinafine -Itraconazole
Tinea corporis	Hx: RFs - occlusive clothing, minor skin trauma, freq skin-to-skin contact PE: Annular/polycyclic scaly plaque Dx: Clinical; KOH prep w/ septate & branching hyphae	
Tinea cruris	Hx: RFs include occlusion & humidity PE: Annular plaque & scaly raised borders; from inguinal folds; pruritic Dx: Clinical; KOH prep w/ septate & branching hyphae	• Localized dz: tx w/ topical (azoles are fungistatic; allylamines & ciclopirox are fungicidal) • Extensive dz, immunosupp, hair follicles: systemic tx -Terbinafine -Fluconazole -Itraconazole
Tinea pedis	Hx: RFs include communal bathing, locker rooms, pools PE: Scaling, erythema, & maceration of interdigital spaces; bacterial superinfxn causes erosions, pruritus, & malador ("athlete's foot")	
Tinea manuum	PE: Scaling of palms, interdigital region, & palmar creases	
Tinea unguium/ onychomycosis	Hx: RFs include nail trauma (tight shoes), immunosupp, DM, communal bathing PE: Toenail varies from discoloration & thickening of proximal, distal/subungal, or superficial portions of nail plate	• Topical tx only for limited dz (<50% distal nailbed), may have poor cure rates: -Ciclopirox (not as monotx) • Systemic tx preferred: -Terbinafine (preferred) -Itraconazole

*Most tx regimens last from 2–6 wk. Onychomycosis can take months to adequately treat, thus pts require f/u w/ their primary provider or dermatologist.

Disposition
- Home w/ primary care or dermatology f/u

Pearl
- Dermatophytid rxn: Delayed-type hypersensitivity rxn to fungal antigens in pts w/ dermatophytosis; pts p/w pruritic papules or vesicles on hands & feet; respond to tx of primary dermatophytosis infxn

Cutaneous Candidiasis/Intertrigo

Definition
- Fungal infxn by *Candida* species (*C. albicans*); predilection for colonizing skin folds (intertriginous areas) where the environment is warm & moist

History & Physical Exam
- Risk factors: Obesity, DM, occlusive clothes, immunosupp, poor hygiene
- Exanthem: Moist, red, shiny patch w/ scalloped borders & satellite macules & pustules, often in intertriginous areas (groin, axilla, pannus folds, gluteal fold, web spaces); can be pruritic, burning, or asx

Physical Findings
- Moist, red, shiny macules/patches w/ scalloped borders, adjacent satellite pustules

Treatment
- Keep dry, topical antifungals (Various preparations: Creams, lotions, powders, w/ or w/o mild steroid combinations; poor data to support 1 type over the other)

Disposition
- Home

HIGH-RISK EXANTHEMS

Pemphigus Vulgaris
Definition
- Rare but potentially life-threatening acute progressive autoimmune (2/2 autoantibodies) bullous dz involving skin/mucosa; mortality 5–10% w/ tx (*Clin Dermatol* 2013;31(4)374–381)
- Idiopathic, but a/w PMH/FH autoimmune dz

History, Physical Exam, & Evaluation
- HX: Subacute-onset (over dys to wks) additive blisters on mucosa & skin (mucosa may precede skin by wks/mos); pain > pruritus; ask about PMH/FH autoimmune dz
- EXAM: Small or confluent flaccid blisters & erosions on erythematous base (+Nikolsky); diffuse, inc on mucous membranes (oropharynx, conjunctiva, anogenital)
- DX: Histologic dx (c/s derm for bx); labs to r/o other causes or complications

Treatment
- Supportive: analgesia, wound care
- Steroids (1 mg/kg/d pred or equiv); c/s derm, ENT, ophthalmology based on lesions
- Role of steroid-sparing tx (MMF, azathioprine, cyclosporine, IVIG, plasma exchange, infliximab) in acute dz unclear, but may help reduce risk of relapse (*Drugs* 2015;75(3):271–284; *J Am Acad Dermatol* 2015;73(2):264–271)

Duration & Disposition
- Duration can be lifelong, or can remit (w/ tx) w/ risk of recurrence
- If rapid progression or extensive dz, admit; c/s derm on all cases in ED

Erythroderma (Generalized Exfoliative Dermatitis)
Definition (*Clin Dermatol* 1993;11(1):67–72)
- Rare but potentially life-threatening acute generalized red rash, affecting >90% TBSA; more common in males; a/w high-output HF
- Idiopathic (25%) or 2/2 meds, malignancy, psoriasis, uncontrolled dermatitis, among others
- Common associated drugs: ACE inh, allopurinol, anticonvulsants, beta-blockers, beta-lactam abx, CCBs, furosemide, minocycline, NSAIDs, sulfonamides, others

History, Physical Exam, & Evaluation
- HX: Subacute-onset (over dys to wks) generalized rash w/ scaling, a/w malaise, chills ± fever; pruritic commonly; always ask about meds, recent infxn sx, PMH/FH inflamm dz & malignancy
- EXAM: Generalized erythema (>90% TBSA; spares palms/soles), progresses to scaling & desquamation; often w/ edema; LAN ± e/o high-output HF, hepatomegaly, splenomegaly
- DX: Elevated ESR, hypoalbuminemia, hyperglobulinemia (2/2 antibodies), mild anemia; may see e/o heme malignancy necessitating additional w/u; consult dermatology

Treatment
- Tx underling cause or d/c causal drug if known
- Supportive: skin moisture, antihistamines, topical steroids; systemic steroids usually warranted (unless c/f SSSS or underlying h/o psoriasis); watch fluid balance (given risk of both dehydration & HF)

Duration & Disposition
- Resolution depends on cause & ability to control/remove it
- Admit, esp if rapid or unstable; consult dermatology

Acute Generalized Exanthematous Pustulosis (AGEP)
Definition
- Rare but life-threatening immunologically-mediated diffuse acute pustular exanthema, often w/ multiorgan dysfxn in ~17% (esp elderly) (*J Am Acad Dermatol* 2015;73(5):843–848)
- Often 2/2 drugs (90%), infxn (parvovirus B19, *C. pneumonia*, CMV), mercury, spider bites (*J Am Acad Dermatol* 2015;73(5):843–848)
- Common associated drugs: Beta-lactam abx, quinolones, sulfonamides, carbamazepine, terbinafine, diltiazem, hydroxychloroquine, others

History, Physical Exam, & Evaluation (*J Am Acad Dermatol* 2015;73(5):843–848)
- HX: Acute-onset (w/ hrs) diffuse pustular rash; often occurs w/i 48 h of starting drug (or longer if not 2/2 abx); pruritic; always ask about meds, recent infxn sx
  - May also have sx of systemic organ involvement: SOB, abd pain, N/V, skin infxn
- EXAM: Numerous small sterile pustules on erythematous base, a/w fever; trunk & intertriginous areas common (rarely mucous membranes); pruritic
  - Assess for systemic dz: pleural effusions/hypoxia, hepatic dysfxn, rarely systemic superinfxn & DIC
- DX: CBC w/ leukocytosis (± eosinophilia), LFTs, ± CXR; c/s dermatology for bx

Treatment
- D/C causal drug or tx underlying infxn
- Supportive: Moist dressings & antiseptic solutions; high-potency topical steroids may help pruritus, but no role for systemic steroids; ± empiric abx if unstable

Duration & Disposition
- 5% mortality, mostly 2/2 superinfxn (*J Am Acad Dermatol* 2013;68(5):709)
- Resolves days after causal drug d/c-ed
- Admit (may need ICU)

Drug Reaction with Eosinophilia and Systemic Symptoms (DRESS)
Definition
- Rare but potentially life-threatening immune-mediated diffuse rash with multiorgan dysfxn
- Common associated drugs: Allopurinol, anticonvulsants, sulfonamides, others

History, Physical Exam, & Evaluation
- HX: Prodrome of pruritus & fever, f/b acute-onset (hrs to dys) diffuse rash; occurs within 2–6 wk of starting drug
- EXAM: Diffuse erythematous morbilliform macules/papules (less commonly erythroderma, pustules, targetoid lesions), can coalesce & become edematous; trunk, extremities, face (can involve mucous membranes)
  - Eval for multiorgan dysfxn: liver (>70% of pts; major source of morbidity/mortality), hematologic, lymphatic, renal, pulm (pneumonitis, ARDS), cardiac (myocarditis), gastroenteritis, meningoencephalitis (*J Am Acad Dermatol* 2013;68(5):693)
- DX: CBC w/ diff (WBC can be >50 k/L; Eos >1.5 k/L; +atypical lymphs), Chem 20 (Cr, lytes, LFTs), Troponin, CXR, dermatology c/s for bx

Treatment (*J Am Acad Dermatol* 2013;68(5):693)
- D/C causal drug
- Supportive: antihistamines, tx underlying organ dysfxn
- Systemic steroids w/ gradual taper over 3–6 mo

Duration & Disposition
- 10% mortality, esp immunosupp (*J Am Acad Dermatol* 2013;68(5):693)
- Resolves months after causal drug d/c-ed
- Admit (may need ICU)

Stevens-Johnson Syndrome (SJS)/Toxic Epidermal Necrolysis (TEN)
Definition (*Am J Clin Dermatol* 2015;16(6):475–493)
Acute generalized mucocutaneous desquamative eruption with various associated causes; immune-mediated but precise mechanism unknown
- Mucous membranes a dz hallmark: 80% cases (first sx in 30%); oropharyngeal, ocular (80% cases), anogenital, GI, endotracheal/bronchial; all w/ severe complications
Differentiation b/w SJS & TEN depends on TBSA desquamated:
- SJS: <10% TBSA w/ detachable epidermis w/ horizontal shear ("+Nikolsky sign")
- SJS/TEN overlap: 10–30% TBSA w/ +Nikolsky
- TEN: >30% TBSA w/ +Nikolsky
Idiopathic (20%), but often a/w meds (most common cause), infxn (*M. pneumoniae*, HSV), less likely food additives, fumigants, malignancy

- Common associated drugs: Allopurinol, anticonvulsants, beta-lactam abx, nevirapine, piroxicam, sulfonamides, others

History, Physical Exam, & Evaluation
- HX: Flu-like prodrome (fever, malaise, HA, sore throat, rhinitis, myalgias) f/b acute-onset (over dys) diffuse rash ± mucosal sx (dysphagia, etc.); pain; always ask about meds (usually w/i 4 wk), recent infxn sx, PMH/FH inflamm dz & malignancy
- EXAM: Diffuse erythematous dusky confluent purpuric macules or patches, rapidly evolve to coalesce & blister (+Nikolsky); often starts on trunk & spreads to extremities (inc palms/soles) & face (inc mucous membranes); eventually generalized sloughing
  - Extent of TBSA w/ +Nikolsky dictates SJS (<10%) vs SJS/TEN (10–30%) vs TEN (>30%)
- DX: CBC, BMP, Lactate & blood cx (esp if hypotensive), derm c/s for bx

Treatment
- Treat underlying cause or D/C causal drug
- Supportive: analgesia, thermoregulation (28–32°; esp important if high TBSA), IVF, airway protection prn, nutritional support (helps healing) wound care (debridement, bacitracin)
- Limited high-quality data supports specific systemic tx modalities:
  - Systemic steroids are standard of care, but have unclear mortality benefit *(Ann Pharmacother 2015;49(3):355–342; J Am Acad Dermatol 2008;58(1):33–40)*
  - High-dose (>2 gk/kg) IVIG in conjunction w/ steroids may reduce hosp LOS by ~3 dys, & dec mortality, benefit strongest in TEN & w/ Asian pts *(PLoS One 2016;11(11):0167120; Int J Dermatol 2015;54(1):108–115)*
  - Cyclosporine may improve survival over IVIG *(J Am Acad Dermatol 2014;71(5):941–947)*
  - TNF inhibitors currently being investigated

Complications
- Mostly from mucosal ulcerations in trachea & bronchi (resp distress), esophagus (GIB, malnutrition), eyes (uveitis, ulceration, blindness), genitourinary (dysuria, retention)
- Sepsis can occur 2/2 superinfxn from skin breakdown

Duration & Disposition
- Mortality 5–30%; TEN prognosis predictable using SCORTEN (see table)
- All patients get admitted; TEN requires burn unit admission
- ED or early inpt c/s to ophthalmology, urology (early foley), ± GI, pulm

Severity of Illness Score for TEN (SCORTEN) *(J Invest Dermatol 2000;115(2):149–153)*			
Point		**Points**	
1	Age >40	1	Epidermal detachment >10% TBSA on day 1
1	HR > 120 bpm	1	BUN >28 mg/dL
1	Comorbid malignancy	1	HCO_3 < 20 mEq/L
Score	**Mortality**	**Score**	**Mortality**
0–1	3.2%	4	58.3%
2	12.2%	≥5	90.0%
3	35.5%		

OTHER EXANTHEMS

Allergic/Urticarial Reactions
Definition
- Acute (can be chronic or recurrent) histamine-mediated exanthem, often due to IgE, direct mast cell activation, complement, or dysmetabolism of arachidonic acid (eg, NSAIDs)
- Triggers: systemic exposures (foods, meds, insect stings, contact w/ external allergens parasites), physical triggers (eg, cholinergic, exercise, pressure, aquagenic, cold, etc.)
- Common associated drugs: ASA, ACE inh, beta-lactam abx, NSAIDs, sulfonamides, others

History, Physical Exam, & Evaluation
- HX: Acute-onset (over mins) diffuse urticaria, ± SOB, N/V, LH; pruritus (no pain); usually occurs within hrs of trigger
- EXAM: Diffuse or localized erythematous wheals, variably sized (mm to cm), round or irregular in shape, can be excoriated 2/2 pruritic nature; occur anywhere on skin
  - Assess for signs of anaphylaxis (wheezing, hypotension)
- DX: Clinical dx; if +myalgias, LFTs to r/o acute hepatitis

Treatment
- D/C causal drug or other trigger
- Antihistamines (H1 & H2), steroids for severe cases, epinephrine if anaphylaxis

Duration & Disposition
- Resolves hours after trigger removed; no mortality risk (unless anaphylaxis)
- Home; RX EpiPen in case recurrence; F/U with allergy for allergen testing &/or desensitization

Serum Sickness & Serum Sickness-like Reactions
Definition
- Acute diffuse immune-mediated (type III hypersensitivity) rash, often 2/2 drug exposure
- Common associated drugs: Barbiturates, beta-lactam abx, fluoxetine, sulfonamides, thiazides, vaccines/anti-serum, others

History, Physical Exam, & Evaluation
- HX: Fever, severe arthralgias, malaise, & acute-onset (over hrs) diffuse rash; pain > pruritus; usually occurs within 2 wk of starting drug
- EXAM: Diffuse urticarial or serpiginous macules & patches (though other morphologies possible), well-demarcated w/ intense red border & central clearing; trunk, face, extremities (no palms/soles); joint ROM limited 2/2 pain
- DX: Clinical dx, no testing indicated

Treatment
- D/C causal drug or other trigger
- Supportive: antihistamines, NSAIDs for pain
- Steroids for severe dz

Duration & Disposition
- Resolves 2–3 wk after trigger removed; no mortality risk
- Home if pain controlled; F/U with allergy

Exanthematous (Morbilliform) Eruption
Definition
- Acute diffuse immune-mediated rash (type IV hypersensitivity) 2/2 drug exposure
- Common associated drugs: Allopurinol, anticonvulsants, beta-lactam abx, NSAIDs, sulfonamides, others

History, Physical Exam, & Evaluation
- HX: May have low-grade fever, f/b acute-onset (over hrs–dys) diffuse rash; pruritus > pain; usually occurs within 2–6 wk of starting drug
- EXAM: Diffuse erythematous macules or papules (but can be pustular or bullous), becoming confluent; viral (morbilliform) appearance; trunk & extremities (no palms/soles & face)
- DX: Clinical; elevated CRP, CBC may have mild eosinophilia (if markedly elevated eosinophils, consider DRESS), LFTs nl (if elevated, consider DRESS)

Treatment
- D/C causal drug (if unknown, d/c all non-necessary drugs); rarely, the causal medication can be continued through the rash if it is essential; discuss with dermatology
- Supportive care: antihistamines
- Steroids for severe dz

Duration & Disposition
- Resolves ~2 wk after med d/c-ed; no significant mortality risk
- Home; F/U with dermatology

Fixed Drug Eruptions
Definition
- Acute but recurrent localized immune-mediated skin eruption 2/2 repeat drug exposure
- Common associated drugs: ASA, NSAIDs, quinine, sedatives, sulfonamides, tetracyclines, others

History, Physical Exam, & Evaluation
- HX: Rash w/o systemic sx; pruritic; occurs within hrs–dys of starting drug; on repeat exposure, lesions occur in same location as prior (new lesions may be present as well)
- EXAM: Solitary or small group of erythematous or hyperpigmented oval macules evolving to plaques (may become brown); pruritus; common sites include lips, extremities, genitals
- DX: Clinical

Treatment
- D/C causal drug (hyperpigmented area may remain)
- Supportive: antihistamines

Duration & Disposition
- Resolves days after med d/c-ed; no significant mortality risk
- Home; F/U with dermatology

Erythema Multiforme

Definition
- Acute (but sometimes recurrent or persistent) diffuse immune-mediated rash which can have mucosal involvement
  - *Erythema multiforme major* – mucosal involvement
  - *Erythema multiforme minor* – no mucosal involvement
- Idiopathic, but can be a/w infxn (90% cases; esp HSV, M. pneumonia, HCV, EBV), meds, malignancy, XRT, inflamm dz (*Int J Dermatol* 2012;51(8):889–902)
- Common associated drugs: Anticonvulsants, beta-lactam abx, NSAIDs, phenothiazines, sulfonamides, others

History, Physical Exam, & Evaluation
- HX: Prodrome (fever, malaise) present in EM major, f/b acute-onset (over dys) diffuse rash (see exam); always ask about meds, recent infxn sx, PMH/FH inflamm dz & malignancy
- EXAM: Diffuse erythematous macules/papules w/ evolving morphology (become targetoid, then polycyclic & annular configuration); trunk, extremities (inc palms/soles), face (mucous memb ~70%) (*Int J Dermatol* 2012;51(8):889–902)
  - Compared to SJS: Less purpuric, less truncal, less painful, less mucosa
- DX: Clinical & histopathologic dx (c/s derm for bx); labs inc HSV PCR/IgM (esp if recurrent episode), ± CXR to r/o causes & complications

Treatment
- Tx underlying cause or d/c causal med if known
- Supportive: antihistamines, analgesia, ± oral anesthetic solutions/antiseptic rinses
- Topical steroids if mild, systemic steroids if severe dz (esp mucosal);
  - Consider long-term valacyclovir in pts if recurrent (*Br J Dermatol* 1995;132(2):267–70)

Duration & Disposition
- Resolves w/i weeks; no significant mortality risk, but can progress to SJS/TEN if offending agent not removed
- Home; f/u w/ dermatology & ophthalmology (if ocular involvement)

Erythema Nodosum

Definition
- Panniculitis (inflam of subcutaneous fat) w/ unknown mechanism; thought 2/2 immune complex deposition in connective tissue (*Clin Dermatol* 2007;25(3):288–294)
- Idiopathic ~30%, infxn ~30% (TB, recent Grp A strep infxn), sarcoidosis ~20%, inflamm dz, malignancy, pregnancy, drugs
- Common associated drugs: Sulfonamides, OCPs/estrogens, others

History, Physical Exam, & Evaluation
- HX: Prodrome (fever, fatigue, malaise, polyarthralgia (symmetric, additive, lg joint), HA, GI sx), f/b acute-onset (over dys to wks) generally-localized rash, ± fever, fatigue, malaise, polyarthralgia (symmetric, additive, lg joint), HA, GI sx; painful; always ask about meds, recent infxn sx, PMH/FH inflamm dz & malignancy
- EXAM: Scattered tender erythematous or purple oval nodules (1–6 cm diam), can coalesce; symmetric & usually anterior tibia (also knees, ankles, thighs, forearms)
- DX: Clinical; labs prn for underlying dz (CBC, ESR/CRP, CXR [r/o e/o Tb, sarcoidosis])

Treatment
- Supportive: NSAIDs for pain
- Short course oral corticosteroids in severe dz

Disposition
- Most cases self-resolve w/i 6 wk, but EN may recur; no significant mortality risk (*Clin Dermatol* 2007;25(3):288–294)
- Home; f/u w/ dermatology or rheumatology

Leukocytoclastic Vasculitis

Definition
- Acute, chronic, or intermittently recurrent immune-mediated (immune complex, ANCA) rash, sometimes w/ systemic organ involvement
- Idiopathic (~50%), or a/w recent infxn (viral [esp HBV/HCV], bacterial, parasites, fungi), inflam dz, meds (see table), illicits, malignancy (*J Am Acad Dermatol* 2003;48(3):311–340)
- Common associated drugs: Allopurinol, abx, anticoagulants (oral), anticonvulsants, NSAIDs, thiazide diuretics, thiouracil, others

History, Physical Exam, & Evaluation
- HX: Acute-onset (over dys) rash; ± systemic sx (fever, arthralgias, GI sx [diarrhea, abd pain], hematuria, hemoptysis); pruritic/burning; always ask about meds, recent infxn sx, PMH/FH inflamm dz & malignancy

- **EXAM:** Diffuse or localized tender palpable purpura or purpuric urticaria, can evolve to coalesce to form plaques or bullae; often lower extremities
- Multiorgan involvement possible: MSK, GI, cardiac, lungs, ocular, kidneys
- **DX:** Clinical; labs to r/o systemic dz (CBC, ESR/CRP, Chem 20, UA, ± CXR)

Treatment
- Tx definitive cause (if known) or d/c causal drug
- Supportive (elevation of legs, compression stockings), antihistamines, analgesia w/ NSAIDs
- Colchicine (± dapsone) if no response to NSAIDs (0.6 mg BID); short-course steroids if still refractory (J Am Acad Dermatol 2003;48(3):311–340)

Duration & Disposition
- Resolves w/i 2 wk if 2/2 drug; if 2/2 underlying dz may persist or recur
- Home if no systemic indications for admx; refer to dermatology & rheumatology

Sweet's Syndrome (Acute Febrile Neutrophilic Dermatosis)
Definition
- Rare presumed immune-mediated acute erythematous skin rash characterized histologically by dense neutrophilic infiltrates (J Am Acad Dermatol 1994;31(4):535–560)
- Idiopathic (~2/3 cases; F>M); malignancy (second most common cause; often undx'ed), inflam dz, infxn (esp URI, GI sx, others), meds, pregnancy (Dermatol Online J 1999;5(1):8)
- Common associated drugs: Vaccines, G-CSF, TMP-SMX, minocycline, others

History, Physical Exam, Evaluation
- **HX:** Acute-onset (over hrs) rash w/ fever (may precede rash), a/w arthralgias, HA; painful
- **EXAM:** Tender, violaceous, well-demarcated papules & plaques (can get central pustules, bullae, or ulcers – esp if paraneoplastic), can evolve to coalesce; common esp on upper body (inc face, mucous memb)
- **DX:** Bx required for dx; elev ESR (>90%), CBC (WBC >8 k in 80%, +bands), anemia, low plts; LFTs, ± CXR; ± imaging to eval for malignancy dx (Dermatol Online J 1999;5(1):8)

Treatment
- Supportive: Analgesia
- Systemic steroids for acute dz; mx agents used for suppressive tx

Duration & Disposition
- Rapid resolution w/ steroids (w/o tx may persist wks to mo); can recur
- Home if pain controlled & stable; f/u w/ dermatology

Photosensitive Reaction
Definition
- Any exanthem appearing in photodistribution after exposure to UV light
  - Drug-related causes: exaggerated sunburn, photosensitive drug rxn (phototoxic, photoallergic), pseudoporphyria
    - Common associated drugs: Diuretics, NSAIDs, phenothiazines, quinolones, sulfonamides, sulfonylureas, tetracyclines, others
  - Not drug-related: porphyria cutanea tarda (PCT), inflamm dz (lupus, dermatomyositis)

History, Physical Exam, & Evaluation
- **HX:** Acute-onset (over hrs) rash localized to sun-exposed areas; h/o UV exposure (tanning booth, phototherapy, sunlight); always ask about meds (usually w/i 4 wk), recent infxn sx, PMH/FH inflamm dz
  - Phototoxic rxn: Onset min–hrs after UV
  - Photoallergic rxn: Onset 24–72 h after UV
  - Pseudoporphyria: Onset hrs after UV
- **EXAM:** Exanthem only present on sun-exposed area, morphologically diverse:
  - Phototoxic drug rxn: Exaggerated sunburn response (erythema, edema ± blistering)
  - Photoallergic drug rxn: Erythema ± eczematous changes
  - Pseudoporphyria: Erythema, tense bulla (± hemorrhagic) & erosions (as opposed to PCT, lacks chronic pigment, hair, or scleroder-mal chgs)
- **DX:** Clinical; further testing prn to r/o PCT or inflamm dz (eg, porphyrins, ANA, etc.)

Treatment
- Supportive: Sun protection (clothing, high-SPF sunscreen), cool compresses, wound care
- Topical steroids, systemic steroids for severe dz
- N-acetylcysteine may speed pseudoporphyria resolution (Br J Dermatol 2000;142(3):580–581)

Duration & Disposition:
- Resolution variable, but drug-induced pseudoporphyria may take months
- Home; F/U w/ dermatology & rheumatology prn to exclude PCT or inflammatory causes

Dermatitis

- Class of skin inflammatory-mediated skin dz marked by similar s/sx: erythema, pruritus, scaling, fissures, varying degrees of lichenification & blistering
- Usually chronic/subacute, but pts may come to ED if bad flare (esp if recent long remission)

Clinical Features and Treatment of Dermatitis		
Condition	Presentation	Treatment
Atopic dermatitis (*J Allergy Clin Immunol* 2013;131:295–299)	Definition: Chronic, relapsing/remitting; mostly children (10–20% of kids; 1–3% of adults), most w/i first 1 yr. RFs: Hx/FH atopy (asthma, allergic rhinitis, food allergies) Triggers: Temp, humidity, irritants, infxn, foods, allergens, stress Exam: Dry pruritic papulovesicular w/ excoriations & serous exudate ± lichenification; in kids often on face, neck, extensor surf; in adults often flexor folds	Skin hydration: Soaking baths f/b moisturizer w/i 10 min Topical Steroids: Low-potency for maintenance, mid- & high-potency for flares Antihistamines: For pruritus; do not use topical agents 2/2 risk of skin sensitization Prevention: Avoid irritants F/U w/ derm: May need tx w/ topical calcineurin inhibitors
Contact dermatitis (allergic) (*Ann Allergy Asthma Immunol* 2006;97:S1–38) Contact dermatitis (irritant) (*Ann Allergy Asthma Immunol* 2006;97:S1–38)	Definition: Inflammatory rxn 2/2 direct contact w/ exogenous agent & subsequent type IV hypersensitivity rxn; in Allergic CD, antigen reacts w/ proteins in skin to cause inflammation; in irritant CD, antigen chemically abrades or damages skin to cause inflammation Triggers: Latex, plant substances, metals (esp nickel), plant resins, soaps, detergents, fragrance, hair products, sunscreen, top meds Exam: Erythematous, papulovesicular w/ varying lichenification, fissuring, scaling, excoriation; often localized to exposed area	Avoid any suspected trigger Sx relief: cold compresses, colloidal baths, emollients Topical steroids: Start w/ high-potency if localized (not on face, genitals), then transition to mid- or low-potency as sx improve Systemic steroids for severe or extensive dz Evaluate & tx superinfxn Antihistamines can be ineffective Refer to dermatology for patch testing
Nummular dermatitis	Definition: Morphologically unique type of atopic dermatitis; can occur older in adulthood; M>F Risk factors: Dry skin, atopy, skin injury/abrasion, poor vascular flow, Vit A containing meds Exam: Round/oval pink/brown pruritic papulovesicular rash w/ serous exudate, evolving to plaque (2–10 cm diam) w/ crust then scale; often on extremities (but can be torso)	See atopic dermatitis
Seborrheic dermatitis	Definition: Dz of the sebum-rich areas (scalp/face/trunk), possibly 2/2 abnl immune response to nl skin fungus (Malassezia); often in infants (cradle cap) & elderly, but also AIDS & Parkinson dz; 20% of pts have h/o dandruff; worse in winter Exam: Pink oily flaking patches of skin on scalp, face (nasolabial folds, eyebrows, ears), chest, flexural skin	Frequent bathing w/ keratolytic shampoos (eg, selenium, zinc-based), reduce oil Antifungal: Ketoconazole shampoo or creams Topical steroids: Low-potency creams (if not on scalp)
Xerotic dermatitis	Definition: Skin dz characterized by changes 2/2 dry skin; common among elderly Exam: Dry skin w/ erythematous superficial cracks & excoriations, often on legs	Skin hydration: Soaking baths f/b moisturizer w/i 10 min Topical Steroids: Low-potency & short duration

Pompholyx	Definition: Subtype of eczema 2/2 edematous fluid accumulation in areas w/ thick epidermis; affecting palmoplantar skin; acute, recurrent, or chronic	Topical steroids: High-potency
		Systemic steroids if severe
	Triggers: a/w atopic & contact dermatitis, drug rxns, stress, id rxn in pts w/ tinea pedis	F/U w/ derm: May need tx w/ topical calcineurin inhibitors
	Exam: Nonerythematous pruritic vesicles or bulla on palms or soles	

Topical Steroid Preparations by Potency (Generic)	
High Potency	**Upper-Mid Potency**
Clobetasol propionate[C,G,O,So]	Fluocinonide[C,G,O]
Betamethasone dipropionate[C,G,O,So]	Betamethasone valerate[O]
	Mometasone furoate[C,O]
Lower-Mid Potency	**Low Potency**
Triamcinolone acetonide[C,O,Sp]	Fluticasone propionate[C,L,O]
Hydrocortisone valerate[C,O]	Hydrocortisone 1%, 2.5%[C,L,O,Sp]
Desonide[C,L,O]	
Special Notes on Administration	
(1) Vehicles: Ointment (O) most soothing for dry skin. Cream (C) most cosmetically acceptable. Lotion (L), gel (G) & solution (So) most ideal for scalp. Spray (Sp) in unique circumstances.	
(2) Avoid high potency or prolonged upper-mid potency for pediatric pts (high absorption), skin folds inc genitals (causes striae), and face (causes atrophy/rosacea/ocular complications).	

ACID–BASE DISORDERS

Approach to the Patient

Diagnostics

• BMP; consider LFTs, CBC, urine electrolytes, ABG/VBG, & serum osmoles

Note: HCO_3 from ABG is calculated & should be w/i 2 mmol/L of BMP total CO_2

Step-wise Approach

• **Step 1:** Is there an acidemia or alkalemia?
  Acidemia: pH <7.36; Alkalemia: pH >7.44

• **Steps 2 & 3:** Is the primary disturbance metabolic or respiratory? Is there compensation?

Assessing Primary Metabolic Disturbances and Physiologic Compensation				
Primary Disorder	**pH**	**pCO₂**	**HCO₃**	**Compensation Formula**
Metabolic acidosis	Low	Low	Low	Decr $pCO_2 = 1.25 \times \Delta HCO_3$
Metabolic alkalosis	High	High	High	Incr $pCO_2 = 0.75 \times \Delta HCO_3$
Acute respiratory acidosis	Low	High	High	Incr $HCO_3 = 0.1 \times \Delta PCO_2$
Acute respiratory alkalosis	High	Low	Low	Decr $HCO_3 = 0.2 \times \Delta PCO_2$
Chronic respiratory acidosis	Nl or low	High	High or nl	Incr $HCO_3 = 0.4 \times \Delta PCO_2$
Chronic respiratory alkalosis	Nl or high	Low	Low or nl	Decr $HCO_3 = 0.4 \times \Delta PCO_2$

• **Step 4a:** Is there an anion gap?

Anion gap acidosis: (Na – (Cl + bicarb)) > 14 (see chart)

Note: Needs to be corrected for albumin; a fall in serum albumin 1 g/dL from the nl value (4.2 g/dL) decreases the anion gap by 2.5 meq/L. Corrected AG = AG + (2.5 × [4.2 – albumin]).

• **Step 4b:** If an anion gap is present, is there an osmolar gap?

Osmolar gap: Measured serum Osm – Calculated Osm >10 mOsm/L, where Calculated Osm = $(2 \times [Na^+])$ + glucose/18 + BUN/2.8 + Ethanol/4.6

• **Step 4c:** If no anion gap is present, what is UAG?

Urinary anion gap: Na + K – Cl

Note: The UAG can help differentiate GI & renal causes of non-AG (hyperchloremic) metabolic acidosis, as base can be lost from the gut or kidney (negative UAG: GI loss [ie, diarrhea, small bowel fistula, ileostomy]; positive UAG: Renal loss, particularly RTA types I & IV)

• **Step 5:** What is the delta ratio, also known as the "delta/delta"?

(AG – nl AG)/(nl HCO₃ – HCO₃), or simply (AG – 12)/(24 – HCO₃)

• If delta/delta >+6, suggests concomitant metabolic alkalosis, or prior compensated respiratory acidosis
• If delta/delta = 0, suggests uncomplicated AG metabolic acidosis
• If delta/delta <–6, suggests concomitant hyperchloremic non-AG metabolic acidosis

Metabolic Acidosis	
Anion Gap Acidosis	**Nonanion Gap Acidosis**
"A CAT'S MUDPILE"	**"FUSED CARD TIP"**
Alcoholic ketoacidosis	**F**anconi syndrome
Carbon monoxide, cyanide	**U**reteroenterostomy
Aspirin	**S**mall bowel fistula
Toluene	**E**xcessive Cl⁻ (NaCl, Ammonium Cl⁻)
Starvation ketoacidosis	**D**iarrhea
Methanol, metformin, methemoglobinemia	**C**arbonic anhydrase inhibitors
Uremia	**A**ddison's dz
DKA	**R**enal tubular acidosis
Paraldehyde, phenformin, propylene glycol	**D**rugs (spironolactone, amiloride, cholestyramine, triamterene)
Isoniazid, iron	**T**oluene (chronic, secondary to RTA)
Lactic Acidosis types A & B	**I**leostomy
Ethylene glycol	**P**ancreatic fistula, parenteral nutrition, posthypocapnia

Osmolar Gap Causes	
Toxic Alcohols:	**Others:**
*Methanol	Acetone
*Ethylene glycol	Mannitol
Isopropyl alcohol	Sorbitol
*A/w anion gap	Glycerol
	Ether trichloroethane

Low Anion Gap (<6)
Lab error
Lithium tox
Bromide tox
Hypoalbuminemia
Paraproteinemias
Severe hypercalcemia/hypermagnesemia

Metabolic Alkalosis	
Pathophysiology	**Differential**
Exogenous HCO_3	-Acute alkali administration: Citrate loads from blood transfusions, acetate loads from TPN, administration of $NaHCO_3$ solution, excessive antacids -Milk–alkali syndrome
NaCl responsive conditions *(urine Cl <10–15 mEq/L)*	-GI loss of H^+: V/D, NGT drainage, adenomas -Renal loss of H^+: Diuretic use -Posthypercapnia
NaCl unresponsive conditions *(urine Cl >15 mEq/L)*	-Volume expansion/hypertensive/mineralocorticoid excess: Hyperaldosteronism, Cushing syndrome, exogenous mineralocorticoid, licorice, renal artery stenosis -Volume contraction/normotensive/2° hyperaldosteronism: Hypokalemia, hypomagnesemia, hypercalcemia/hypoPTH, Bartter's syndrome, Gitelman's syndrome -Volume expansion/hypertensive/hypoaldosteronism: Liddle's syndrome

Respiratory Acidosis	
Pathophysiology	**Differential**
Central respiratory depression	Drugs (opioids, sedatives), brainstem infarct, high C-spine injury, obesity hypoventilation syndrome (ie, Pickwickian syndrome)
Nerve or muscular disorders	Paralysis, muscular dystrophy or other myopathies, myasthenia gravis, toxins (ie, organophosphate, snake envenomations), Guillain–Barré, ALS
Airway issues	Upper airway obstruction, laryngospasm, bronchospasm
Respiratory issues	Asthma, COPD, CHF, pneumonia, ILD, aspiration, ARDS, inadequate mechanical ventilation
Chest wall trauma	Flail chest, PTX, hemothorax, diaphragmatic paralysis, kyphoscoliosis

Respiratory Alkalosis	
Pathophysiology	**Differential**
Cardiac, respiratory	Pulmonary edema, pulmonary embolism, restrictive lung dz, mechanical hyperventilation
Psychiatric, neurologic	Hyperventilation syndromes (eg, anxiety, pain, stress), meningoencephalitis, tumor, trauma, CVA
Infection	Fever, pneumonia, sepsis
GI	Liver failure
Meds, other	Salicylates, hyperthyroidism, high altitude, anemia, pregnancy

Treatment and Disposition
- Both will largely depend on severity & underlying etiology of the disorder
- Limited role for bicarbonate in the absence of hemodynamic collapse

ABNORMAL ELECTROLYTES

Hyponatremia

Definition
- Na <135, excess of water relative to sodium, usually from elevated ADH; generally not symptomatic at Na >125

History
- Most sxs are nonspecific: Fatigue, weakness, muscle cramps, thirst, or postural dizziness. Severe sxs include confusion, agitation, delirium, lethargy, somnolence, coma, or szs.
- Other helpful historical features include h/o CHF, cirrhosis, renal dz, cancer, adrenal or pituitary dysfxn, recent GI surgery, thiazide or loop diuretics use, alcoholism

Physical Exam
- Look for signs to assess pt fluid status:
  - Hypervolemia: Elevated JVP, peripheral edema, crackles, ascites, anasarca
  - Hypovolemia: Tachycardia, hypotension, dry mucous membranes, oliguria, poor skin turgor, IVC collapsibility
- Look for signs of profound hyponatremia: Lethargic, disoriented/abnl sensorium, depressed reflexes, hypothermic, pseudobulbar palsy, Cheyne–Stokes respiration

Diagnostics
- **Labs:** BMP, FSG, urine electrolytes (Na, Cr, Osm), serum Osm, albumin
- VBG w/ stat sodium & Osm may provide more rapid turnaround
- **Corrected Na$_{glucose}$ = Serum Na + [0.016 × (serum glucose − 100)]** up to 400 mg/dL
- for glucose >400 mg/dL, 4 mEq/L should be added to every additional 100 mg/dL

Step-wise Approach to Hyponatremia
- **Step 1:** What is the serum osmolality?

Causes of Hyponatremia by Serum Osmolality		
Hypertonic HypoNa	**Isotonic HypoNa**	**Hypotonic HypoNa**
Hyperglycemia	Lab/blood draw error	Etiology based on volume status.
Mannitol	Hyperparaproteinemia	*See Step 2
Glycerol	HL	⇓
Sorbitol	Post TURP (bladder irrigation w/ osmotic solutions)	
Nl serum osmolality = 275–290 mosmol/kg		

- **Step 2:** What is the pt's volume status? Hypervolemic, euvolemic, or hypovolemic?
- **Step 3:** What are the urine Na, urine Osm, & FeNA values?
  - **Fractional Excretion of Sodium = FeNa = (Na$_{urine}$ × Cr$_{serum}$)/(Na$_{serum}$ × Cr$_{urine}$)**

Assessing Causes of Hypotonic Hyponatremia by Volume Status and Urine Analysis				
Volume Status	**Urine Na**	**Urine Osm**	**FeNa**	**Etiology**
Hypervolemic	>20		>1%	Renal failure
	<10		<1%	CHF, cirrhosis, nephrosis
Euvolemic		>100		SIADH, *hypothyroidism, glucocorticoid deficiency
		<100		Psychogenic polydipsia (>12 L fluid/d), low solute (beer potamania, tea/toast diet, dilution of infant formula)
		Variable		Chronic malnutrition (anorexia), pregnancy
Hypovolemic	>20		>1%	Renal losses: Diuretic use, osmotic diuresis, salt-wasting nephropathy, mineralocorticoid deficiency, nonoliguric ATN
	<10		<1%	Extrarenal losses: Vomiting, diarrhea, NGT drainage, 3rd spacing (pancreatitis, SBO), sweating

*Pneumonia, asthma, COPD, SCLC, pneumothorax, trauma, CVA, hemorrhage, tumors, infection, hydrocephalus, antipsychotics/antidepressants, chemo, vasopressin, postoperative.

Treatment
- Asymptomatic or mild sxs of hyponatremia: Correct serum Na at ≤0.5 mEq/L/h
- Severe manifestations of hyponatremia: RAPID correction serum Na at 2 mEq/L/h × 2–3 h OR until sxs resolve

IV Fluid Management		
Total Body Water (TBW) = Weight (kg) × 0.6 (use 0.5 if female or elderly, 0.6 for infants)		
Rate of Infusion (cc/h) = $\dfrac{1000 \times [\text{TBW} \times (\text{desired Na} - \text{serum Na})]}{[\text{Na(mmol/L)}_{\text{infusate}} \times \text{time(h)}]}$		
Infusate concentrations:		
LR: 130 mmol/L	NS: 154 mmol/L	3% NS: 513

Requires checking serum Na *(& Glu) q1h

- Euvolemic hyponatremia
  - Asymptomatic: Free water restrict (500–1000 mL/day)
  - Symptomatic: See above
- SIADH
  - Free water restrict + treat underlying cause
  - Caution if using hypertonic or nl saline esp if IVF Osm < urine Osm, serum sodium may worsen (higher Osm will draw out fluid)
  - Consider lithium or demeclocycline – nephrogenic DI (NEJM 2007;356:2064)
- Hypovolemic hyponatremia
  - Volume replete w/ nl saline, as above (once dehydration resolved, stimulation of ADH will decline & Na will correct)
- Hypervolemic hyponatremia
  - Free water restrict (0.5–1.5 L/d)
  - Increase arterial volume: W/ vasodilators (Nitro), loop diuretics; consider albumin in cirrhosis
  - Severe hyponatremia: Consider diuresis + Na replacement

Disposition
- Home: Mild asymptomatic hyponatremia
- Admit: Symptomatic, comorbidities, elderly. May require ICU admission if severe.

Pearl
- Rapid correction >10–12 mEq/L/d may result in central pontine myelinolysis (dysarthria, szs, quadriparesis due to focal myelin destruction in pons & extrapontine areas)

Hypernatremia
Definition
- Na >145, usually from free water loss or sodium gain (eg, infusion of hypertonic fluid)
- Appropriate response to hypernatremia is increased free water intake stimulated by thirst & renal excretion of a minimal volume of maximally concentrated urine as regulated by ADH

History
- Mild sxs include increased thirst or polyuria
- Severe sxs: AMS (irritability, lethargy, confusion, delirium, coma)
- RFs: Elderly, infants, debilitated. Endocrine pathology; cardiac, renal, liver dz; psychiatric disorder (see Etiology of Central and Nephrogenic Diabetes Insipidus); MEDS (see below chart), living situation (access to free water).

Physical Exam
- Look for signs to assess pt fluid status:
  - Hypervolemia: Elevated JVP, peripheral edema, crackles, ascites, anasarca
  - Hypovolemia: Tachycardia, hypotension, dry mucous membranes, oliguria, poor skin turgor, IVC collapsibility
  - Severe hypernatremia: Lethargy, muscle spasticity, tremor, hyperreflexia, respiratory paralysis, ataxia

Diagnostics
- **Labs:** BMP, FSG, urine electrolytes (Na, Cr, Osm), serum Osm, albumin
- VBG w/ stat sodium & Osm may provide more rapid turnaround
- **Corrected Na$_{glucose}$** = Serum Na + [0.016 × (serum glucose − 100)] up to 400 mg/dL
  - For glucose >400 mg/dL, 4 mEq/L should be added to every additional 100 mg/dL

Step-wise Approach to Hypernatremia
- **Step 1:** What is the serum osmolality?
  - Nl serum osmolality = 275–290 mosmol/kg
- **Step 2:** What is the pt's volume status? Hypervolemic, euvolemic, or hypovolemic?
- **Step 3:** What are the urine Na & urine Osm values?

Assessing Causes of Hypernatremia by Volume Status and Urine Analysis			
Volume Status	**Urine Na**	**Urine Osm**	**Etiology**
Hypervolemic	>20		**Increased Sodium Absorption:** Cushing dz, adrenal hyperplasia, exogenous steroids, mineralocorticoid excess
Euvolemic		<300	Complete DI (central & nephrogenic)*
		300–600	Partial DI (central & nephrogenic)*
		>600	**Exogenous Sodium Intake:** Hypertonic saline, sodium bicarb tablets, sea water ingestion, concentrated infant formula
Hypovolemic	>20	300–600	**Renal Water Losses:** Loop diuretic, osmotic diuresis (mannitol, urea)
	<20	>600	**Extrarenal Water Losses:** Vomiting, diarrhea, NGT drainage, szs, exercise, severe burns, fever, 3rd spacing **Decreased Water Intake:** Defective thirst mechanism, dementia, AMS, infancy, intubation

*Central DI: Congenital, trauma/surgery, tumors, hypothalamic deficiency, pituitary deficiency, hypoxic encephalopathy, anorexia, idiopathic. Nephrogenic DI: Congenital, drugs (lithium, amphotericin, demeclocycline, foscarnet, cidofovir), hypercalcemia, severe hypokalemia, protein malnutrition, polycystic kidney dz, sickle cell, Sjögren, amyloid, pregnancy.

Treatment

IV Fluid Management*
Free water deficit (Liters) = Total Body Water × [1 − (140/serum Na)]
Total body water (TBW) = Weight (kg) × 0.6 (use 0.5 if female or elderly; 0.6 for children)
Hourly maintenance (mL/h) = Free Water Deficit (mL)/24 h
Rate of Infusion (cc/h) = $\dfrac{1000 \times [\text{TBW} \times (\text{serum Na} - \text{desired Na})]}{[\text{Na}]_{\text{infusate}} \times \text{time (h)}}$

Infusate concentrations
D$_5$W: 0 mEq   ¼ NS: 38 mEq   ½ NS: 77 mEq

*Requires checking serum Glucose & Na q1h. Rate of Na correction should NOT exceed 0.5 mEq/L/h to avoid cerebral edema. Urine output: >0.5 cc/kg/h.

- Hypervolemic hypernatremia
  - Treat underlying disorder
  - Replace free water deficit (as above)
- Euvolemic hypernatremia
  - Replace free water deficit (as above)
  - Treat underlying etiology
  - Central DI: Vasopressin 10 U SQ
- Hypovolemic hypernatremia
  - Restore volume 1st then replace free water deficit (as above); add 40 mEq KCl IV to fluid replacement once pt is urinating

Disposition
- Home: Mild hypernatremia which can be corrected in <24 h
- Admit: Likely admit

Hypokalemia
Definition
- K$^+$ <3.5 mEq/L (ie, decreased intake, shift into cells, loss); 98% of potassium is intracellular

Hypokalemia Differential	
Pathophysiology	**Differential**
GI	Poor oral intake; diarrhea, vomiting, & NG tube drainage
Endocrine	High insulin levels, hyperaldosteronism, alkalosis, DKA, Cushing dz, hypomagnesemia
Renal	Renal tubular acidosis (type 2), renovascular dz, Bartter syndrome, Liddle syndrome
Meds/toxins	Thiazide & loop diuretics, insulin, β-2 agonists, α-antagonists, amphotericin B, laxative abuse, exogenous mineralocorticoid use, massive blood transfusions, barium tox, toluene tox

History
- Usually not symptomatic until K^+ <3 mEq/L.
- Nausea, vomiting, weakness, fatigue, myalgia, muscle cramps.
- Pts at highest risk for electrocardiac cx of hypokalemia include those w/ acute ischemia, prolonged QT syndrome, & those taking digoxin

Physical Exam
- Paresthesias, depressed reflexes, proximal muscle weakness, ileus
- Severe hypokalemia: Hypoventilation, spasm, paralysis, rhabdomyolysis, myoglobinuria
- ARF, polymorphic VT, asystole

Diagnostics
- **Labs:** BMP, UA, urine electrolytes, urine Osm; consider blood gas, CPK, serum Osm
- Urine K^+ <15 mmol/d suggests extrarenal, while urine K^+ >15 mmol/d suggests renal etiology
- Transtubular K^+ concentration gradient (TTKG) is helpful, but rarely used in the ED: **TTKG = $(Plasma_{Osm} \times Urine_K)/(Plasma_K \times Urine_{Osm})$**

Note: Hypokalemia w/ TTKG >4 suggests renal K^+ loss due to distal K^+ secretion

- **ECG:** T-wave flattening/inversion, ST depression, U-waves, prolonged QT/QU interval; may also see PR prolongation, decreased voltage, QRS widening, atrial/ventricular dysrhythmias

Treatment
- ED
  - Potassium replacement: Potassium chloride, Potassium bicarbonate, Potassium phosphate

> (Drop 1 mEq/L = 200–400 mEq total body loss)
> Mild (K^+ >2.8 mEq/L): 40 mEq K^+ PO q4–6h
> Moderate/severe: 40 mEq K^+ PO q4h (if tolerating oral) + KCl 10 mEq/h IV, recheck K^+ q4h

  - Treat underlying cause
  - Replace Mg as needed (*Note: Concurrent Mg & K^+ deficiency could lead to refractory K^+ repletion)
  - Goal K^+ = 4 mEq/L in pts at highest risk
- Home
  - Counsel pts to increase dietary intake of K^+ (dried fruits, nuts, avocados, wheat germ lima beans, vegetables [spinach, broccoli, cauliflower, beets, carrots], fruits [banana, kiwi, etc])
  - Discuss w/ PCP: Decrease diuretic dose; start/substitute for K^+-sparing med (βB, ACE, ARB, K^+-sparing diuretic)
  - Potassium replacement: KCl 20 mEq PO QD for prevention; KCl 40–100 mEq PO QD for tx

Disposition
- Home: Mild hypokalemia w/ close f/u to recheck labs
- Admit: Moderate/severe hypokalemia, acid–base abnormalities, arrhythmia, severe sxs

Pearl
- Avoid dextrose solutions (stimulate insulin & inward shift of K^+)

Guideline: Cohn JN, Kowey PR, Whelton PK, Prisant LM. New guidelines for potassium replacement in clinical practice. Arch Intern Med. 2000;160:2429–2436.

Hyperkalemia

Definition
- K+>5 mEq/L (ie, K+ release from cells, decreased renal losses, iatrogenic)

Hyperkalemia Differential	
Pathophysiology	**Differential**
Endocrine/metabolic	Hypoaldosteronism, DKA, other acidoses
Renal	Renal insufficiency, end-stage renal failure, renal tubular acidosis (type 4), diabetic nephropathy, Gordon's syndrome
Other	Tumor lysis syndrome, hemolysis, rhabdomyolysis, *pseudohyperkalemia (hemolyzed blood sample, prolonged tourniquet), exercise
Meds	NSAIDs, ACE−, ARBs, heparin, TMP–SMX, pentamidine βBs, digoxin poisoning, K+ sparing diuretics, exogenous KCl supplements, cyclosporine, *succinylcholine

*Pseudohyperkalemia should be suspected in o/w asymptomatic pts w/o underlying causes. Repeated K+ should be obtained prior to initiating tx in such cases.

History
- Weakness, muscle cramps, paresthesias, nausea, palpitations. Meds (see *Differential table*).

Physical Exam
- Paresthesias, tetany; assess fluid status
- Severe hyperkalemia: Flaccid paralysis, hypoventilation, PEA arrest, or asystole

Diagnostics
- Labs: BMP; consider blood gas w/ stat K+, UA, urine electrolytes, urine Osm, CPK
- ECG: Early: Peaked & symmetric T waves, flattened P waves, PR prolongation, 1° AVB. Late: Widening/slurring of QRS → sinusoidal waveform → VFib or asystole

Hyperkalemia Treatment			
Intervention	**Dose**	**Onset**	**Effect**
Calcium gluconate OR Calcium chloride***	1–2 amps IV	Few minutes	Stabilizes cell membrane; used in pts w/ cardiac conduction abnormalities (no direct effect on K+)
Bicarbonate	1–2 amps	15–30 min (up to 2 h)	Transient K+ into cells in exchange for H+ (may ↓ K+ 0.47 mmol/L)
Albuterol (β-agonist)	10–20 mg inh or 0.5–2.5 mg IV	30–90 min	Transient K+ into cells (↓ K+ 0.3–0.99 mmol/L)
Insulin + D50W	10 U IV + 1 amp D50W	15–30 min, lasts 2–4 h	Transient K+ into cells (↓K+ 0.45–1 mmol/L)
Kayexalate***	30–90 g PO/PR	90 min for PO, 30 min for PR	Decreases total body K+ by exchanging Na for K+ in gut
Diuretics (Furosemide)	≥40 mg IV	30 min	Decreases total body K+
HD (emergent)			Decreases total body K+ (pts w/ cardiac cx or new/worsened renal failure)

*Standard teaching is not to use calcium in digitalis tox → hypercalcemia may potentiate the tox; however, recent data shows that this may be inaccurate.

**Calcium chloride contains 3 times more calcium ion, onset in seconds to minutes & lasts 30 min, but much more caustic to veins than Calcium gluconate.

***May cause intestinal necrosis in pts w/ postoperative ileus; may also worsen pulmonary edema in pts w/ fluid overload; data on its efficacy at reducing total body potassium is poor.

Treatment
- Continuous cardiac monitoring
- Treating underlying cause
- Check electrolytes every 2–4 h until normalized

Disposition
- Home: Only if mild, stable hyperkalemia with good outpatient f/u
- Admit: Most pts will require admission; may require ICU admission

Pearls

- Think "ABCD" (albuterol, bicarbonate, calcium, dextrose/insulin, dialysis, diuretics)
- Combination therapy is proven more efficacious than any therapy alone
- HD is the most rapid & effective way of lowering plasma K^+

Hypocalcemia

Definition

- Ca <8.5 mg/dL (2 mmol/L) OR ionized Ca <4.5 mg/dL (1.1 mmol/L); 50% bound to albumin, 40% is free, 10% complexed to anions

Hypocalcemia Etiology		
Pathophysiology	**PTH**	**Differential**
Endocrine	↓	Hypoparathyroidism [familial, autoimmune, infiltrative, iatrogenic: Surgery, neck irradiation], DiGeorge syndrome, hypomagnesemia
Vit D deficiency	↑	Nutritional/sunlight deprivation; malabsorption; drugs (anticonvulsants, rifampin, ketoconazole, 5-FU/leucovorin); genetic; renal insufficiency (impaired production)
Renal	↑	Chronic renal failure, ARF (elevated phosphorous)
Neoplasm	↑	Osteoblastic metastases, tumor lysis (elevated phosphorous)
Other	↑	Pancreatitis, multiple blood transfusions, rhabdomyolysis, burns, prematurity, pseudohypoparathyroidism

History

- Weakness, muscle cramps, paresthesias, irritability, depression, tetany, AMS. Meds (see *Differential* table).

Physical Exam

- Paresthesias; Chvostek sign (tap over facial nerve causing facial twitching); +Trousseau sign (inflate a BP cuff to 20 mmHg above systolic BP over bicep × 3 min to cause carpal spasm); may also see psychosis, szs, ↑ ICP, bronchospasm, laryngospasm

Diagnostics

- Labs: BMP w/ Ca/Mg/Phosphorus testing. Check ionized calcium level, albumin, consider PTH for continued inpt w/u:

Corrected Ca = measured serum calcium (mg/dL) + [0.8 × (4-serum albumin (g/dL))]

- ECG: *Prolonged QTc*, heart blocks, ventricular dysrhythmias, torsade

Treatment

- Asymptomatic: Oral elemental Ca (1–3 g/d in divided doses)
- Symptomatic: [10% Calcium gluconate (1–2 g IV over 20 min) OR 10% Calcium chloride (1–2 g IV diluted in 100 cc D_5W to decrease tissue irritation)], ± Vit D, ± Mg (50–100 mEq/d)

Disposition

- Home: Asymptomatic, w/ oral regimen described above & PCP f/u in 5–7 d to recheck electrolytes
- Admit: Severe hypocalcemia, comorbid conditions, HD unstable

Hypercalcemia

Definition

- Ca >10.5 mg/dL; usually asymptomatic at levels up to 11.5 mg/dL

Hypercalcemia Etiology		
Pathophysiology	**PTH**	**Differential**
Excess PTH prod	↑	1° hyperparathyroidism* (adenoma, hyperplasia, rarely adenoCa), 3° hyperparathyroidism (renal insufficiency), FHH
Vit D excess	↓	Sarcoidosis, TB, histoplasmosis, Wegener granulomatosis, Vit D intoxication, lymphoma
↑ bone resorption	↓	Hyperthyroidism, immobilization
Neoplasm*	↓	PTHrP-producing solid tumors (squamous cell, renal bladder), lytic lesions (breast, myeloma), Paget dz
Other	↓	Meds (lithium, Vit A, thiazides, Ca-based antacids), massive dairy, consumption (milk–alkali syndrome), TPN, endocrine d/o (adrenal insufficiency, VIPoma)

*Most common causes of hypercalcemia.

History

- Polyuria, polydipsia, dehydration, nausea, vomiting, depression, confusion, coma, AMS; abdominal pain, anorexia, constipation, bone pain, Meds (see *Differential table*)
- May cause pancreatitis, nephrolithiasis, pathologic fractures thus suspect hypercalcemia in pts presenting w/ sxs consistent w/ these diagnoses

Physical Exam

- General weakness, epigastric tenderness, depressed deep tendon reflexes, coma

Diagnostics

- Labs: BMP w/ Ca/Mg/Phosphorus testing, ionized Ca, lipase (if considering pancreatitis), urine electrolytes, albumin (see corrected Ca equation above), consider PTH
- ECG: *Shortened QTc*, PR prolongation, QRS widening; rarely BBB, sinus bradycardia or high-degree AV block

Treatment

- Address/treat underlying causes

Hypercalcemia Acute Treatment			
Intervention	Dose	Onset/Duration	Effect
NS	4–6 L/d	Hours	Promote calcium excretion (Ca can drop 2 mEq)
Furosemide	20–60 mg IV q6h	Hours	Promotes calcium excretion; hold if intravascularly dry
Bisphosphonates (pamidronate, zoledronic acid, alendronate)	Variable	Days	Inhibit osteoclasts (esp useful in malignancy), caution in renal failure pt
Hypercalcemic antidote (calcitonin, plicamycin)	Calcitonin: 4 IU/kg q12h Plicamycin: 25 mcg/kg IV over 4 h	Hours, lasts days	Direct RNA inhibitor, may develop tachyphylaxis
Hydrocortisone	200–300 mg IV QD	Days	Useful only for Vit D toxic pts, multiple myeloma, sarcoid & lymphoma pts
HD			Useful in renal failure pts

Disposition

- Home: Mild stable hypercalcemia
- Admit: Most will need admission until resolution

Pearl

- Hypercalcemia = stones, bones, moans, abdominal groans, & psychiatric overtones

Hypomagnesemia
Definition

- Mg <0.7 mmol/L

Hypomagnesemia Differential	
Pathophysiology	Differential
Cardiac	CHF
GI	V/D, NGT suctioning, malabsorption
Renal	Chronic renal failure (causing tertiary hypoparathyroidism)
Endocrine	Hyperaldosteronism, Vit D deficiency
Other/Meds	Alcoholism, pregnancy, thiazide & loop diuretics, aminoglycosides, amphotericin, gentamicin, pentamidine, tobramycin

History

- Weakness, AMS, muscle cramps. Meds (see *Differential table*).

Physical Exam

- Tetany, Chvostek/Trousseau signs, papilledema, hyperreflexia

Diagnostics

- Labs: BMP w/ Ca/Mg/Phosphorus testing, ionized Ca, albumin, consider PTH for continued inpt w/u.
- ECG: Similar to hypokalemia & hypocalcemia (prolonged intervals, T-wave flattening, widening of QRS, U waves)

Treatment
- Address underlying cause
- Magnesium replacement: 50% magnesium sulfate 2–4 g (16.6–33 mEq) IV over 30 min. Oral form may cause diarrhea (eg, magnesium citrate, milk of magnesia).
- Alcoholics: Consider thiamine; phosphorous & potassium replacement as needed

Disposition
- Home: Mild hypomagnesemia
- Admit: Severe hypomagnesemia w/ other associated electrolyte abnormalities (potassium, calcium), comorbid conditions

Pearl
- Most exogenously administered Mg will be excreted in urine; full Mg replacement takes days

Hypermagnesemia
Definition
- Mg >3 mEq/L

Hypermagnesemia Differential	
Pathophysiology	**Differential**
GI	Chronic constipation, bowel obstruction
Renal	Acute or chronic renal failure
Autoimmune/endocrine	DKA, adrenal insufficiency, hyperparathyroidism, hypothyroidism
Other/Meds	Hemolysis, lithium, exogenous Mg infusions, opioids, anticholinergics, tumor lysis syndrome, milk–alkali syndrome, rhabdomyolysis

History
- Nausea, vomiting, lethargy, weakness, AMS; depends on level (renal insufficiency, GI motility disorder, adrenal insufficiency, hyperparathyroidism), Meds (anticholinergic, narcotic, lithium)

Physical Exam
- Depends on level
  - Mg >3 mEq/L: N/V cutaneous flushing
  - Mg >4 mEq/L: Hyporeflexia
  - Mg >5 mEq/L: Hypotension
  - Mg >9 mEq/L: Respiratory depression, shock, coma
  - Mg >10 mEq/L: Asystole

Diagnostics
- Labs: BMP w/ Ca/Mg/Phosphorus testing, ionized Ca, albumin
- ECG: QRS widening, QT prolongation, prolonged AV conduction → complete block

Treatment
- Calcium:
  - Immediate: Calcium gluconate IV or Calcium chloride (see *Hypocalcemia*)
  - Continuous: 10% Calcium gluconate 2–4 mg/kg/h if indicated
- Diuretics: Loop diuretics + aggressive hydration (improve excretion)
- Dialysis: Particularly for pts in renal failure

Disposition
- Home: Asymptomatic, stable
- Admit: All need admission until sxs & lab values have normalized

Pearls
- Magnesium abnormalities are often seen w/ K⁺ or calcium abnormalities
- Check serial DTRs to assess toxicity in preeclamptic pts receiving Mg

Hypoglycemia
Definition
- Glucose <60 mg/dL; however, clinical hypoglycemia is any plasma glucose level low enough to cause sxs or signs c/w hypoglycemia (see below). Usually <55 mg/dL causes sx.
- Whipple's triad: Sign/sxs of hypoglycemia, low plasma glucose, resolution of sx when plasma glucose is raised

Hypoglycemia Differential	
Pathophysiology	**Differential**
Medications*	Insulin, sulfonylureas (glyburide, glipizide, glimepiride), Meglitinides (repaglinide, nateglinide), alcohol
GI	Liver failure, post-gastrectomy/gastric bypass
Renal	ARF
Endocrine	Hypothyroidism, insulinoma (including MEN-1), hypopituitarism, adrenal insufficiency, insulin autoimmune hypoglycemia (Ab to insulin or its receptor)
Other	Sepsis, starvation, accidental/surreptitious/malicious hypoglycemia

*Most common cause of hypoglycemia.

History

- Neurogenic/autonomic sxs: Agitation, tremor, diaphoresis, palpitations, pallor, hunger
- Neuroglycopenic sxs: Fatigue, HA, AMS, lethargy, somnolence, coma, sz
- Take detailed med hx (see *Differential table*); consider new meds, med dose changes, incorrect use, intentional/accidental overdose, OTC/naturopathic meds, AKI
- Diabetics: Inquire recent FSG values (if taken), last meal, dietary changes, excess exercise
- ROS of contributing causes: Fever, chills, cough, abdominal pain, diarrhea, urinary sx, etc.
- RFs: Diabetics (esp on insulin), alcoholics, infants, elderly, s/p gastric bypass, critically ill

Diagnostics

- Labs: FSG, BMP; consider infectious w/u (CBC, UA, CXR)

*In o/w healthy, nondiabetics, consider LFTs, TSH, insulin, β-hydroxybutyrate, proinsulin, & C-peptide (low in exogenous insulin, high in insulinoma or sulfonylureas) in consultation w/ an endocrine specialist

- Serial glucose assessments may be necessary when prolonged hypoglycemia is expected in pts unable to communicate (eg, dementia, delirium, comatose, infants)

Treatment

- Glucose replacement:
  - PO: Glucose paste/tablets (20 g), fruit juice, soft drinks, candy, a meal, etc.
  - IV: 1 amp D_{50}; infusion may be needed
  - IM: 0.5–1 mg IM or SC glucagon (may cause N/V)

Disposition

- Home: Identifiable cause, does not need further monitoring
  - Prompt f/u w/ primary care or endocrinologist should be arranged
  - Pts should keep a glucose diary & should become concerned about the possibility of developing hypoglycemia when self-monitored glucose levels fall rapidly or is no greater than 70 mg/dL
- Admit: Long-acting hypoglycemic agents, unable to tolerate POs, HD unstable

Pearls

- βBs can mask adrenergic signs of hypoglycemia
- Efforts should be made to contact pt's primary physician or endocrinologist

Guideline: Cryer PE, Axelrod L, Grossman AB, Heller SR, Montori VM, Seaquist ER, Service FJ. Evaluation and management of adult hypoglycemic disorders: An Endocrine Society clinical practice guideline. *J Clin Endocrinol Metab.* 2009;94:709–728.

HYPERGLYCEMIC EMERGENCIES (DKA/HHS)

Criteria for Diabetic Ketoacidosis (DKA) and Hyperosmolar Hyperglycemic State				
	DKA (glucose >250 mg/dL)			**HHS (glucose >600 mg/dL)**
	Mild	**Moderate**	**Severe**	
Arterial pH	7.25–7.30	7–<7.24	<7	>7.3
Serum bicarbonate (mEq/L)	15–18	10 to <15	<10	>18
Urine ketone	+	+	+	Small
Serum ketone	+	+	+	Small
Serum osmolality	Variable	Variable	Variable	>320 mOsm/kg

| | DKA (glucose >250 mg/dL) | | | HHS (glucose >600 mg/dL) |
	Mild	Moderate	Severe	
Anion gap	>10	>12	>12	Variable
Mental status	Alert	Alert/drowsy	Stupor/coma	Stupor/coma

Adapted from: Kitabchi AE, Umpierrez GE, Miles JM, Fisher JN. Hyperglycemic crises in adult patients with diabetes. Diabetes Care. 2009;32(7):1335–1343.

Diabetic Ketoacidosis and Hyperosmolar Hyperglycemic State

Definition
- See above for consensus diagnostic criteria. DKA characterized by uncontrolled hyperglycemia, metabolic acidosis, & increased ketone body concentration. HHS characterized by profound hyperglycemia & serum hyperosmolality, nl arterial pH & bicarbonate, & AMS.
- Marked by insulin deficiency & increased counter-regulatory hormones
- HHS generally occurs in Type II diabetes; DKA generally occurs in Type I diabetes, but may occur in Type II diabetes w/ stressors:

5 I's of DKA	
Etiology	Cause
Insulin deficiency	New-onset T1DM, failure to take enough insulin
Infection*	Pneumonia, UTI, cellulitis, etc.
Inflammation	Pancreatitis
Intoxication	Alcohol, drugs
Iatrogenesis	Glucocorticoids, thiazides, sympathomimetics, antipsychotics
Other	AMI, CVA, eating d/o in pts w/ T1DM

*Most common precipitating factor.

History
- DKA often more acute in onset, c/w HHS which evolves over days to weeks
- Polyuria, polydipsia, N/V, dehydration, weight loss, abdominal pain, visual changes, AMS
- Take detailed med hx (see *Differential table*); consider new meds, med dose changes, incorrect use, intentional/accidental overdose, OTC/naturopathic meds, insulin pump use
- ROS of contrib causes: Fever, chills, cough, abdominal pain, diarrhea, urinary sx, depression
- RFs: Insulin pump users

Physical Exam
- Appears dry, Kussmaul respiration, lethargy, coma; abdominal tenderness (ileus)

Evaluation
- Labs: FSG, BMP (elevated anion gap acidosis, pseudohyponatremia, total body K^+ generally depleted despite lab value), Ca/Mg/Phosphorus, urine/serum ketones, β-hydroxybutyrate, nitroprusside test, UA, CBC, lactate, lipase, LFTs, serum osmolality, VBG, urine hCG; ABG if HD unstable or comatose; blood cultures, urines cultures if clinically indicated

Equations
Anion gap (AG) = (Na − (Cl + bicarb))
Corrected AG = AG + (2.5 × [4.2 − albumin])
Calculated Osm = (2 × [Na^+]) + glucose/18 + BUN/2.8 + Ethanol/4.6
Corrected Na = Serum Na + [0.016 × (serum glucose − 100)]
(up to 400 mg/dL; for glucose >400 mg/dL, 4 mEq/L should be added to every additional 100 mg/dL)

- ECG: If older than 30 yr
- Imaging: CXR (r/o infection); may need abdominal CT or U/S if clinically indicated

Treatment
- Supportive: Continuous cardiac monitoring, 2 large-bore IVs
- Electrolyte monitoring: Glucose fingerstick q1h; BMP, Ca/Mg/Phosphorus, VBG q2–4h

Acute Treatment	
Medication	**Dose/Frequency**
IV hydration***	NS bolus + NS 15–20 cc/kg/h (adjust for dehydration & cardiovascular status); usually 1–1.5 L during 1st hour →Continue NS 250–500 cc/h if corrected Na low →Δ IVF to ½ NS 250–500 cc/h if corrected Na nl or high →Δ IVF to D5 ½ NS 150–250 cc/h when glucose ≤200 mg/dL
Insulin	0.1 U/kg (regular insulin) IV push × 1, followed by 0.1 U/kg/h Persistent anion gap: Continue drip Resolution of anion gap: Change to SC insulin (overlap IV w/ SC by 1–2 h) →When glucose ≤200 mg/dL in DKA & ≤300 mg/dL in HHS, reduce insulin infusion to 0.02–0.05 U/kg/h IV, or Δ to rapid acting insulin at 0.1 U/kg q2h
Electrolyte repletion	Potassium: Goal to maintain K+ 4–5 mEq/L →Add 20–40 mEq/L IVFs if serum K+ <4.5 (insulin promotes K+ entry into cells, but careful w/ renal pts) →Hold insulin & give K+ 20–40 mEq/h if K+ <3.3 HCO_3: If cardiac unstable or pH <7 Phosphate: Replete if <1 (20–30 mEq/L KPhos added to IVF)

*After volume resuscitation, choice of fluid replacement will depend on hemodynamics, hydration status electrolytes, etc.

**IVF volume should be used w/ caution in pts w/ cardiac or renal impairment.

Adapted from: Kitabchi AE, Umpierrez GE, Miles JM, Fisher JN. Hyperglycemic crises in adult patients with diabetes. *Diabetes Care.* 2009;32(7):1335–1343.

Disposition
- Home: None
- Admit: All pts will require admission, may need ICU monitoring

Pearls
- ~10% of the DKA population may present w/ glucose ≤250 mg/dL
- An initial insulin bolus may not be necessary as some pts respond to fluid resuscitation
- Consider increasing continuous insulin dose if glucose does not decrease 50–75 mg/dL/h
- Tx w/ SC rapid-acting insulin q1–2h is an effective alternative to IV regular insulin
- Cx: Hypoglycemia, hypokalemia, fluid overload, cerebral edema

THYROID EMERGENCIES

Hypothyroidism/Myxedema Coma
Definition
- Hypothyroidism is characterized by insufficient production of thyroid hormone by the thyroid gland. Cretinism is a form of hypothyroidism found in infants.
- Hypothyroidism can be classified on the basis of its time of onset (congenital or acquired), the level of endocrine Dysfxn (1° [thyroid] or 2° [pituitary or hypothalamic]), & its severity (subclinical, clinical, severe [myxedema coma])
- Myxedema coma is a rare, extreme expression of severe hypothyroidism. Myxedema coma typically occurs in pts who develop systemic illness superimposed on previously undiagnosed hypothyroidism.

Hypothyroidism Differential	
	Cause
Endocrine	Hashimoto (autoimmune thyroiditis, subacute thyroiditis (de Quervain's thyroiditis), lymphocytic thyroiditis (postpartum thyroiditis), hypothalamic or pituitary failure, iodine deficiency
Iatrogenic	Surgical removal & XRT
Meds/toxins	Radioactive iodine (therapeutic or environmental), amiodarone, lithium, stavudine, interferon α, polybrominated/polychlorinated biphenyls, resorcinol (textile workers)
Other	Congenital hypothyroidism (endemic iodine deficiency, thyroid gland dysgenesis, defective thyroid hormone biosynthesis); hemochromatosis

Adapted from: Roberts, CG, Ladenson PW. Hypothyroidism. *Lancet.* 2004;363(9411):793–803.

Factors Precipitating Myxedema Coma	
• Infection (sepsis, PNA, UTI) • CVA • CHF • Hypothermia • GIB	• Trauma, burns • Metabolic disturbances (hypoglycemia, hyponatremia, acidosis, hypercapnia, hypercalcemia) • Meds (anesthetics, sedatives, opioids, amiodarone, lithium, withdrawal of L-thyroxine) • Ingestion of raw bok choy

Adapted from: Klubo-Gwiezdzinska J, Wartofsky L. Thyroid emergencies. *Med Clin N Am*. 2012;96(2):385–403.

History
- Hypothyroidism: Weakness, fatigue, myalgias, HA, depression, cold intolerance, weight gain, constipation, menorrhagia, dry skin, brittle hair, hoarseness
- Myxedema coma: Severely altered mental status/coma
- Meds (see *Differential table*)
- RFs: Postpartum women, family h/o autoimmune thyroid disorders, prior H&N surgery or irradiation, other autoimmune disorders (ie, Type 1 DM, adrenal insufficiency, autoimmune polyendocrine syndrome types 1 & 2 etc.), Down's syndrome, Turner's syndrome

Physical Exam
- Hypothyroidism: Obese, delayed DTRs, diastolic HTN, dry, thick skin SQ tissue (myxedema), bradycardia, pl/pericardial/peritoneal effusion, hypothermia, hypotension, hypoventilation, altered sensorium
- Myxedema coma: Hypothermia & severely altered mental status/coma are hallmark
- Vitals/Pulm/CV: Hypothermia, hypoventilation, hypoxia, hypotension, or bradycardia
- HEENT: Facial swelling, periorbital edema, macroglossia
- Neuro: Lethargy → comatose, cerebellar signs, poor memory & cognition, delayed reflexes
- Psych: "Myxedema madness" disorientation, paranoia, depression, hallucinations, etc.

Evaluation
- Labs: TFTs (TSH elevated); BMP (hyponatremia, hypoglycemia), CBC (anemia); consider T4, free T4, T3, antimicrosomal Ab, antithyroid peroxidase Ab, antithyroglobulin Ab
  - ↑TSH, ↓ free T4 confirms primary hypothyroidism of any cause
  - ↑TSH, ↓ free T4, +antithyroid abs confirms Hashimoto thyroiditis
  - variable TSH, ↓ free T4 consistent w/ secondary hypothyroidsm disorders
  - mild ↑TSH, nl free T4, & subtle sxs consistent w/ subclinical hypothyroidism
- ECG: Myxedema-bradycardia, AV block, low voltage, flattened/inverted T-waves, prolonged QTc, atrial/ventricular dysrhythmias.
- Bedside cardiac u/s: Pericardial effusion/tamponade may be seen in myxedema

Treatment (Only Start Empiric Treatment if Severely Symptomatic/Coma)
- Thyroid replacement: (Start in ED if severely symptomatic/coma)
- Levothyroxine: 5–8 mcg/kg IV × 1, then 50–100 mcg QD; consider synthetic T3 5–10 mcg IV q8h (b/c peripheral conversion impaired, but is more arrhythmogenic)
- Adrenal replacement: Hydrocortisone 100 mg IV × q8h (decreased reserve in coma)

Disposition
- Home: Discuss w/ PCP prior to starting any thyroid medications; usual starting dose of Levothyroxine 1.8 µg/kg PO QD (required repeat TFTs at 4–6 wk)
- Admit: All pts w/ severe hypothyroidism/myxedema; may require ICU admission

Thyrotoxicosis/Hyperthyroidism/Thyroid Storm
Definition
- Thyrotoxicosis is a disorder of excess thyroid hormone
- Hyperthyroidism specifically describes overproduction & secretion of excess of free thyroid hormones: Thyroxine (T_4), triiodothyronine (T_3), or both
- Thyroid storm/crisis is a rare, extreme expression of severe thyrotoxicosis
- Precise criteria for thyroid storm have been defined (*Endocrinol Metab Clin North Am* 1993;22: 263–277)

	Differential
Thyrotoxicosis w/ Hyperthyroidism	
Endocrine	*Graves' dz, **toxic multinodular goiter, **solitary toxic adenoma, TSH-secreting pituitary adenoma
Neoplasm	Metastatic follicular thyroid carcinoma, struma ovarii, choriocarcinoma (hCG secretion)
Other/Meds	Amiodarone, iodine, & radiographic contrast agents
Thyrotoxicosis w/o Hyperthyroidism	
Thyroiditis	Early Hashimoto (autoimmune thyroiditis), subacute thyroiditis (de Quervain's thyroiditis), lymphocytic thyroiditis (postpartum thyroiditis), acute infectious thyroiditis, drug-induced thyroiditis (amiodarone, lithium, interferon α), radiation thyroiditis
Other	Exogenous thyroid hormone, "Hamburger" thyrotoxicosis, infarction of thyroid adenoma

*Most common cause of hyperthyroidism caused by autoantibodies to & stimulation of TSH receptors.
**Next most common causes of hyperthyroidism caused by autonomous overproduction of thyroid hormone secondary to activating mutations in TSHR or gene for functional autonomy, respectively. Adapted from: Franklyn JA, Boelaert K. Thyrotoxicosis. *Lancet.* 2012;379(9821):1156–1166.

Factors Precipitating Thyroid Storm	
• Infection (sepsis)	• Trauma (including vigorous thyroid palpation), burns
• Sz	• Postthyroidectomy
• PE	• Metabolic disturbances (hypoglycemia, DKA)
• Parturition	• Meds (amiodarone, radioactive iodine tx, iodinated contrast,
• Emotional stress	thyroxine/triiodothyronine OD, ASA OD, withdrawal of PTU/methimazole)

Adapted from: Klubo-Gwiezdzinska J, Wartofsky L. Thyroid emergencies. *Med Clin N Am* 2012;96(2):385–403.

History
- Neck fullness, double vision, restlessness, anxiety, palpitations, sweating, heat intolerance, tremor, weight loss, diarrhea, irregular menses, periodic paralysis, lethargy, hair thinning/loss
- Thyroid storm: AMS (delirium, agitation, coma), sz, fever, tachycardia, N/V, diarrhea
- Meds (see *Differential table*; assess h/o hyperthyroidism)

Physical Exam
- Thyrotoxicosis: Cachexia, diaphoretic, agitation, tremor, tachycardia, AFib, systolic HTN, widened pulse pressure
- Thyroid storm: Hyperthermia & severely AMS are hallmark
- Vitals/Pulm/CV: Hyperthermia, hyperventilation, tachycardia
- GI: Nausea, vomiting, diarrhea, diffuse abdominal pain (may mimic acute abdomen)
- Neuro: AMS (delirium, agitation, coma), sz
- Psych: Disorientation, paranoia, psychosis, etc.

Evaluation
- Labs: TSH (low) w/ elevated free T4 (if TSH low & free T4 nl, free or total T3 concentration should also be measured to identify potential T3 toxicosis; consider thyroxine-binding globulin in pregnancy); BMP/Ca/Mg/Phosphorus, LFTs, UA, urine hCG; consider TRH or thyroid peroxidase
- ECG: Tachycardia, supraventricular ectopy, AFib

Treatment (Only Start ED Treatment if Severely Symptomatic/Thyroid Storm)
- Thyrotoxicosis: Therapies include antithyroid meds (methimazole/PTU), radioiodine, surgery
- Thyroid storm: βB → PTU or methimazole → iodine or lithium → steroids w/ supportive care
  - βB: Propranolol or esmolol (improve α-adrenergic activity & tachycardia)
    - Propranolol 1 mg IV over 10 min, then 1–3 mg boluses q3h
    - Propranolol 60–80 mg q4h if taking PO
    - Esmolol 250–500 mcg/kg loading dose, then 50–100 mcg/kg/min
  - PTU: Blocks hormone synthesis, inhibits peripheral conversion of T4 to T3
    - Loading dose of 500–1000 mg, then 250 mg q4h
    - Preferred to methimazole, particularly if pregnant & 1st trimester
  - Methimazole: Blocks hormone synthesis
    - Dose 20 mg q4h (60–80 mg/d)
    - Pts should receive baseline CBC & LFTs prior to tx

- Iodine: Blocks thyroid hormone release but give >1 g after PTU (can potentiate thyroid storm if given before)
  - Potassium iodide 5 drops (0.25 mL or 250 mg) PO q6h
  - For iodine allergic pts, can use lithium carbonate 300 mg 6 h
- Steroids: Hydrocortisone 100–300 mg IV bolus, then 100 mg IV × q8h (can decrease conversion of T4–T3)
- Consider plasmapheresis & therapeutic plasma exchange (Graves' dz)
- Supportive care: Hyperpyrexia – APAP as needed; avoid aspirin (can increase T3 conversion)
- Treat underlying precipitant (often infection)

Disposition
- Home: TSH low but no severe sxs: F/u w/ PCP or endo RE: outpt meds ± surgery.
- Admit: All pts w/ severe hyperthyroidism. Pts w/ thyroid storm require ICU admission.

Guideline: Bahn Chai RS, Burch HB, Cooper DS, et. al. Hyperthyroidism and other causes of thyrotoxicosis: Management guidelines of the American Thyroid Association and American Association of Clinical Endocrinologists. Thyroid. 2011;21(6):593–646.

ADRENAL INSUFFICIENCY

Definition
- Condition in which the adrenal glands, do not produce adequate amounts of steroid hormones, primarily cortisol, but may also include impaired aldosterone production
- Primary adrenal insufficiency (Addison's dz) refers to pathology of the adrenal cortex, where secondary adrenal insufficiency may occur as a result of pituitary or hypothalamic dzs.

Adrenal Insufficiency Differential	
	Cause
Infiltrative dz	Tuberculosis, CMV, histoplasmosis/cryptococcosis/blastomycosis, amyloidosis, sarcoidosis, histiocytosis AIDS (opportunistic dz)
Vascular*	Hemorrhage, thrombosis, necrosis (meningococcemia, sepsis, **APLAS)
Endocrine	Autoimmune adrenalitis (alone or as component of autoimmune polyglandular syndromes types 1 & 2), pituitary failure
Neoplasm	Metastatic dz (lung, breast, kidney), lymphoma, pituitary tumor (primary or mets), craniopharyngioma, hypothalamic tumors
Meds	Ketoconazole, etomidate, rifampin, anticonvulsants, megestrol, glucocorticoid withdrawal
Other*	Trauma (esp head trauma, burns) postpartum pituitary necrosis (Sheehan's syndrome), empty sella syndrome, pituitary radiation/surgery

*Causes of acute onset adrenal insufficiency.
**APLAS: Antiphospholipid antibody syndrome.
Adapted from: Oelkers W. Adrenal insufficiency. NEJM. 1996;335(16):1206–1212.

- Dysfxn of the hypothalamic–pituitary–adrenal axis in critical illness is termed critical illness-related corticosteroid insufficiency (CIRCI)

History
- Weakness, fatigue, anorexia, nausea, vomiting, presyncope, craving for salt
- Meds (see *Differential* table); also elicit if pt is on chronic steroids at baseline

Physical Exam
- Orthostatic hypotension, hyperpigmentation, vitiligo

Evaluation
- Labs: BMP (may see hypoglycemia, hyponatremia, hyperkalemia, acidosis), CBC (may see mild normocytic anemia, lymphocytosis, & eosinophilia); send serum cortisol/ACTH level for inpt w/u
  - Serum cortisol >25 µg/dL in a pt requiring intensive care likely rules out adrenal insufficiency
  - CIRCI is best diagnosed by a delta cortisol (after 250 µg cosyntropin) of <9 µg/dL or a random total cortisol <10 µg/dL
  - ACTH stimulation test is rarely used in the ED
- Imaging: Consider head MR (assess pituitary), adrenal CT

Treatment (Only Start ED Treatment if Symptomatic/Hypotensive)
- Steroids: Hydrocortisone 100 mg IV bolus, followed by continuous infusion at 10 mg/h; may also give 200 mg/d in 4 divided doses
- IV hydration: Volume resuscitation w/ nl saline
- Steroids (particularly, hydrocortisone) should be considered in the management strategy of pts w/ septic shock, particularly those pts who have responded poorly to fluid resuscitation & vasopressors (SBP <90, despite IVF & vasopressors)

Disposition
- Home: Stable, already on meds
- Admit: All pts w/ new onset adrenal insufficiency; may require ICU admission if concomitant infection or HD unstable

Pearls
- Acute adrenal insufficiency should be suspected in the presence of fluid & pressor-refractory hypotension, esp in a pt w/ signs & sxs as noted above
- Pts w/ known adrenal insufficiency & concomitant febrile illness should be instructed to increase their home dose of steroid by 2–3 times until recovery to prevent possible adrenal crisis. Stress dose steroids can be given in the ED prior to disposition.

Consensus: Marik PE, Pastores SM, Annane D, et al. Recommendations for the diagnosis and treatment of corticosteroid insufficiency in critically ill adult patients: Consensus statement from an international task force by the American College of Critical Care Medicine. *Crit Care Med* 2008;36:1937–1949.

DEHYDRATION

Approach
- Careful hx: Understand whether pt has had excessive fluid loss or inadequate intake
- Attempt to quantify fluid deficit
- Check FSG to r/o hypoglycemia, electrolytes

Dehydration Differential	
Pathophysiology	**Differential**
Cardiac	Arrhythmia (1f)
Endocrine	Adrenal insufficiency, DI, DKA, SIADH, thyroid Dysfxn
Infectious	Encephalitis (4b), meningitis (4b), Lyme dz (4h), sepsis (16b), syphilis (4)
GI	Bowel obstruction, diarrhea, gastroenteritis, intestinal volvulus, vomiting, GIB
FEN/GU	Electrolyte disturbances, renal insufficiency
Neurologic	GBS, myasthenia gravis, ALS, stroke, migraine
Hematologic/oncologic	Metastatic dz
Toxic	Drug induced
Environmental	Hyperthermia
Psychiatric	Anorexia, bulimia, laxative abuse, psychosis

History
Excessive fluid loss (V/D, sweating, polyuria, diuretic/laxatives, bowel regimen), inadequate intake (debilitated, institutionalized, NM d/o, H&N pathology), altered thirst mechanism (intoxication, systemic illness, malignancy, antipsychotic use)

Findings
↑ HR w/ standing (Δ >20 bt/min lying → standing) 75% sens & spec; skin tenting, dry MM

Evaluation
CBC (hemoconcentration), BMP (↓ bicarb, ↑ BUN/Cr, abnl Na, K), ECG abnl
UA: Ketones, hyaline casts, spec grav >1.02: Uroconcentration, >1.03 = Severe dehydration

Treatment
Initial fluid resuscitation w/ NS or LR (avoid NS if concern for hyponatremia), then tailor to electrolyte abnlty/pathology (labor: Nonglucose IVF, malnourishment: D5 NS)
nl LV fxn: 2–3 L NS, follow clinical sxs, VS, UOP
Compromised LV fxn: 500 cc/h, watch pulmonary status (O₂ sat, SOB)
Consider antiemetic if N/V contributes to dehydration

Disposition
Home once dehydration adequately treated unless concerning electrolyte abnormalities, pt able to maintain hydration status
Consider care coordination/placement if pt lives alone & unable to hydrate self

Pearls
Up to 30% of healthy pts are orthostatic w/o dehydration (βBs, autonomic Dysfxn (DM))
Oral rehydration w/ glucose to facilitate intestinal absorption of Na & water if pt tolerates, "recipe" is 2 tbl sugar: 0.5 tsp salt: 1 quart water; ½ dilute apple juice also effective
Healthy adults tolerating PO rarely require IVF & PO rehydration is usually adequate

Types of Dehydration		
	Losses	**Mechanism**
Hypotonic	Na loss > water loss	Diuretics
Isotonic	Na loss = water loss	Vomiting, diarrhea
Hypertonic	Na loss < water loss	Fever, sweating, faulty thirst mechanism

Degrees of Dehydration			
Degree	**Fluid Deficit**	**Sxs**	**Signs**
Mild	30 cc/kg (3%)	Thirst, fatigue	Slight tachycardia, ↓ UOP
Moderate	50–60 cc/kg (5–6%)	Dry mucous membranes, ↓ skin turgor, symptomatic when standing	Tachycardia, ↓ BP, flat neck veins
Severe	70–90 cc/kg (7–9%)	Symptomatic when lying down, ↓ mentation	Supine ↓ BP, ↑ HR, skin tenting, delayed cap refill

Composition of Resuscitation Fluids					
1 L Fluid	Glucose (g/L)	Sodium (mEq/L)	Chloride (mEq/L)	Potassium (mEq/L)	mOsm/L
NS	0	154	154	0	308
Ringer's lactate	0	130	109	4	272
D₅W	50	0	0	0	278
D₅W ½ NS	50	77	77	0	432
3% NS	0	513	513	0	1026

BITES AND STINGS

Approach
- Treat anaphylaxis; give tetanus prophylaxis
- Consider x-ray for underlying fx or FB
- Assess for joint space violation, copious wound irrigation/wash out w/ NS; if heavily contaminated, do not close
- 24–48 h wound check for high-risk bites, esp in kids or unreliable pts
- National Poison Control Center (PCC): (800) 222-1222

HUMAN & ANIMAL BITES

Human
History
- Laceration near MCP joint during altercation should be considered a human bite ("fight bite"); bacteria spread along tendon sheath deep into hand

Evaluation
- Consider x-ray to assess for fracture, air in joint, tooth fragments; no serology needed
- Extend & explore periarticular MCP joint injuries, including in that position that injury occurred

Treatment
- Preferred regimen: Amoxicillin/Clav acid) 875/125 mg BID × 5–10 d
- Alternatives: Doxycycline or TMP-SMX or pen VK or fluoroquinolone or cefuroxime PLUS clindamycin or metronidazole
- If late/complicated/needs admit, IV ampicillin/sulbactam 1.5 g q6h
- Delayed 1° closure if closure needed

Disposition
- Scheduled strict f/u in 24–48 h

Pearl
- Eikenella (most common), Staph/Strep species found in mouth, anaerobes

Cat
Evaluation
- Consider x-ray to assess for fracture, air in joint, tooth fragments
- Extend & explore joint injuries including in the position that injury occurred

Treatment
- Amoxicillin/Clav Acid 875/125 mg BID, cefuroxime 500 mg BID or doxycycline 100 mg BID
- Delayed 1° closure only if cosmetically needed; 80% of cat bites become infected!

Disposition
- Scheduled strict f/u in 24 h

Pearls
- Pasteurella multocida most common organism
- Consider cat-scratch dz if pt has tender LAD 1 wk after bite/scratch
- Very high infection rate despite abx use
- Consider rabies prophylaxis (rabies immunoglobulin + vaccine) if unknown cat (4i)

Dog
Evaluation
- Consider x-ray to assess for fracture, air in joint, tooth fragments

Treatment

- Amoxicillin/Clav acid 875/125 mg BID or clindamycin 300 QID + ciprofloxacin 500 mg BID
- 1° closure after copious irrigation possible except on hand/foot; only 5% become infected

Disposition

- Scheduled strict f/u in 24 h

Pearls

- Polymicrobial infections
- Consider rabies prophylaxis if unknown dog as above w/ cats (4i)

SNAKE BITES

Crotalinae/Pit Vipers (Rattlesnakes, Copperheads, Water Moccasins)

History

- Pain & swelling around fang marks, attempt identification of snake if possible

Findings

- Local (pain, swelling, ecchymosis), systemic (↓ BP, ↑ HR, paresthesias), coagulopathy (↓ PLTs, ↑ INR, ↓ fibrinogen), pulmonary edema, acidosis, rhabdomyolysis, neuromuscular weakness if Mojave rattlesnake

Evaluation

- Consult PCC/toxicologist; CBC, BMP, coags w/ fibrinogen & split products, CK, T&C, x-rays to r/o retained fang; watch compartment pressures

Treatment

- Remove rings, constrictive clothing, general wound care, tetanus
- Antivenom (Crotalidae) if systemic effects or coagulopathy; surgical assessment if compartment syndrome; supportive care; no proven benefit w/ abx or steroids

Disposition

- D/C if absence of any findings 8–12 h post bite envenomation in healthy adults, 12–24 h in children/elderly, 12–24 h if concerns for Mojave rattlesnake
- ICU admission if antivenom given

Pearls

- Avoid oral or mechanical suction of wound, tourniquets, incision, & suction
- 25% of bites are "dry strikes" (no effect); pit vipers identified by 2 fangs

Grades of Pit Viper Envenomation (Dynamic)		
Grade	**Signs/Sxs**	**Vials of Antivenom**
Mild	Local pain, edema. No signs of systemic tox. nl labs.	None
Moderate	Severe local pain, edema <50 cm around wound. Systemic tox: N/V. Labs abnl (↓ Hct, ↓ PLTs).	4–6
Severe	Generalized petechiae/ecchymosis, compartment sx, bleeding, ↓ BP, AMS, renal dysfxn, markedly abnl coags	Initial dose 8–12

Elapidae/Coral Snake (Micrurus fulvius)

History

- Bitten by brightly colored snake (black, red, & yellow bands), primarily in tx, FLA

Findings

- Neurotoxic effects from venom: Tremor/sz, ↑ salivation, respiratory paralysis, bulbar palsy (dysarthria, diplopia, dysphagia), usually less local tissue damage than Crotalinae

Evaluation

- Consult PCC/toxicologist; CBC, BMP, coags/DIC eval not usually indicated, consider pulmonary fxn testing

Treatment

- Consult PCC before giving antivenom as higher risk for allergic rxn; surgical assessment if concern for compartment syndrome; supportive care (esp respiratory support)

Disposition
- 12–24 h observation; ICU admission if antivenom given or respiratory compromise

Pearl
- True coral snakes have red on yellow banding, nonvenomous snakes have red band on black background: "Red on yellow: Kill a fellow. Red on black: Poison lack."

SCORPION BITES

Scorpion (Centruroides exilicauda)
History
- Burning & stinging w/o visible injury at bite site

Findings
- Usually no visible local injury; possible systemic effects include roving eye movements (pathognomonic), opisthotonos, ↑ HR, diaphoresis, fasciculations
- Mydriasis, nystagmus, hypersalivation, dysphagia, restlessness
- Severe envenomation may cause pancreatitis, respiratory failure, coagulopathy, anaphylaxis

Evaluation
- "Tap test": Exquisite tenderness w/ light tapping in exilicauda stings; consult PCC/toxicologist
- CBC, BMP, coags, LFTs, CK, ECG

Treatment
- Most bites are self-limited, provide supportive care
- BZD for muscle spasm/fasciculations, pain control, tetanus, reassurance
- If severe systemic sxs, 1–2 vials scorpion antivenom; avail from AZ PCC

Disposition
- Admission for observation; ICU admission if antivenom given

Pearl
- Only C. exilicauda (bark scorpion) found in Western US produces systemic toxicity

---

SPIDER BITES

Brown Recluse (Loxosceles reclusa)
History
- Pt may not remember bite & initially have no pain; pain & pruritus develops over 2–8 h
- Severe rxn: Immediate pain & blister formation, necrosis & eschar over next 3–4 d
- Loxoscelism: Systemic rxn 1–3 d after envenomation; N/V, f/c, muscle/joint aches, sz, rarely renal failure, DIC, hemolytic anemia, rhabdomyolysis

Findings
- Necrotic blister w/ surrounding erythema, petechiae

Evaluation
- Consult PCC/toxicologist, surgery/plastics consult for lesion >2 cm
- CBC, BMP, coagulation profile, UA

Treatment
- No antivenom; wound care, tetanus, supportive care (eg, hydration, abx, transfusion, HD), local debridement
- May consider dapsone 50–100 mg BID to prevent necrosis, hyperbaric O_2, steroids (all are controversial)
- Dapsone causes hemolysis, hepatitis; monitor LFTs, check G6PD level

Disposition
- Admission for observation

Pearl
- Located in S. Central & SW (desert) of US; violin-shaped marking on back

Black Widow (Latrodectus mactans)
History
- Immediate pain, then swelling, possible target-shaped lesion, can have unexplained severe abd/back pain, muscle cramps w/i 1 h
- Pain may continue intermittently for 3 days, is often a/w muscle weakness & spasm for wk to mo

Findings
- Severe rxns: HTN, respiratory failure, abd rigidity, fasciculations, shock, coma

Evaluation
- CBC, BMP, CK, coagulation profile, UA, abd CT (r/o acute abdomen), ECG

Treatment
- Antivenom if severe rxn: 1–2 vials over 30 min (after cutaneous test dose)
- Wound care, tetanus, supportive care: BZD, analgesia

Disposition
- Consider admission for observation & pain control

Pearls
- Painful abd muscle cramps can mimic peritonitis
- Red hourglass-shaped marking on spider's abdomen

HYMENOPTERA (BEE, WASP, STINGING ANT)

History
- Immediate pain & swelling at site of bite

Findings
- Local & systemic signs of allergic rxn can occur

Treatment
- Treat anaphylaxis/allergic rxn; local rxn treated w/ cleansing, ice packs, & elevation
- If present, stinger should be removed immediately by scraping it from the wound (bees)

Disposition
- Close wound care f/u; prescribe epinephrine auto-injectors in cases of anaphylaxis

Pearls
- The more rapid onset of sxs, the more severe the rxn; IgE-mediated allergic rxn
- Rapid onset: 50% D in 30 min, 75% in 4 h; usually see fatal rxn following prior mild rxn
- Delayed rxn similar to serum sickness can present 10–14 d after a sting/bite

---

JELLYFISH STINGS

History
- Swimming in seawater w/ jellyfish

Findings
- Painful papular lesions & urticarial eruptions last min to h
- Systemic rxns rare; vomiting, muscle spasm, paresthesias, weakness, fever, respiratory distress, Irukandji syndrome: Rare, severe chest/abd/back pain, HTN, GI sx

Evaluation
- CBC, BMP, CK, coagulation profile, ECG

Treatment
- Analgesia, supportive care
- Tentacles should be removed w/ forceps; nematocysts should be scraped off w/a knife/blade after dusting w/ talcum powder & covering w/ shaving cream
- Analgesia & after nematocyst removal wash w/ hot (40°C) salt water (helps w/ pain)
- Antivenom available for serious systemic effects (cardiopulmonary arrest, severe pain) from the Commonwealth Serum Laboratory in Melbourne, Australia

Disposition
- D/C if mild & pain controlled, admission for observation o/w

Pearls
- Box jellyfish are severely toxic, can induce respiratory & myocardial arrest in min
- Use seawater/acid/vinegar (not urine!) to wash; freshwater causes nematocysts to fire

OCCUPATIONAL EXPOSURE

Approach
- Institutional guidelines vary regarding occupational exposures of HC workers to bodily fluids
- Refer to CDC/local experts for recs on postexposure prophylaxis (PEP)
- National Clinicians' Postexposure Prophylaxis Hotline (PEPline): (888) 448-4911

History
- Any percutaneous injury, mucous membrane exposure, or exposure of nonintact skin to any blood & other bodily fluids considered potentially infectious
- RFs: High-risk procedures, use of equipment w/o newer safety designs, failure to follow universal precautions

Findings
- Physical examination nl; should be documented for future reference

Evaluation
- Consent & test source pt for HIV, HBsAg, Hep C Ab (direct viral assays not rec)
- Test HC worker for HIV & Hep C Ab, draw HBsAb titers if unknown immune status
- Check serum hCG, CBC, BMP, LFTs, & UA before starting prophylaxis
- If source pt is HIV+, ID consult for appropriate regimen based on source pt's regimen

Treatment
- HIV: 2 drug regimen (Combivir) × 4 wk; 3 drug regimen (Nelfinavir) for high-risk exposures
- Hep B: Start vaccination series if unvaccinated, Hep B immune globulin (HBIG) if HBsAg+
- Multiple doses HBIG w/i 1 wk of exposure provides 75% protection from infection
- Hep C: CDC does not recommend use of interferon or ribavirin for HCV exposure
- Consider interferon & ribavirin tx as soon as HCV seroconversion is documented

Disposition
- F/u w/ ID specialist; fully inform risks & benefits of tx & nontx

Pearls
- ~80% ↓ rate of transmission w/ immediate initiation (w/i 2 h) of HIV PEP
- Rates of occupational transmission after percutaneous exposure
- HIV + source pt: 0.3%; Hep B + source pt: 5–20%; Hep C + source pt: 1–10%

Antiretrovirals for HIV Exposure		
Name	Regimen	Side Effects
Combivir [Zidovudine (AZT)/Lamivudine (3TC)]	1 tablet (300 mg AZT, 150 mg 3TC) every 12 h	HA, malaise, fatigue, nausea, diarrhea, myalgias
Nelfinavir (Viracept)	1 tablet (250 mg) TID	Diarrhea, nausea, rash, fatigue, stomach cramps

Occupational Exposure Risk Assessment	
Low-risk Exposure	High-risk Exposure
Instrument used for giving injection	Instrument visibly contaminated w/ source pt blood, directly placed in pt vein/artery
Superficial puncture in employee	Deep puncture in employee
Splash or mucosal exposure in employee	Terminal source pt (high viral load)

From Centers for Disease Control and Prevention. Updated U.S. public health service guidelines for the management of occupational exposures to HBV, HCV, and HIV and recommendations for postexposure prophylaxis. MMWR Recomm Rep 2001;50(RR-11):1–67.

BURNS

Approach
- Early airway assessment, determine need for intubation (soot in airway, edema, voice Δ, deep facial burns, ↓ O_2 sat; transfer to burn center if intubated)
- 100% O_2 or O_2 by NRB mask until CO (10e) & other inhalation tox assessed
- Evaluate for concomitant trauma (fall, blast injury); maintain c-spine precautions
- Start IVF resuscitation early (almost universally required)
- Keep room warm to ↓ insensate losses

History
- How burn occurred (explosion? closed space?), duration of exposure, type of burn

Findings
- Assess burn

Evaluation
- Mental status on extrication, assess degree of burn, % of total body surface area
- Check CO level (10e), CBC, BMP, lactate, ABG, LFTs, coags, tox, T&S, UA, CXR

Treatment
- Early & generous analgesia: Morphine IV q5–10min titrated to pain
- Airway management: Intubate early
  - Toxic inhalation (cough, dyspnea, carbonaceous sputum, soot in oropharynx): Intubate or perform fiberoptic airway exam early; delay could cause ↑ airway edema → airway compromise, difficult/impossible intubation
- If >15% TBSA, aggressive IVF resuscitation, 2 LBIV through unburned skin
  - Parkland formula calculates IVF requirement in 1st 24 h after burn:
    - 4 mL × weight (kg) × BSA (2nd- & 3rd-degree burns)
    - Give ½ over 1st 8 h, other ½ over next 16 h; use LR to avoid NAGMA w/ NS
- Urinary catheter placement: Target urine output: 30–50 mL/h
- Burn mgmt: Irrigate w/ NS, remove debris, clothing, jewelry, & ruptured blisters (prevent future infection)
  - Apply silver sulfadiazine (antipseudomonal) ointment to denuded areas
  - Bacitracin only on face (silver sulfadiazine may cause discoloration)
  - Immediate escharotomy for full-thickness circumferential burns that compromise distal neurovascular status or significantly ↓ chest compliance
- Tetanus prophylaxis, no role for steroids or immediate IV abx

Disposition
- Admit 2nd-degree burns 10–20% BSA (or 5–10% if <10 y/o), circumferential or if meet criteria below

Pearls
- Burns often progress in severity, watch for worsening burns
- Remove tar (asphalt burns) w/ mineral oil
- Consider cyanide w/ industrial/closed space fires, check lactate, treat w/ hydroxocobalamin

Burn Clinical Findings by Degree	
Degree	**Clinical Findings**
1st: Epidermis	Painful, erythematous, indurated area w/o blisters
2nd: Dermis	Blisters, painful, erythematous or mottled, indurated
3rd: Full-skin thickness	Charred, leathery, mottled/white, painless
4th: Full-tissue thickness	Includes SQ tissue, muscle, fat, blood vessels & nerves, to bone. Catastrophic.

Criteria for Transfer to Burn Unit
Burns >20% BSA (or >10% if age <10 or >50)
3rd-degree burns >5% BSA or 2nd-degree burns >20% BSA
Burns involving face, eyes, ears, hands, feet, or perineum
Burns a/w significant electrical, chemical, inhalational, or traumatic injury
Burns suspected to be related to abuse
Burns to pts w/ special psychosocial or rehabilitative care needs

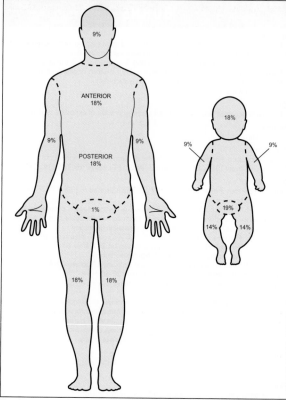

Figure 10.1 Reprinted with permission from: Mick NW, Peters JR, Egan D, et al. *Blueprints Emergency Medicine*. Philadelphia, PA: Lippincott Williams & Wilkins; 2006.

CARBON MONOXIDE POISONING

Approach
- Early airway assessment, determine need for intubation (AMS)
  - 100% O_2 or O_2 by NRB mask until CO assessed
- Pulse oximetry not useful b/c it will detect carboxyhemoglobin (COHgb) as oxyhemoglobin

History
- Exposure to CO from combustion, faulty heating, closed-space fire, defective automobile exhaust; often multiple people exposed/symptomatic
  - Mild poisoning: Frontal HA, N/V, DOE, dizziness/confusion
  - Severe exposure: Syncope, coma, or sz

Findings
- Mild confusion progressing to agitation, sz, coma
- May have subtle psychomotor abnormalities: Ataxia, muscle rigidity, tachycardia, hypotension, retinal hemorrhage, ↓ visual acuity, cyanosis, or pallor
- Neurologic findings primarily cerebellar: Dysmetria, ataxia, etc.

Evaluation

- ABG alone not useful b/c pO_2, a measure of dissolved O_2, will be nl; check ABG for COHgb via co-oximetry
  - Level is weakly correlated w/ tox but it confirms significant exposure
  - Level of <10–15% may be nl in smokers
  - Higher risk for myocardial injury: Check ECG esp if baseline CAD, risk fx, or high CO
- Assess for suicidal gesture; may need psychiatry consult

Treatment

- O_2 via NRB (60% O_2) at least, ideally deliver 100% O_2
- Airway management: If AMS, hypoxemia or shock → intubate
- Cardiac monitoring; admission if dysrhythmia or e/o ischemia on ECG
- Hyperbaric O_2 tx controversial but recommended by Undersea & Hyperbaric Med Society, potential long-term neuro sequelae benefit
- Fetal Hgb has higher affinity for CO than adult Hgb; lower threshold for hyperbaric O_2 in pregnant women

Disposition

- Admission based on level & clinical findings; D/C asymptomatic pt w/ HbCO <10%

Pearls

- CO is the most common cause of D from acute poisoning & fires; reversibly binds Hb more avidly than O_2 → functional anemia
- May see delayed neurologic sequelae (personality Δ, HA, sz, parkinsonian Δ) 2–40 d after exposure; virtually universally resolve w/i 6 mo
- Half-life of COHgb: 300 min on RA, 90 min on 100% NRB, 30 min hyperbaric

Indications for Hyperbaric O_2 in CO Poisoning
Transient or prolonged unconsciousness (syncope, coma)
CO level >25–40%
Persistent neurologic disturbances
Cardiovascular Dysfxn
Severe acidosis
Pregnancy w/ CO level >20% or signs of fetal distress

DYSBARISM

Background

- Atmospheric pressure at sea level = 760 mmHg = 14.7 psi: 1 atm
  - Each descent of 33 ft under water ↑ pressure by 1 atm
- Dive tables & computers set standards for rate & depth of ascent to avoid dysbarism

Approach

- Careful hx: Length, depth, # of dives, interval btw dives, comorbid dz, sinus pain during dive, intoxication, onset of sxs, dive relative to decompression limits
- Divers Alert Network, Duke University: (919) 684-8111, 24-h med advice

DECOMPRESSION SICKNESS (DCS)

History

- Improper dive time, depth, & ascent; sx can develop during or after (1–24 h) ascent, longer if air travel

Findings

- Fatigue, AMS, visual defects, lingual pallor, tachypnea, tachycardia, N/V, ↓ UOP, sz, neuro Δ, joint pain, lymphedema, pruritus

Evaluation

- Cardiac monitor, CBC, CMP, O_2 sat, tox screen, CO level, coags, CXR, head CT

Treatment

- 100% O_2 (NRB mask), place pt in L lateral decub & mild Trendelenburg, hyperbaric O_2, IVF (UOP 1.5 mL/kg/h) for recompression
- Goal of recompression to ↓ mechanical obstruction of air bubbles, ↑ tissue O_2 delivery
- Sx tx: Intubation (inflate cuff w/ saline), needle decompression, sz control

Disposition
- Ground transport, or low-flying air transport (cabin pressure <1000 ft)
- Admit to institution w/ hyperbaric O_2 capability

Pearls
- Spectrum of illness: Formation of small nitrogen gas bubbles in blood & tissues
- Depends on location & degree of bubble formation
- ↑ freq w/ longer & deeper dives, comorbid illness (COPD, CAD, PFO, asthma)
- Residual paralysis, myocardial necrosis, other ischemic injuries possible; early recognition & tx imperative
- Wait >12–48 h btw diving & flying, no diving for 7 d after DCS I, 28 d after DCS II

Types of Decompression Sickness	
Type I: Pain "the bends"	• Extremity/joint pain w/o localized tenderness or erythema • Skin: Pruritus, rash, mottling or marbling of skin, violaceous rash • Lymphatics: Venous stasis • Inflate BP cuff to 150 mmHg over affected joint; if relieves pain, confirms dx
Type II: CNS or pulm gas embolism	• Pulmonary sxs: Pleuritic pain, respiratory distress, nonproductive cough • Hypovolemic shock: Tachycardia, postural hypotension, cyanosis • Nervous system: Mimics spinal cord trauma; ext weakness & paresthesias, moves proximally, focal neuro deficit, plegia, AMS, sz

MIDDLE EAR BAROTRAUMA

History
- Usually occurs on descent; ↑ pain w/ ↑ water pressure on TM, equilibration via Eustachian tubes, rupture occurs b/w 5 & 17 ft → pain relief; vertigo, N/V, hearing loss

Findings
- Reversible Bell palsy from increased pressure to facial nerve in severe cases

Evaluation
- Concomitant eval for inner ear barotrauma

Treatment
- Nasal vasoconstrictor drops/spray to open fluid from middle ear; antihistamines, analgesia, pinch nose & swallow to displace fluid through Eustachian tube

Disposition
- ENT f/u in 2 wk

Pearl
- No benefit w/ abx; use occlusive earplugs when diving/showering until TM healed

Other Dysbarisms	
Inner ear barotrauma	• Occurs during descent; nausea, vertigo, tinnitus, hearing loss • Insufflation in ear canal using otoscope produces nystagmus • Conservative mgmt, 1 wk bed rest, no Valsalva
Nitrogen narcosis	• "Rapture of the deep" from ↑ tissue nitrogen concentration • Euphoria, false sense of well being, confusion, loss of judgment, disorientation, inappropriate laughter, ↓ motor control, paresthesias • Start around 100 ft, resolves w/ ascent
Facial barotrauma	• Neg. pressure generated in airspace created by mask over face • If pt doesn't force exhale through nose, get conjunctival edema, petechial hemorrhages over face, subconjunctival hemorrhages
Arterial gas embolism (AGE)	• "The chokes" occur when diver doesn't exhale properly during ascent • Sudden onset stroke sxs in 10 min of surfacing, dyspnea, hemoptysis • Look for PFO, shouldn't dive again, emergent recompression
PTX/Pneumomediastinum	• Results from barotrauma, seen on CXR • Pleuritic pain, dyspnea, subcutaneous emphysema/crepitus • Unless hemodynamic compromise or tension, not life-threatening

ELECTRICAL INJURY

Background
- Current: Measure of amount of energy flowing through an object; in amperes (A)

Approach
- Early & continuous cardiac monitoring for dysrhythmias
- Evaluate for concomitant trauma (fall, injury); maintain c-spine precautions
- Divided in low voltage <500 & high voltage

History
- Usually obvious & reported (eg, occupational injury of electrician, home handyman); pt reports minor shock (tingling) related to home appliance use
- "3rd rail" contact from light-rail mass transportation system
- Toddler w/ burns to corners of mouth (chewing) or hands (playing w/ socket)
- Bimodal distribution w/ most pts <6 or adult workers

Findings
- VF more common w/ low voltage AC, asystole w/ high voltage AC or DC
- Respiratory arrest via chest wall paralysis or respiratory center of brain possible
- Skin wounds may appear minor & entry/exit wounds may be present (examine bottoms of feet for exit); may be more severe than they appear due to deep-tissue injury
- Long-bone fx, scapular fx, shoulder dislocation, spinal fx from mechanical trauma caused by whole body tetanic contractions or trauma of being blown back
- Perforated TMs, delayed cataracts in 6% of pts

Evaluation
- ECG, CBC, BMP, cardiac enzymes (rhabdomyolysis), UA (myoglobin)

Treatment
- Resuscitate, eval for trauma, immobilize c-spine, continuous cardiac monitoring
- High-volume IV crystalloid (NS, avoid K-containing fluids)
- Urinary catheter placement: Target urine output: 0.5–1 mL/kg/h
- If rhabdomyolysis ($\uparrow$ CK, +UA dip), maintain high UOP until urine dip neg.
- Goal serum pH 7.45–7.55
  - Alkaline urine (pH > 6.5) to $\uparrow$ excretion of acidic myoglobin by $\uparrow$ solubility; D_5W + 150 mEq $NaHCO_3$ OR D5 ¼ NS or D5 ½ NS + 100 mEq $NaHCO_3$
  - Diuresis w/ Lasix 20–40 mg IV or mannitol 25 g IV (then 12.5 g/kg/h) prn
- Treat wounds the same as thermal burns (10 d)
- Compartment pressures ± fasciotomy if sx of compartment syndrome
- Splint injured extremities in best "position of fxn" to minimize contractures

Disposition
- If asx & nl exam, can be D/C
- If mild cutaneous burns & nl ECG, nl urine dip, observe for 2 h, then D/C
- ECG Δ, myoglobinuria, entry/exit burns, partial/full thickness burns: Admit burn center

Pearls
- Electrical injuries are often minor, but may be more serious than they 1st appear. If any concern, observe for 6–12 h.
- Pediatric oral "bite" burns may develop delayed labial artery bleed at 2–3 wk

Types of Current	
Direct current (DC)	Occupational, high voltage: Current flows in 1 direction only; most pts are "blown" from this exposure & suffer blunt trauma
Alternating current (AC)	Home, low voltage: 3× more dangerous than DC of same voltage due to continuous muscle contraction/tetany from current alternating direction of flow; pt "can't let go"
Arc injury	Pt trapped in electrical arc b/w 2 objects; mostly serious b/c of $\uparrow$ risk of blunt trauma & temp as high as 2500–5000°C causing burn

HIGH-ALTITUDE ILLNESS

Background
- Caused by acute exposure to hypobaric hypoxia (low PO_2) usually above 8K ft
- Altitude illness is generally considered as a progressive spectrum from AMS to HACE
- Acclimatization allows body to minimize effects of hypoxia; ↑ RR (↓ $PaCO_2$), ↑ CO, ↑ hematopoiesis & 2,3-DPG production (favors O_2 release to tissues)
- Takes 5–7 d for full effect; inherent acclimatization ability varies by individual

Approach
- O_2, descent, symptomatic relief; HAPE can be fatal w/i h unless treated

History
- Rapid ascent to altitude >8K ft, risk increased by exertion, past h/o altitude illness
- Flu-like sxs, "hangover," HA, fatigue, DOE, sleep disturbance, N/V, dizziness, paresthesias
- Sxs manifest 6–12 h after ascent, subside in 1–2 d or may progress to HAPE, HACE
- Watch for sxs of HAPE (dry cough, fever, SOB at rest) or HACE (ataxia, emesis, LOC)

Findings
- Depends on severity of altitude illness
- HAPE: Tachycardia, tachypnea, rales/wheeze, fever, orthopnea, pink/frothy sputum
- HACE: AMS, ataxia, sz, slurred speech, stupor, coma, D from brain herniation

Evaluation
- Clinical Dx
- HAPE: CXR (patchy infiltrates), US (comet tails), pulse oximetry (relative hypoxia)
- HACE: Head CT neg., MRI (white matter Δ showing ↑ edema)

Treatment
- Descent! If unable: O_2, symptomatic relief, bed rest
- Hyperbaric O_2 chamber: Used as temporizing measure until descent
- Meds: Unclear benefit but low risk:
  - Acetazolamide: 125–250 mg PO q12h; for ppx start 1d prior to ascent
  - Dexamethasone: 8 mg PO × 1, then 4 mg PO q6h
- In HAPE:
  - Nifedipine (pulm vasodilation): 10 mg PO q6h, SR 30 mg PO q8–12h (<90–120 mg/d)
  - Inhaled β-agonist (Salmeterol; clears alveolar fluid): Inhalation q12h
  - PDE-5 inhibitors (tadalafil, sildenafil) have shown efficacy in HAPE ppx & can be considered in tx: Tadalafil 10 mg q12h, sildenafil 50 mg q8h

Disposition
- Admit if hypoxic, dyspnea at rest; prognosis excellent for survivors

Pearls
- Avoid abrupt ascent, spend 1–2 nights at intermediate elevation, descend to sleep
- Underlying medical conditions (COPD, CAD, HTN, SSD, pregnancy) affected more
- Consider other causes of sxs: PNA (HAPE does not usually cause fever), PE, SDH, CVA
- Descent is the mainstay of any tx

Summary of High-Altitude Illnesses			
Dz	Signs & Sxs	Altitude & Course	Tx
AMS	Viral illness, HA + GI upset, insomnia, fatigue, lightheaded, Lake Louise Scoring system	8–10K ft; onset 6–12 h, peak 1–2 d, duration 3–5 d	Acetazolamide, O_2, Ibuprofen, avoid further ascent
HAPE	SOB at rest, fatigue, HA, anorexia, cyanosis, rales, tachypnea, tachycardia	>14500 ft; onset 2–4 d, resolution 1–2 d after descent	O_2, descent, rest, nifedipine; hyperbaric if severe
HACE	HA, ataxia, slurred speech, AMS (hallucinations), insomnia, stupor, coma	>12K ft; onset 1–3 d, peak 5–9 d, resolves 3–7 d after descent	O_2, descent, rest; dexamethasone; hyperbaric if severe
High altitude retinal hemorrhage	Usually asymptomatic, sometimes central scotoma	>17500 ft; ?onset/ peak; resolves 1–3 wk	No emergent tx

HYPOTHERMIA

Background
- Multiple classifications of hypothermia based on severity & etiology

Approach
- Careful hx: Determine etiology of hypothermia: Environmental exposure vs. medical
- Environmental hypothermia can occur even in the absence of freezing weather (malnourished pt, elderly)
- Many medical etiologies: Hypothyroidism (myxedema coma), hypoglycemia, hypoadrenalism, sepsis, hypothalamic lesion (eg, 2/2 trauma, tumor, stroke), dermatologic conditions that prevent heat conservation (burns, erythrodermas)
- If unresponsive, check BS/give D50, give naloxone 2 mg

History
- Environmental exposure, drug use, trauma, comorbid illnesses

Findings
- Based on degree of hypothermia (table below)

Evaluation
- Obtain core temp (bladder, rectum, esophagus: All may be inaccurate)
- Cardiac monitor, CBC (Hct ↑ 2% for every 1° ↓ temp), CMP (↑ K bad sign), tox screen, coags, CXR, lipase (cold-induced pancreatitis), CK, UA (rhabdo), ABG, head CT
- ECG shows Osborn waves (J pt deflection in same direction as QRS), <32°C/90°F
- Interval prolongation (PR, QRS, QT), AF w/ slow ventricular response (common)

Treatment
- Rewarm as per table below; intubate as needed, remove wet clothing
- Maintain horizontal position, avoid movement, limit manipulation to essential tasks. However, this should not prevent CPR or other critical interventions.
- Monitor ECG, check for pulse q1min; chest compressions may cause ventricular dysrhythmias, perform only if no pulse
- If no cardiac activity, start CPR
  - VF or VT: Defibrillate up to 3 times
  - Core temp <30°C, cont compressions/rewarming, no ACLS meds/shock until >30°C
  - Core temp >30°C, ACLS protocol w/ meds/shock, allow longer time b/w doses
  - Cont resuscitation until core temp >32°C/90°F
    - Consider hydrocortisone 250 mg IV or levothyroxine 250–500 µg if doesn't rewarm w/ above

Disposition
- Based on severity of hypothermia (table below)

Pearls
- Hypothermic bradycardia is refractory to atropine since not vagally mediated; no indication for temporary pacing
- Core temp afterdrop: Peripheral vasodilation from rewarming extremities may cause return of cooler peripheral blood to core
- Consider femoral line placement if needed to avoid cardiac stimulation (vs. IJ, SC)
- "You're not dead until you're warm & dead"; aggressively rewarm before stopping efforts

Classifications of Hypothermia		
	Physiologic Response	**Clinical Presentation**
Mild (90–95°F, 32–35°C)	Increased: HR, BP, CO, RR, metabolic activity, shivering, cold diuresis	Dizziness, lethargy, confusion, amnesia, apathy, dysarthria, nausea, ataxia, loss of fine-motor skills
Moderate (86–90°F, 30–32°C)	Decreased: HR, BP, CO, RR, metabolic activity, cold diuresis, shivering stops	Delirium (paradoxic undressing), stupor, pupillary dilatation, ↓ reflexes
Severe (<86°F, <30°C)	Decreased: HR, BP, CO, RR, metabolic activity, no shivering	Unresponsive, fixed & dilated pupils, rigid, very cold skin, coma, pulm edema; ↑ risk of ventricular fibrillation & asystole

Rewarming Strategies by Severity of Hypothermia			
	Rewarming Strategy	Tx	Disposition
Mild (90–95°F, 32–35°C)	Passive rewarming (PR)	Warm blankets, heat lamps, ACLS if cardiac arrest	Likely D/C
Moderate (86–90°F, 30–32°C)	PR, active external rewarming (AER) to trunk only	Hot water bottles (45–65°C) to axilla & groin, ACLS for cardiac arrest	Admit, cardiac monitoring
Severe (<86°F, <30°C)	PR, AER, active internal rewarming	Warm IVF (NS 45°C), warm humidified O_2 (45°C), If cardiac arrest, shock (no ACLS meds); CP bypass/pl lavage, central venous "radiator" cath	Admit, likely ICU

FROSTBITE

History
- Cold exposure, numbness of body part → loss of sensation

Findings
- Distal body part most commonly affected (fingers, nose, toes, ears)
- Caused by both immediate cell D from cold & delayed injury from inflammatory response
- Skin initially white, waxy, insensate → erythematous, edematous, painful 48–72 h after rewarming → bleb formation, devitalized tissue demarcation over weeks

Evaluation
- Check core temp to look for systemic hypothermia
- Superficial: Areas of pallor & edema, local anesthesia, potentially clear blisters, erythema, no tissue loss
- Deep: Hemorrhagic blisters, eschar, if severe extends to muscle/bone, mummification

Treatment
- Handle tissue gently, keep extremity elevated, sterile/nonadherent dressing
- Rapid rewarming of frozen extr in gentle warm water bath (40–42°C), ROM exercise in bath, avoid water temp falling outside of range; 30 min if superficial/60 min if deep
- Consider intra-arterial tPA in severe cases
- Topical aloe vera q6h
- Aspirate & débride clear blisters, only aspirate (do not débride) hemorrhagic blisters to avoid desiccation, infection of deeper tissues
- Tetanus prophylaxis, consider ppx abx
- Early surgical intervention not indicated other than escharotomy for circumferential limb lesions (very uncommon)

Disposition
- Refer to burn service; consider admission for 24–48 h to observe for progression

Pearls
- Long-term cx: Cold insensitivity, paresthesias, nail loss, joint stiffness
- Avoid refreezing, if unable to maintain warmth to affected part (e.g. prehospital) do not rewarm

HYPERTHERMIA

Background
- Spectrum of heat-related illnesses including heat rash, cramps, syncope, stroke

Approach
- Careful hx: Determine etiology of hyperthermia: External (environmental) or internal (toxic/metabolic) factors, environmental hypothermia can occur even in absence of exertion (malnourished pt, chronically ill, elderly)
- Look for medication related hyperthermia: MH, NMS, SS
- Use rectal thermometer to determine core temperature

Heat Cramps

History
- Brief, intermittent, severe muscle cramping usually following cessation of strenuous activity. Often in abd or calf muscles.

Findings
- Euthermic, clinical signs of dehydration

Evaluation
- BMP ($\downarrow$ Na, $\downarrow$ Cl), urine lytes optional ($\downarrow$ urinary Na & Cl from sweating)

Treatment
- Oral salt or electrolyte repletion tablets or sports drinks; IV hydration rarely required

Disposition
- Home after observation for sx relief

Pearl
- Related to electrolyte deficiency; electrolyte enhanced sports drinks may be helpful although may cause diarrhea due to the high sugar content

Heat Edema

History
- Swollen feet/ankles after long periods of sitting/standing due to hydrostatic pressure, vasodilation & orthostatic pooling → vascular leak, interstitial fluid accumulation
- No underlying hepatic, lymphatic, cardiac, or venous dz

Findings
- Euthermic, B LE pitting edema w/o signs of CHF or renal failure

Evaluation
- BMP, UA for proteinuria, CXR for pulm edema, ECG for e/o LVH, RH strain

Treatment
- Elevate lower extremities, provide support hose
- No evidence that diuretics help

Disposition
- Home after reassurance, PCP f/u

Pearl
- Dx of exclusion

Heat Rash (Prickly Heat, Miliaria, Lichen Tropicus)

History
- Sweat gland blockage w/ localized inflammatory response
- Often seen in pts newly arrived to subtropical/tropical areas or during heat waves

Findings
- Euthermic, erythema w/ pruritic vesicles, primarily in intertriginous areas, then becomes anhidrotic
- Occasionally will become superinfected, usually *Staph*

Evaluation
- None

Treatment
- Treat pruritus: Diphenhydramine 25–50 mg PO or hydroxyzine 25 mg PO
- Desquamate skin w/ chlorhexidine antibacterial soap or salicylate-containing topical scrub

Disposition
- Home, PCP f/u

Pearl
- Avoid routine talcum powder application, which may block sweat glands

Heat Syncope

History
- Syncopal event in warm/humid weather or following strenuous activity
- Heat → vasodilation → peripheral intravascular blood pooling, $\downarrow$ central venous return

Findings
- Euthermic, nl exam

Evaluation
- EKG, eval for other causes of syncope (see *1c*)
- Syncope/presyncope sx should resolve w/i 30 min, if not consider further w/u

Treatment
- PO or IV hydration

Disposition
- Home, PCP f/u

Pearl
- Dx of exclusion, diagnose only in young healthy pts w/ no cardiac dz

Heat Exhaustion
History
- Gradual onset, extreme fatigue in warm/humid weather following strenuous activity, profuse sweating, dizziness, N/V; often pale w/ cool, moist skin
- Inadequate PO intake

Findings
- Mild hyperthermia, may reach 40°C (104°F), nl mental status

Evaluation
- BMP for electrolyte imbalance, UA (rhabdomyolysis uncommon)

Treatment
- IV hydration (PO if pt tolerates), replace w/ NS (or alternate w/ ½ NS if ↑ Na)

Disposition
- Observation w/ continued hydration until normothermic w/ good UOP

Pearl
- No value w/ fever-reducing medications

Heat Stroke
History
- Acute onset when compared to heat exhaustion
- Classic: Occurs during heat waves, affects susceptible pts: Elderly, chronically ill, scleroderma, CF, burns, alcoholics, homeless, mentally ill, on diuretics or anti-chol
- Exertional: Occurs in pts who are overwhelmed by heat overproduction: Athletes, military recruits, thyroid storm, pheochromocytoma, sympathomimetic overdose

Findings
- Hyperthermia >41°C/106°F, CNS Dysfxn: Confusion, disorientation, delirium
- Classic: Anhidrotic, tachypnea
- Exertional: Diaphoretic until "sweat gland fatigue"
- Muscles usually flaccid in HS, if rigid consider NMS, etc.

Evaluation
- BMP (electrolyte imbalance, ↓ blood sugar), LFTs (hepatic damage common), coags (DIC possible but uncommon), CK & UA (rhabdo common in exertional heat stroke)

Treatment
- Aggressive fluid resuscitation: Cooling procedures → vasoconstriction, can ↑ BP so may need to guide fluid status by UOP, IVC US, CVP, etc.
- Rapid cooling indicated, ↓ by 0.2°C/min → 39°C/102.2°F to avoid overshooting
- Ice water immersion: Can ↓ core temp in 10–40 min
- Evaporation: Spray water mist & use fan, maintains cutaneous vasodilation, avoids heat generation by shivering, 7× more efficient than ice packing but 2× as fast
- Adjunctive cooling strategies: Strategic ice packs near large blood vessels (ant neck, axilla, groin), ice water gastric lavage at NS 200 mL/h
- Mannitol 50–100 g IV ↑ renal blood flow, ↓ cerebral edema
- Treat rhabdo w/ IVF, HD if anuric, tx coagulopathy w/ FFP

Disposition
- Admit for ongoing tx & cooling

Pearls
- Avoid alcohol sponge baths, dantrolene
- Avoid antipyretics (APAP damages liver, salicylates aggravate bleeding)

- Avoid α-adrenergic drugs (promote vasoconstriction, ↑ hepatic/renal damage, CO same)
- Avoid atropine/anticholinergics that ↓ sweating; use BZD to stop shivering
- Avoid neuroleptics (chlorpromazine): ↓ sz threshold, interfere w/ thermoregulation, etc.

INTERNAL HEAT EMERGENCIES

Malignant Hyperthermia (MH)

History
- Acute ↑ body temp after administration of inhaled anesthetic or succinylcholine
- Genetic abnlty of skeletal muscle sarcoplasmic reticulum → inappropriate Ca release → severe tetany & spasm (heat); often FH of adverse rxn to anesthesia

Findings
- Acute hyperthermia after anesthetic, hypercapnia (early sign), muscular rigidity, masseter muscle spasm, acidosis, tachycardia, rhabdomyolysis

Evaluation
- Check core temp, electrolytes, CK

Treatment
- Stop offending agent, increase ventilation rate, dantrolene 2.5 mg/kg bolus IV, repeat doses of 1 mg/kg until sxs subside; MH protocols

Disposition
- Usually occurs in OR, admission for supportive care

Pearl
- MH hotline: 1-800-MH-HYPER (1-800-644-9737), ask for "Index Zero"

Neuroleptic Malignant Syndrome (NMS)

History
- Antipsychotic use (phenothiazines, butyrophenones, thioxanthenes, lithium, TCAs); recent initiation or dose ↑ (⅔ of cases in 1st wk)
- Anti-Parkinson medication withdrawal
- Dopamine receptor blockade → severe muscle spasticity & dystonia, heat overproduction

Findings
- Triad: Hyperthermia, muscular rigidity (lead pipe), autonomic Dysfxn
- AMS, dyskinesia, tachycardia, dyspnea, diaphoresis, dysphagia, tremor, incontinence

Evaluation
- UA for myoglobin, CK for rhabdomyolysis, ↑WBC, Chem, tox

Treatment
- Stop offending agent, mainstay is supportive tx: IVF, BZDs
- May consider dantrolene (as for MH), whole body cooling w/ evaporating fans
- Dopamine antagonists (bromocriptine 2.5 mg PO q8h, amantadine 200 mg PO q12h)
- Treat rhabdomyolysis w/ IVF, alkaline urine (pH > 6.5) to ↑ myoglobin excretion
- Keep Na in IVF close to 154 mEq/L; add NaHCO₃

Disposition
- Admission; mortality 10–20%

Pearl
- NMS hotline: 1-888-667-8367

Serotonin Syndrome (SS)

History
- Drug & food interactions: MAOI + tyramine (found in aged cheese, wine, etc.); caused by excessive serotonin activity in spinal cord & brain

Findings
- Hunter criteria: Combination of clonus, hyperthermia, agitation, diaphoresis, ocular clonus, hyperreflexia, tremor, hypertonia
- Diarrhea, cramps, hypersalivation (similar to NMS), autonomic Dysfxn

Evaluation
- UA for myoglobin, CK for rhabdomyolysis, CBC, Chem, tox
- Clinical dx, must confirm h/o 2 serotonergic agents, r/o toxic, metabolic, infectious cause

Treatment
- Stop offending agent, supportive tx, whole body cooling, treat rhabdo w/ IVF**
- BZD: May require high doses
- Dantrolene not recommended: May ↑ central serotonin metabolism & production
- Nonsp serotonin inhib: Cyproheptadine 12 mg PO then 2 mg PO q2h

Disposition
- Admission; most resolve w/ no sequelae in 24–36 h after starting tx

Pearl
- Pts must stop MAOI for 6 wk prior to starting SSRI

Differentiating NMS and Serotonin Syndrome		
	NMS	**SS**
Etiology	• A/w neuroleptic use • Idiosyncratic rxn to therapeutic doses	• A/w serotonergic agents • Manifestation of tox; often from combination of 2 serotonergic drugs
Timing	• Slow onset (days → weeks) • Slow progression (24–72 h)	• Rapid onset & progression
Sxs	• Bradykinesia, lead-pipe rigidity	• Hyperkinesia, less rigidity
Tx	• BZD • Dantrolene • Dopamine antagonists	• BZD • Serotonin inhibitors • NOT dantrolene

LIGHTNING INJURY

Background
- Acts as direct current → asystole; heart's intrinsic automaticity usually restarts in SR but CNS injury & concussion may cause respiratory arrest w/ secondary cardiac arrest

Approach
- Early & continuous cardiac monitoring for dysrhythmias
- Evaluate for concomitant trauma (fall, injury); maintain c-spine precautions
- Reverse triage in field: Lightning victims that appear dead should get CPR as pts can be pulseless w/ fixed, dilated pupils & still have good survivability

History
- Usually obvious, reported lightning strike near pt; often witnessed collapse

Findings
- TM rupture, transient vasospasm (cool ext), symp nervous system instability
- Various burn patterns
  - Linear: Caused by steam production during flashover (charge passes over surface of body only) where sweat accumulates
  - Punctate: Multiple cigarette-like burns
  - Feathering: Not actual burns; electron showers make a ferning pattern on skin (Lichtenberg figures)
  - Thermal: Usually from burnt clothing
- Ocular pathology: Corneal lesions, hyphema, vitreous hemorrhage, retinal detachment, cataracts develop long term
- Keraunoparalysis: Transient paralysis that can occur, likely 2/2 vasospasm, LE > UE, usually resolves in hours, still will need eval for true spinal cord pathology 2/2 trauma

Evaluation
- ECG, CBC, BMP, CK (rhabdomyolysis), UA (myoglobin), head CT if unresponsive

Treatment
- Resuscitate, eval for trauma, immobilize c-spine, continuous cardiac monitoring
- High-volume IV crystalloid (NS); same tx as electrical injury (10f)
- Urinary catheter placement: Target urine output 1–1.5 mL/kg/h (200–300 mL/h)
- If rhabdomyolysis (↑ CK, +UA dip), maintain high UOP until urine dip neg.
- Treat wounds the same as thermal burns (10 d), tetanus, wound care, etc.
- Splint injured extremities in best "position of fxn" to minimize contractures & edema

Disposition
- If asx & nl exam, can be discharged; good prognosis if survive in field
- ECG Δ, myoglobinuria, entry/exit burns, partial/full thickness burns: Admit to burn center

Pearl
- Lightning causes ~50–300 Ds in US each year, 25–30% of lightning strike victims die, of those that survive ~75% have permanent disability

DROWNING

Background
- AHA guidelines suggest a broad definition of drowning to include D from drowning, near drowning (no longer used!), wet drowning, etc.
- Definition: Respiratory impairment from being submerged under a liquid
- >4000 drowning Ds annually in US; toddlers & teenage boys at greatest risk
- Freshwater vs. saltwater vs. chlorinated pool water: No difference, theoretical diff only
- 1° insult to lung; water moves across alveolar–capillary membrane, destroys (freshwater) or washes out (salt water) surfactant → hypoxia
- Diving reflex = immersion of face in water <68°F, blood shunts from periphery → brain & heart → apnea, bradycardia, hypothermia → ↓metabolic demand prevents/delays severe cerebral hypoxia

Approach
- Careful hx: Possible diving (cervical spine or head) injury vs. 1° drowning, intoxicants, comorbidity, submersion time, water temp, initial rescuer response (ACLS)
- Extricate pt, remove wet clothing, ABCs, ACLS, intubation as appropriate
- Bedside glucose or D50 if AMS
- Cervical spine immobilization if suspicion for head or neck injury (diving, pool accident)

History
- Submersion event

Findings
- Variable presentation (awake, coma, cardiac arrest)
- Wheezes/rales/rhonchi, ecchymosis/crepitus/other signs of trauma on exam

Evaluation
- CBC, BMP, LFTs, tox, CXR may show pulmonary edema or aspiration 2–6 h after event, CT head & c-spine if concern for trauma, AMS

Treatment
- ABCs, intubation or supplemental O_2, CPR, ACLS, Foley placement
- Measure core temp, treat for hypothermia if indicated to temp 30°C/86°F
- Ventilator PEEP 5–10 mm H_2O to ↓ intrapulmonary shunting

Disposition
- Admission for continued tx, watch for signs of ARDS/VALI
- May develop pulm Δ even after mild submersion, observe asx pts for at least 8 h

Pearls
- Prophylactic abx & steroids not indicated
- Artificially induced hypothermia does not improve outcome

BOTULISM

Background
- Caused by neurotoxin produced by anaerobic gram-positive rod *C. botulinum*
  - Spore-forming bacterium found in soil & water, particularly in CA, UT, PA
- Blocks ACh release at neuromuscular jxn & autonomic ganglions (nicotinic receptors)

Approach
- Early airway management & ventilatory support
- Contact CDC Botulism center (404-639-2206/3311) for antitoxin, BabyBIG from CA

History
- 3 main etiologies: Infant, foodborne, or wound; also potential for bioterrorism
- Infant: Consumption of unpasteurized honey or likely exposure to endemic spores (feeding through a nipple dropped on the ground, sucking on fingers after playing in dirt)
- Foodborne (adult): Ingestion of food contaminated w/ spores, usually home-canned goods
- Wound: Spores infiltrate skin wounds, germinate, & release tox into the bloodstream

Findings
- Weakness, flaccid paralysis, respiratory arrest, autonomic dysfxn; CN affected 1st
- Infant: Weak cry, poor sucking, flaccid/hypotonic muscles
- Foodborne (12–36 h) & wound (several days): Autonomic dysfxn, descending symmetric motor paralysis, nl sensorium

Evaluation
- None needed prior to intervention
- Collect serum, stool, wound, & food samples for CDC testing

Treatment
- ABCs, intubation or supplemental O_2
- Administer antitoxin 1 vial IV to adults & children
- Infants need only supportive care, no antitoxin

Disposition
- Admission to ICU for ventilatory support

Pearls
- Consider botulism in all infant sepsis workups
- Artificially induced hypothermia does not improve outcome
- AGs, magnesium contraindicated as they potentiate neuromuscular blockade
- Recovery of strength may take ~4 mo; may require respiratory support for months

ANAPHYLAXIS AND ANGIOEDEMA

Approach
- Eval & treat anyone w/ potential anaphylaxis immediately; can deteriorate rapidly
  - Anaphylaxis median time to resp/card arrest: 5 min (2/2 drug), 15 min (2/2 venom), 30 min (2/2 food) *(Curr Opin Allergy Clin Immunol 2013;13(3):263)*

Definition
- Anaphylaxis – acute-onset occasionally life-threatening IgE-mediated rxn causing multisystem Dysfxn: skin (eg, urticaria), mucosa (eg, angioedema), GI (eg, n/v), respiratory (eg, bronchospasm), circulatory (eg, hypotension, syncope), neuro (eg, AMS)
  - Absence of cutaneous sx rare *(J Allergy Clin Immunol 2005;115:S485)*
- DDx: anaphylactoid rxn, angioedema, neurocardiogenic syndromes, malignancies a/w flushing (eg, carcinoid), scombroid toxicity, systemic mastocytosis, other causes of shock or respiratory collapse *(J Allergy Clin Immunol 2005;115:S485)*

Anaphylaxis & Anaphylactic-like Syndromes	
Pathophysiology	Definition
Anaphylaxis	IgE-mediated rxn → urticaria, hypotension, & bronchospasm (mx causes; requires repeat exposure but not always known)
Anaphylactoid rxn	Non-IgE-mediated rxn, can appear identical to anaphylaxis, but doesn't require prior exposure (eg, iodine-contrast)
Angioedema	Subdermal/submucosal edema, typically of the face, airway, & GI tract (eg, 2/2 ACEI, C1-esterase deficiency, idiopathic)

History
- Sx: sudden-onset is key; sx can involve many organ sx – hives, swelling of tongue/throat, hoarseness, dyspnea, N/V, abd cramps, presyncope
- Assess recent exposures: Foods (nuts, egg, shellfish), meds (abx, NSAIDs, vancomycin, iodine contrast; ACEi for angioedema), enzymes (insulin, trypsin, etc), airborne allergens (pollen, mold), venoms (bees, fire ants, snakes), exercise-induced, latex, idiopathic
- Check PMH for atopy, hypersensitivity syndromes, or hereditary angioedema

Physical Exam
- Urticaria, conjunctival injection, diffuse erythema, facial or oropharyngeal swelling, drooling, hoarseness, stridor, wheezing, ↓BP

Evaluation & Treatment
- Labs not routinely indicated; consider serum tryptase during acute event esp if idiopathic or dx uncertain (tryptase elevation sp but insensitive for IgE-mediated rxns)

Tx	
Type of rxn	Tx Approach
Most allergic rxns	Remove allergen
	H1-blocker: Diphenhydramine 25–50 mg PO or IV
	H2-blocker: Ranitidine 150 mg PO or 50 mg IV
	Prednisone 60 mg or Methylprednisolone 125 mg IV
Anaphylaxis *(J Allergy Clin Immunol 2005;115:S485; Ann Emerg Med 2006;47:373)*	Intubation: Consider early, consider fiberoptic/awake
	All txs for allergic rxn (IV)
	IVF bolus
	Epinephrine: (Repeat prn, ± infusion) IM: 0.3–0.5 mg (1:1000) IV: 0.1–0.25 mg (1:10000) if severe (IM is safer) Neb: 0.5 mL 2.25% epi in 2.5 mL NS (No IV) Epi gtt: 1–4 µg/min (titrate to stability)
Angioedema *(Ann Allergy Asthma Immunol 2007;98:383; NEJM 2008;359:1027)*	C1 esterase deficiency: FFP
	ACEI-induced: Stop ACEI, give icatibant if available (reduces time to resolution) *(NEJM 2015;372(5):418)*.
	Stable: Fiberoptic eval ± intubation
	Unstable: Cricothyrotomy

- H1-blocker + H2-blocker > H1-blocker alone for urticaria *(NEJM 2004;351:2203)*
- Epi IM vs. SC: IM preferred → more rapid absorption *(J Allergy Clin Immunol 2001;108:871)*
- Epi IM vs. IV: IM preferred → safer *(World Allergy Organ J 2015;8(1):32)*
- Epi & cardiac dz: Place on monitor → epi is relatively contraindicated w/ CAD, but mortality of anaphylaxis w/o epi >> mortality from arrhythmia 2/2 epi
- Epi vs. glucocorticoids: Epi first-line in anaphylaxis; glucocorticoids best for delayed sx, but evidence on acute benefit inconclusive *(Cochrane 2012;4:CD007596)*

Disposition
- Home: pts w/ either local rxns (w/o airway involvement) or delayed-presentation generalized rxn (w/o airway involvement)
  - Provide EpiPen Rx (esp if unknown cause) & allergist f/u
- **Biphasic rxns:** may occur in up to 20% of cases; median onset 11–15 h after initial sx resolve; risk reduced if 2/2 food, & increased if 2/2 drug or idiopathic; higher risk if initially hypotensive (*Immunol Allergy Clin North Am* 2007;27(2):309; *J Allergy Clin Immunol Pract* 2015;3(3):408; *Ann Allergy Asthma Immunol* 2015;115(4):312)
  - Risk of clinically important biphasic rxn small (<0.5%) (*Annals Emerg Med* 2014;63(6):736)
- Consider observation if required epi or if high risk for biphasic rxn; however, there is no clear data on recommended duration of observation, & early d/c may be appropriate (*Allergy* 2014;69(6):791)
- Admit to ICU: Severe anaphylactic rxn (mx epi, epi gtt, airway compromise)

Pearls
- ACEI can cause angioedema at any time, independent of length of use
- PCN allergy: IgE-mediated allergy confers low (~1%) risk of cross-reactivity w/ cephalosporins; however, avoid if rxn is severe (*NEJM* 2006;354:601)

ONCOLOGIC EMERGENCIES

See also Chapter 1 (Cardiac tamponade), Chapter 2 (Respiratory distress, Hemoptysis), Chapter 5 (Altered mental status, Seizure, Brain tumor, CNS infections), Chapter 9 (SIADH, Hypercalcemia), Chapter 12 (Cauda equine syndrome)

NEUTROPENIC FEVER

Overview (*Clin Infect Dis* 2011;52(4):e56)
- **Definition:** Fever (single temp >38.3°C *or* temp >38°C for 1 h) + Neutropenia (ANC <500 or predicted <500 w/i 24 h or "functional neutropenia" [eg, AML])
- **Approach:** Early IV access, IVFs, & abx; most pts will not end up having identifiable infxn (only 20–30%), but those who do can deteriorate quickly
- **Etiology:** Infxn found in 20–30% (bacteremia in 10–25%); fungal infxn rare unless neutropenia >1 wk; consider also trauma, drugs (chemo)

Differential for Fever in Neutropenic pt	
Category	**Source**
Bacterial	HEENT (sinusitis, mucositis, otitis, pharyngitis), Pulm (PNA, TB, pneumonitis), GI (colitis, mucositis, hepatobiliary), GU (UTI, pyelo), cardiac (endocarditis), neuro (meningoencephalitis, epidural abscess), skin (cellulitis, line-related infxn, abscess [inc perianal])
Viral	Influenza (in epidemics), RSV, other viral pathogens, HSV, CMV, EBV
Fungal	Candidiasis, aspergillosis (most common life-threatening)
Drug-related	Many chemo agents can cause immune-mediated febrile rxns

History
- Date of fever onset & last chemo (ANC nadirs 10–14 d after chemo); thorough ROS
- Assess RFs warranting inpt care: MASCC score (*see Disposition*)

Physical Exam
- Examine skin, mouth, lung, abdomen, catheter/surgical sites, perirectal area (No DRE)

Evaluation
- CBC w/ diff, Chem 20, coags, UA/urine cx, blood cx (at least 2 + any catheter port if present), ± CXR if resp sx
- ±Additional labs: Coags, culture (stool/sputum/peritoneal/CSF)
- Imaging: Consider imaging of chest, abdomen/pelvis, sinuses, brain

Low-risk Criteria for Neutropenic Fever	
Adults (*J Clin Oncol* 2000;18:3038)	Age <60, minimal sxs, no ↓ BP, solid tumor, No COPD, No fungal infection, No dehydration
Pediatrics (≤16 y/o) (*J Clin Oncol* 2000;18:1012)	Monocyte ≥100, No comorbidity, nl CXR

Treatment (*Clin Infect Dis* 2011;52(4):e56)
- Empiric tx depends on risk level (*see above*): low-risk (PO, outpt) vs. high-risk (IV, inpt)
  - Low risk: Ciprofloxacin + (amoxicillin/clavulanate or clindamycin [if PCN allergic])
    - If no RFs, mortality & tx failure w/ oral tx = similar to iv tx (*Cochrane* 2013;10:CD003992)

- High risk: Antipseudomonas (ceftazidime, cefepime, carbapenem [not ertapenem])
  - If PCN-allergic: levofloxacin + aztreonam or AG
  - If cx: Can add AG or quinolone for additional GNR synergy
  - If line-infxn, PNA, hypotension: Add vancomycin
  - If MDRO, consider carbapenem (if ESBL), vancomycin (if MRSA), linezolid (if VRE)
- Antifungals generally not indicated except if strong hx, shock, or recent HSCT

Disposition

- Admit all high-risk pts; low-risk pts can be d/c-ed only if close outpt f/u guaranteed
- CISNE score may outperform MASCC Risk Index in identifying low-risk pts who present to ED for eval (Ann Emerg Med 2015;PMID 28041827)

Multinational Association for Supportive Care in Cancer (MASCC) Risk Index				
Criteria	Pts	Predictive Performance of Fever Resolution w/o Serious cx		
No or mild sxs	5			
No hypotension (SBP > 90 mmHg)	5	Total Pts	PPV (%)*	
No active COPD (O$_2$, steroids, bronchodilators)	4			
No solid tumor or hx of previous fungal infxn	4	≥17	84	
No dehydration	3	≥19	86	
Moderate sx burden	3	≥20	90	
Outpt status	3	≥21	91	
Age <60 yr	3	≥22	94	

*PPV of fever resolution w/o med complications. J Clin Oncol 2000;18(16):3038.

Clinical Index of Stable Febrile Neutropenia (CISNE)					
Criteria	Pts	Rate of Adverse Outcome by Points			
ECOG performance status ≥2*	2	Outcome	Total Points		
Stress-induced hyperglycemia	2		0 (%)	1–2 (%)	≥3 (%)
Active COPD	1	Med Cx.	1.1	6.2	36.0
Chronic cardiovascular dz	1	Bacteremia	9.1	9.0	15.5
Mucositis NCI grade ≥2**	1	Mortality	0.0	0.0	3.1
Monocytes <200/μL	1				

J Clin Oncol. 2015;33(5):465. *ECOG Performance Status: 0 (fully active, able to carry on all predisease performance w/o restriction), 1 (restricted in physically strenuous activity but ambulatory & able to carry out work of a light or sedentary nature), 2 (ambulatory & capable of all self-care but unable to carry out work activities; up & about more than 50% of waking hours), 3 (capable of only limited self-care; confined to bed or chair more than 50% of waking hours), 4 (completely disabled; cannot carry on any self-care; totally confined to bed or chair). Source: Am J Clin Oncol 1982;5:649. **NCI Mucositis Grades: 0 (none), 1 (painless ulcers, erythema, or mild soreness in absence of lesions), 2 (painful erythema, edema, or ulcers but eating/swallowing possible), 3 (painful erythema, edema, or ulcers requiring IV hydration), 4 (severe ulceration or requiring parenteral or enteral nutritional support or prophylactic intubation). Source: Cancer 2004;100(9 Suppl):1995.

TUMOR LYSIS SYNDROME

Overview (NEJM 2011;364(19):1844; Oncology 2011;25(4):378)

- **Definition:** ≥2 metabolic abnltys (>25% ↑ K, ↑ PO$_4$, ↑ Ca, ↑ uric acid) w/i 3 d before or 7 d after the start of chemo, AND e/o AKI (GFR ≤ 60), arrhythmia, or sz
- **Etiology:** Rapid destruction neoplastic cells → release of nucleic acids, K, PO$_4$ → uric acid (from nucleic acids), AKI (2/2 uric acid), ↓ Ca (2/2 PO$_4$)
- Typically 48–72 h after starting cytotoxic cancer tx, a/w large, rapidly proliferating, tx-responsive tumors (esp acute leukemia, NHL, Burkitt)
- **Approach:** Obtain ECG immediately (look for signs ↑ K), & put on cardiac monitor

History

- Diverse sx (need high index of suspicion prior to labs): Lethargy, edema, CHF, hematuria, cardiac dysrhythmia, sz, muscle cramps, tetany, syncope, sudden D
- Assess last chemo, but may be presenting signs of malignancy

Evaluation (NEJM 2011;364(19):1844)

- Serial Chem 10 (↓ Ca, ↑ PO$_4$, ↑ BUN/Cr, ↑ K), ↑ uric acid (draw on ice), ↑ LDH (marker of tumor proliferation), UA (urine pH), CBC w/ diff, VBG, Foley or close UOP measurement

Treatment (NEJM 2011;364(19):1844)

- Correct electrolyte d/o (↑ K, ↑ PO$_4$, ↓ Ca), except: use Ca tx in hyperK cautiously (may worsen CaPO$_4$ crystals in kidneys & worsen AKI) (see also Chapter 9)

- Maintain UOP > mL/kg/h: IVF ± loop diuretic PRN
- Reduce uric acid: allopurinol (prevents uric acid formation) or rasburicase (more effective; breaks down existing uric acid); give rasburicase in consultation w/ oncology
  - Rasburicase (compared to allopurinol): lowers mean peak PO_4 & uric acid, less AKI, reduces need for HD; superior in mx trials
- Avoid $NaHCO_3$ for urine alkalinization: ↓ uric acid crystals, but also ↑ $CaPO_4$ crystals
  - Consider only if no rasburicase available AND nl serum PO_4
- HD: If persistent ↑ K, severe acidosis, volume overload, uremia, severe ↑ PO_4 or ↓ Ca

Disposition
- Admit (floor vs. ICU, depending on severity)

SUPERIOR VENA CAVA SYNDROME

Overview
- **Definition:** Intrinsic/extrinsic SVC obstruction causing upstream high venous pressures
- **Etiology:** Malignancy (eg, lung, mediastinum) in 90%, thrombosis (eg, a/w implantable device), rarely TB & syphilitic aortitis *(NEJM 2007;356(18):1862)*

History
- Subacute onset (usually wks) of facial swelling ± laryngeal edema (cough, hoarseness, stridor), cerebral edema (HA, confusion), or ↓ venous return (hypotension)
- Severity of sx, acuity of worsening, & type of malignancy dictate intervention & urgency

Physical Exam
- Check for facial/oropharyngeal edema, JVD, abnml lung sounds, neuro deficits

Evaluation
- Chem 10, CBC, CXR, CT Chest (w/ IV contrast) ± CT Head (r/o ICH), bedside echo

Treatment *(NEJM 2007;356(18):1862; Crit Care Med 2012;40:2212)*
- Elevate head of bed (decrease ICP), intubate if impending airway obstruction
- If 2/2 malignancy: Chemo, XRT, Endovascular stenting (if no tissue dx)
  - Glucocorticoids commonly used to reduce swelling, but uncertain benefit
- If 2/2 thrombosis: anticoagulation (if concurrent HA: r/o ICH first), remove line if able
- If cerebral edema or airway obstruction: c/s Rad-Onc, Interventional Radiology from ED

Disposition
- Admit for expedited w/u (eg, bx) & tx

NEUTROPENIC ENTEROCOLITIS (TYPHLITIS)

Overview *(World J Gastroenterol 2017;23(1):42)*
- **Definition:** Rare life-threatening dz of neutropenic pts, characterized by mucosal injury, bowel edema & distention, bacterial translocation; cecum ± ileum & other colon
- **Approach:** Early IV access, IVF, abx, surgical consultation

History
- Abd pain (RLQ or diffuse), diarrhea, fever; ± N/V, distention, GIB
- Onset corresponds to WBC nadir (10–14 d after chemo)

Physical Exam
- Always assess for rebound tenderness; No DRE given neutropenia

Evaluation
- CBC, Chem 20, lactate, blood cx, CT A/P (bowel thick/dilated, pneumatosis), ±Upright abd XR if CT delay (can show intramural gas) or c/f perforation (subdiaphragmatic air)

Treatment *(World J Gastroenterol 2017;23(1):42)*
- Supportive: IVF, analgesia, antiemetics, NGT for bowel decompression
- Early abx as for neutropenic fever (see above); add flagyl if hx or c/f Cdif
- May need surgical intervention if e/o perforation or bowel necrosis

Disposition
- Admit, may need ICU

HYPERVISCOSITY SYNDROME *(Emerg Med Clin N Am 2014;32:495)*

Overview
- **Definition:** Rise in serum viscosity 2/2 proteins, causing low-flow & prolonged bleeding
- Most common in Waldenström macroglobulinemia (leading cause; can be presenting sx), multiple myeloma, acute leukemia (2/2 cellular proteins)
- **Approach:** Early IV access, IVF, abx, surgical consultation

History
- Classic triad: mucosal bleeding, visual deficits, focal neuro signs; can also see CHF, pulm edema, AKI, confusion

Physical Exam
- Assess mucosal bleeding, fundoscopic exam, neuro findings

Evaluation
- CBC w/ diff, Chem 20, lactate ± NCHCT (if neuro sx), BNP, Troponin, CXR

Treatment
- Supportive: IVF
- Consultation w/ oncology for emergent plasmapheresis or expedited chemotx

Disposition
- Admit, may need ICU

SICKLE CELL DISEASE

Overview
- **Pathophysiology:** Recessive β-globin mutation → structurally abnl HbS → deoxygenated form polymerizes → RBC sickles → hemolysis/microvascular occlusion → tissue ischemia

Acute Presentations of SCD	
Acute anemia	**Aplastic crisis:** reduced marrow production (eg, parvo B19) combined w/ short existing RBC half-life **Splenic sequestration:** sequestration of RBCs in spleen **Hyperhemolytic crisis:** 2/2 hemolysis
Vaso-occlusive crisis (VOC)	Can manifest as pain, tissue infarction (stroke, renal necrosis, aseptic necrosis, hepatic); priapism
Acute chest syndrome (ACS)	Resembles PNA; fever, dyspnea, hypoxia, CXR infiltrates; 13% will require mechanical vent; mortality up to 9%; 80% occur w/ VOC (Chest 2016;149(4):1082)

- **Approach:** Initiate empiric IVF & analgesia early, can decompensate quickly; maintain high index of suspicion for infection from encapsulated organisms 2/2 functional asplenia

History & Physical Exam
- **HX:** Assess location, duration, & severity of pain; similarity to prior crises; infectious sx
- **PE:** Assess joint ROM in areas affected; respiratory status; neuro deficits; priapism

Evaluation
- CBC w/ diff (compare to baseline), Chem 20 (↑ bili in hemolysis), reticulocyte count (↑ in hemolysis or sequestration; ↓ in aplastic crisis), LDH (elevated), ABG (if hypoxic)
- Imaging as directed by sx: CXR (if CP or c/f ACS), x-ray/MRI (osteomyelitis or avascular necrosis), CTA chest (PE); CTA/MRI (stroke)

Treatment

Acute tx in SCD (Chest 2016;149(4):1082)	
Aplastic crisis	pRBC transfusion
Hyperhemolytic crisis	pRBC transfusion if hemodynamic compromise
Splenic sequestration	pRBC transfusion
VOC	O₂, IVF, Analgesia (check pain plan w/ outpt hematologist if possible), pRBC transfusion if below baseline
Acute chest syndrome	O₂, IVF, Abx (CTX/azithromycin), exchange transfusion; pRBC transfusion if delay to exchange transfusion
Acute stroke	O₂, IVF, exchange transfusion; pRBC transfusion if delay to exchange transfusion
Other severe organ injury (eg, hepatic)	O₂, IVF, pRBC transfusion, discuss exchange transfusion w/ hematology
Sepsis (any cause)	Broad-spectrum abx, esp if indwelling line

Chronic
- Hydroxyurea: ↑ HbF & ↓ pain crises, frequency & duration of hospitalizations, & risk of acute chest syndrome (NEJM 1995;1332:1317), ↓ mortality (NEJM 2003;1289:1645)

Disposition
- Home: If pain controlled, no e/o hemolysis; close hematology f/u
- Admit: Any acute cx as detailed above

ABNORMAL BLEEDING

Overview
- Etiology & tx depend on nature of problem (plt count, plt fxn, clotting time, combo)

Differential Dx for Abnl Bleeding	
1° Problem	Potential Causes
↓ plt count	ITP, HUS/TTP, DIC, HELLP syndrome (if pregnant), SLE, HIT, splenic sequestration (eg, NHL, myelofibrosis, cirrhosis), bone marrow failure (eg, aplastic anemia, heme malignancy), massive transfusion/dilution, chronic systemic dz
↓ plt fxn	vWD, meds (eg, ASA/NSAIDs, clopidogrel, GP IIb/IIA inhibitor), chronic systemic dz (eg, uremia, cirrhosis, leukemia/MDS)
↓ clotting cascade	DIC, meds (eg, coumadin, DOACs), factor deficiency (eg, hemophilia), chronic systemic dz (eg, malnutrition, cirrhosis), massive transfusion/dilution

History & Physical Exam
- Bleeding syndromes can present in many organ systems, including several at once:

Hx			
System	Manifestation	System	Manifestation
HEENT	Gingival bleeding, epistaxis	GU	Hematuria, menorrhagia
CNS	ICH, epidural hematoma	MSK	Hematoma, hemarthrosis
Pulm	Hemoptysis	Skin	Petechiae, purpura, ecchymosis
GI	Hematemesis, melena, hematochezia		

- Physical exam may suggest sp bleeding problem:
  - Petechiae: ↓ plt count
  - Purpura: ↓ plt count, ↓ plt fxn, problem w/ blood vessels or connective tissue
  - Ecchymosis: ↓ clotting cascade, problem w/ connective tissue, trauma

Evaluation
- CBC w/ diff, Chem 7, Coags; consider LFTs, peripheral blood smear, DIC panel (fibrinogen, D-dimer, LDH, haptoglobin), direct Coombs

IMMUNE THROMBOCYTOPENIA

Overview
- **Definition:** Immune Ab-mediated destruction of PLTs (PLT count <100 k/μL); either 1° (idiopathic) or secondary (2/2 virus, meds, autoimmune dz, pregnancy, vaccine)
  - Common associated meds: quinine, antimicrobials (linezolid, rifampin, vancomycin, sulfa), anticonvulsants (phenytoin, VPA, carbamazepine), thiazides, H2-blockers, NSAIDs/tylenol, chemotx (NEJM 2007;357(6):580)
- Dx of exclusion: r/o TTP/HUS, HIT, hematologic d/o (eg, malignancy, MDS, HIV)

History & Physical Exam
- Acute/subacute petechiae ± e/o bleeding (see above; assess for ICH, GIB, etc.); always ask about new meds, recent infectious sx, pregnancy

Evaluation (Blood 2010;115(2):168)
- CBC w/ diff (↓ plt count, otw nml), peripheral smear (no schistocytes), Coags (nml), T+S
- HIV/HCV recommended on all pts to r/o alt cause, H. pylori can be associated as well
- If dx confirmed or highly suspected: obtain baseline IgG/A/M levels, direct antiglobulin

Treatment (Blood 2010;115(2):168; NEJM 2007;357(6):580)
- Adults: If asx, tx rarely indicated if PLTs >50k & no bleeding, trauma, or surgery
- Children: Manage mild cases expectantly, treat if PLTs <20k or active bleeding

Tx for ITP		
Adults	No bleeding, Plt >50k	May manage expectantly; close f/u
	No bleeding, Plt <50k	Prednisone (0.5–2 mg/kg/d until plts), OR dexamethasone (40 mg/d), OR IV methylprednisolone (1 g/kg/d) if severe
		IVIG (1 g/kg/d) × 1–2 d
		Anti-D Ig (Rh+ pts only) (75 µg/kg/d)
	Bleeding, Plt <50k	Combine tx above, transfuse
Children	No bleeding, Plt <20k	Steroids: Prednisone 4 mg/kg/d PO × 4 d
		Anti-Rh(D) Ig: 75 µg/kg IV × 2 d
		IVIG: 0.8–1 g/kg IV × 1 dose
	Bleeding, Plt <20k	Combine tx above, transfuse

- Transfuse platelets as per guidelines below (see Transfusion section)
- Steroids: 50–75% response, often by 3 wk
- IVIG: Equivalent but quicker remission compared to steroids; consult w/ hematology
- Anti-D Ig: As effective as IVIG, but shorter infusion, longer response; consult w/ hematology
- Second-line tx should be discussed w/ consultant: azathioprine, cyclosporine, cyclophosphamide, dapsone, mycophenolate, rituximab, splenectomy, others
  - No role for plasmapheresis in tx of ITP

Disposition
- Home: If no active bleeding, PLTs >20k
- Admit: Any pt w/ PLTs <20k &/or active bleeding
- Long-term relapse is common (>70%) despite tx modality (NEJM 2007;357(6):580)

HEPARIN-INDUCED THROMBOCYTOPENIA (HIT)

Overview
- **Definition:** TCP (<150k) or 30–50% drop in plt count after starting heparin
  - More common w/ unfractionated heparin, but occurs as well w/ LMWH
- **Pathogenesis:** Heparin-dependent IgG binds PF4 → plt activation → ↑ thrombosis
  - Thrombosis causes sx in 50% pts: PE, DVT > limb ischemia, stroke > MI

History & Evaluation
- Can have sx of TCP (if plts very low), thrombosis (even w/ nl plt count), or be incidental discovery; very rarely causes bleeding
- Usual occurrence 5–10 d after starting heparin, more rapid onset if recent heparin exposure
- Anti-PF4 enzyme assays highly se, poorly sp (good NPV); combine lab testing w/ clinical probability (hi, med, low) based on: Δ plt count (>50%, 30–50%, <30%), timing (5–10 d, >10 d, <4 d), thrombotic cx, & alternative causes (yes, possible, no)

Treatment (NEJM 2006;355:809; NEJM 2001;344:1286)
- STOP heparin + any device/flush that contains heparin (even if thrombotic cxs)
- Initiate nonheparin a/c (even if no thrombosis): argatroban (first-line), bivalirudin, lepirudin
  - Avoid vitamin-K antagonists, as will decrease protein C → ↑ thrombosis
- Avoid PLT transfusions unless bleeding or high risk of bleeding
- Recurrence w/ future heparin may be low if neg. for PF4 Ab >100 d after Dx

Disposition
- Admit for monitoring & intravenous anticoagulation

HEMOLYTIC-UREMIC SYNDROME (HUS) & THROMBOTIC THROMBOCYTOPENIC PURPURA (TTP)

(NEJM 2006;354(18):1927; NEJM 2014;371(7):654)

Overview
- **Definition:** Systemic (TTP) or intrarenal (HUS) microvascular occlusive d/o 2/2 PLT aggregation → MAHA + TCP
- **Pathogenesis:** TTP a/w ADAMTS13 dysfxn (ADAMTS13 normally cleaves vWF, resultant inability to cleave vWF → plt activation → microthrombi); HUS a/w E. coli O157:H7

History & Physical Exam
- TTP: Acute/subacute, can be subtle & non-sp (classic pentad rare); adults > children
  - MAHA: Vague sx (abd pain, nausea, weakness) 2/2 diffuse microvascular thrombi
  - TCP: e/o bleeding, skin findings (petechial, purpura)
  - Neuro sx: AMS, stroke, szs; neuro sx present only 50%
  - AKI: Can be mild
  - Fever: Uncommon, low-grade when present); no other cause
- HUS: Acute-onset, bloody diarrhea & abd pain, f/b TCP & renal failure
  - Classic triad: MAHA + TCP + Renal failure
- Always ask about triggers: HUS (contaminated food), TTP (meds, systemic dz, HSCT)

Evaluation
- CBC w/ diff (↓ Hct, ↓ Plt), Chem 20 (↑ Cr, ↑ LFTs), peripheral smear (schistocytes), coags (nml), ↑ LDH, ↓ haptoglobin, fibrinogen, D-dimer, UA

Treatment (NEJM 2006;354(18):1927; NEJM 2014;371(7):654)
- Consult hematology, consider renal consult early
- TTP: Plasma exchange (↑ survival @ 6 mo, 78%), FFP (if delay to plasma exchange), Steroids (prednisone 1–2 mg/kg/d, methylprednisolone 1 g/d, data on efficacy limited)

- HUS: Supportive; pts commonly need dialysis
- Do not give PLTs → ↑ microvascular thrombosis

Disposition
- Admit, may require ICU
- Risk of relapse is low in acquired TTP, but can occur even years after initial episode
- HUS in kids often resolves w/o long-term renal dz (but >45% mortality in adults)

DISSEMINATED INTRAVASCULAR COAGULATION (DIC)

Overview
- **Definition:** Acquired life-threatening consumptive coagulopathy a/w diverse dz
- **Pathogenesis:** Widespread activation of coagulation → thrombosis of small/midsized vessels → organ dysfxn, ↓ PLTs/coagulation factors → bleeding & thromboembolism

Causes of DIC	
Cancer (top cause)	Solid tumors, hematologic malignancy, metastasis
Infectious dz	Sepsis, viremia
Trauma	Severe trauma, burn, head injury, fat embolism
Obstetrics	Amniotic fluid embolism, abruptio placentae, HELLP syndrome
Immunologic	Severe allergic rxn, transfusion rxn, tpx rejection, autoimmune dz

History, Physical Exam, Evaluation
- Underlying systemic dz is necessary for dx (see above)
- Assess for s/sx of bleeding, end-organ damage
- CBC w/ diff (↓ PLTs [usually <100]), ↑ PT, ↑ PTT, ↑ D-dimer, ↓ fibrinogen, ↑ LDH, ↑ Fibrin degradation products, e/o end-organ damage (↑ lactate, ↑ Cr); imaging PRN by sx
- Different scoring systems used to help in dx of DIC (Thromb Haemost 2011;105(1):40)

Treatment
- Treatment of underlying disorder is mainstay of tx
- Transfuse if bleeding, risk of bleeding, or need for procedure: PLTs (if bleeding + plt <50k, or plt <20k), FFP (if INR >1.5; beware large doses may be required [15–30 mL/kg]), cryoprecipitate (if fibrinogen <1.5 g/dL despite FFP), prothrombin complex concentrate (if bleeding & FFP delayed/not possible [eg, volume])
- Heparin/LMWH if thromboembolism predominates (LMWH may be superior to UH)

Disposition
- Admit to ICU

VON WILLEBRAND DISEASE (vWD)

Overview
- **Definition:** Most common inherited bleeding d/o caused by ↓ vWF (↓ quantity [type 1, 3] or fxn [type 2]); vWF carries factor VIII & enables plt adhesion/aggregation; rarely acquired
- **Etiology:** Precursor vWF cleaved by ADAMTS13 (see TTP above) → circulating vWF activated by vascular damage → vWF binds collagen → plt aggregation → ↓ vWF leads to ↓ plt aggregation & ↑ factor VIII degradation

History & Physical Exam
- Mucocutaneous bleeding, menorrhagia, bruising, epistaxis, hemarthrosis, hematomas
- 5–20% of pts w/ menorrhagia will have vWD (sometimes requiring TAH)
- Most pts aware of their hx (60–80% will have bleeding after surgery)

Evaluation
- CBC w/ diff, T&S, coags (↑ PTT); ↓ vWF Ag, ↓ vWF activity, ↓ factor VIII activity

Treatment
- Desmopressin (DDAVP): Most useful in Type 1 vWD, where sufficient & functional vWF exists in noncirculating form; DDAVP causes endothelial release of vWF & ↑ circulating vWF levels (no chg in overall vWF); efficacy variable; dose 0.3 µg/kg IV
- vWF replacement: most useful in Type 2 or 3, where endogenous vWF either dys-fxnal or absent; options in include cryoprecipitate (requires up to 8–12 bags), plasma-derived vWF/factor VIII concentrate (Humate-P), or recombinant vWF + factor VIII
- Life-threatening bleeds: Important to increase levels of both vWF & factor VIII
- Adjunct tx: Antifibrinolytic amino acids (eg, TXA); high-quality data lacking

Disposition
- If severe or significant bleeding, admx; if d/c, f/u w/ hematology

HEMOPHILIA A/B

(BMJ 2012;344:e2707; Haemophilia 2013;19(1):e1)

Overview
- Definition: X-linked (males) d/o 2/2 ↓ factor VIII (hemophilia A) or factor IX (hemophilia B)

Hemophilia Dz Severity		
Severity	**Factor Concentration (% of nml)**	**Manifestations**
Mild	5–40 IU/dL	Spontaneous IM bleeding
Moderate	1–5 IU/dL	Severe bleeding w/ minor trauma
Severe	<1 IU/dL	Severe bleeding w/ major trauma

History & Physical Exam
- Bleeding (GI, GU, mucosa), hematoma, hemarthroses, bruising

Evaluation
- CBC, nml INR, ↑ PTT, T&S, Imaging PRN

Treatment
- Minor bleeds: desmopressin/DDAVP (0.3 μg/kg IV, 150 μg IN kids/300 μg IN adults) increases factor VIII concentration 3–5 × 2/2 release of vWF; transexamic acid (25–50 mg/kg/d); DDAVP for hemophilia A, TXA for hemophilia A/B
- Moderate–Severe bleeds: factor VIII/IX concentrate based on extent of deficiency; refer to product-sp dosing instructions (Haemophilia 2013;19(1):e1)
  - If severe (eg, ICH), give factor even prior to diagnostic testing
  - If pts have developed inhibitors to factor VIII, consider use of factor VIIa or prothrombin complex (bypass factor VIII in clotting cascade)

TRANSFUSIONS

See Chapter 18 for transfusions in trauma.

Overview
- **Approach:** Obtain type/screen for any pt suspected of needing transfusion

Transfusion Product Sp	
Irradiated	Use for pts w/ cellular immunosuppression (eg, neonates, HSCT, congenital immune def); destroys donor T-cells (↓ GVHD)
Leuko-reduced	Use for tpx pts or pts requiring mx transfusions; removes WBCs (↓ infxn [eg, CMV], ↓ rejection against donor product)
Washed	Use for pts w/ hx of transfusion allergic rxns; removes plasma components (↓ allergic rxns); very time intensive
Pheresis	Single-donor (vs. pooled-donor); refers to platelet transfusion

Packed Red Blood Cell Transfusion (Ann Intern Med 2012;157:49)
- **When to give:** restrictive strategies ↓ adverse events, mortality (Cochrane 2012;(4):CD002042)
  - All pts: Hgb ≤7, Hgb >7 + acute, ongoing, or significant sx
  - Cardiovascular dz: Hgb ≤8, Hgb >8 + acute, ongoing, or significant sx
- **What to give:** always obtain T&S in anyone who may need transfusion
  - Emergent transfusion: O neg. blood to females, O positive to males
  - In massive transfusion (expected >10 U PRBC/d), give FFP & PLTs as well
- **How much to give:**
  - Neonates: ↑ Hgb by 3 g/dL for 10–15 mL/kg of PRBCs
  - Adult: ↑ Hgb by 1 g/dL or Hct by 3%, for each 1 U PRBCs
- **What to monitor:**
  - Electrolytes: esp if large volume PRBC (↑ K, ↓ Ca)
  - O₂: Pts w/ CHF may require concurrent diuresis

Platelet Transfusion
- **When to give:**
  - PLT < 10K: regardless of s/sx of bleeding or comorbidities
  - PLT < 20K: non-bleeding but high risk if deteriorates (eg, chronically ill, high-risk onc)
  - PLT < 50K: active bleeding or need for invasive procedure
  - PLT < 100K: need for ophthalmologic or neurosurgical procedure
- **How much to give:** ↑ PLTs by 5000–10000 for each 1 U PLTs

Fresh-Frozen Plasma Transfusions (Transfusion 2010;50(6):1227)
- **When to give:** Mass transfusion (see Trauma section); reversal of warfarin; coagulopathy (eg, DIC); TTP/HUS (if delay to plasmapheresis); replacement of factor deficiencies

- **How much to give:** 10–20 mL/kg will ↑ coagulation factors by 20–30% (1U FFP = 200 mL); consider giving concurrent diuretic if e/o or known hx of CHF

Cryoprecipitate Transfusions
- How much to give: fibrinogen level <1 g/dL; factor XIII deficiency; hemophilia or vWD
- How much to give: 1 U/5–10 kg body weight to maintain fibrinogen >1 g/L

ANTICOAGULATION REVERSAL

Approach
- Hold further doses of anticoagulant
- Supportive care: Gastric lavage or activated charcoal (if overdose w/i 1 h), apply pressure to site of bleeding if possible, transfuse (as indicated)
- Agent-sp reversal: If significant/life-threatening bleeding (eg, ICH, hemoptysis, GIB) or need for emergent procedure/surgery

Reversal of Common Anticoagulants		
Antiplatelet agent	Minor bleed	Weigh risks/benefits of holding antiplatelet
	Severe bleed	Hold antiplatelet agent Consider plt transfusion (though new data suggests may cause harm in case of ICH)[1,2]
Heparin		Protamine (1 mg/90–100 U heparin in last 2–3 h; max 50 mg)[2]
LMWH		Protamine may be partially (60–80%) effective (dosing above)[2] Andexanet may be effective (under study)[3]
Warfarin[4]	INR <5 No bleeding	Decrease or omit single warfarin dose F/U for INR check w/i 48–72 h
	INR 5–9 No bleeding	Omit 1–2 warfarin doses Vitamin K 2.5 mg PO × 1 if risk for bleeding F/U for INR check w/i 24–48 h
	INR >9 No bleeding	Hold warfarin (until F/U INR recheck) Vitamin K 5 mg PO × 1 F/U for INR check w/i 12–24 h
	INR >1.5 Serious bleed	Hold warfarin Vitamin K 5–10 mg IV (risk of anaphylactoid rxn) Prothrombin clotting complex (25–50 IU/kg) FFP (10–20 mL/kg) only if PCC unavailable
DOAC	Dabigatran	Idarucizumab reverses bleeding w/i minutes[5] 4-factor PCC may have effectiveness
	Rivaroxaban	4-factor PCC may have effectiveness Andexanet may be effective (under study)[6]
	Apixaban	4-factor PCC may have effectiveness Andexanet may be effective (under study)[6]
	NOTE: At time of publishing, several additional DOACs & reversal agents are under investigation. Data is limited.	

[1]Lancet 2016;387(10038):2605. [2]American College of Chest Physicians Evidence-Based Clinical Practice Guideline on Antithrombotic and Thrombolytic Therapy (8th ed.). [3]Hematol Oncol Clin North Am 2016;30(5):1085. [4]Circulation 2012;125(23):2944. [5]NEJM 373(25):2413. [6]NEJM 2015;373(6):511.

Pearls
- Irreversible antiplatelet agents inhibit life of platelet (7–10 d)
- Vitamin K takes 6 (IV) to 24 (PO) hours to reverse warfarin; IV may cause anaphylactoid rxn in rare instances (push slowly over 30 min)
- 4F-PCC superior to FFP, may have fewer adverse events (Lancet 2015;385(9982):2077)
  - Adverse events: w/ 4F-PCC mostly 2/2 thrombosis; w/ FFP mostly 2/2 volume

TRANSFUSION COMPLICATIONS

Approach
- Always obtain consent if possible before giving a transfusion
- If e/o rxn: Stop transfusion, check bag, label, & send remaining products to blood bank
  - May be possible to resume transfusion in mild allergic rxn only (see below)
- If febrile, obtain CBC, smear, direct Coombs, UA, gram stain, BCx (pt & product)

Common or Critical Transfusion rxns		
Rxn	Incidence*	Note
Febrile (nonhemolytic)	1:100	Recipient Ab against donor cytokines; dx of exclusion **HX:** Fever, discomfort ± transient HTN **TX:** Antipyretics, monitor to r/o infxn (septic tfusion) or hemolysis (acute hemolytic rxn)
Allergic	1:1000	Histamine-mediated; more common w/ platelet tfusion
Anaphylactic	1:10,000	**DX:** Pruritus, urticaria ± angioedema, e/o anaphylaxis **TX:** H1B; if anaphylaxis then add H2B, glucocorticoids, IM epi; can restart transfusion if sx were local only & full resolution (stop if recurs) **Pearls:** If hx of tfusion allergic rxn, consider washed products & H1B premed; no role for steroid premed
Febrile (acute hemolytic)	1:10,000	Blood product error (eg, ABO incompatibility, incorrect preparation): can be immune or nonimmune **DX:** Fever (first sign) → flank pain, AKI, hemoglobinuria, anemia, DIC, shock w/i 24 h **TX:** If fever, monitor for other sx; IVF/diuretics for UOP **Pearls:** Differs from delayed hemolytic rxn (1:2.5K [1:10 in SCD]; 2/2 Abs against non-ABO groups; occurs 1 wk after tfusion; dx by Hgb not rising as expected, +Coombs; ↑ Bili; no tx needed)
TRACO (transfusion-associated circulatory overload)	1:10,000	Excess volume/rate of tfusion, ↑ risk if hx of CHF, CKD, large volume or rapid rate (eg, hemorrhage) **DX:** SOB, ↑ BNP, ↑ CVP, pulm edema w/i 6 h of tfusion **TX:** O₂, diuresis, NIPPV prn, restart tfusion slowly **Pearl:** Give diuresis w/t fusion high-risk for TRACO
TRALI (transfusion-related lung injury)	1:100,000	Proposed etiology: donor Abs bind recipient WBCs → pool in pulm capillaries → ↑ permeability → edema **DX:** SOB, ↓ O₂, CXR w/ b/l infiltrates; fever/hypothermia, hypotension/HTN; w/i 72 h of tfusion **TX:** Supportive (O₂, low tidal-volume vent if intubated)
Septic	1:100,000	Infected blood product, most common w/ platelets **DX:** Fever, rigors, hypotension; +BCx (pt & product) **TX:** Broad-spectrum abx (inc antipseudomonal)
Viral infection	Variable	HBV (1:250K), HCV (1:1.6M), HIV (1:1.8M)

*Incidence estimates are per unit transfused; rounded to nearest factor of ten. *Lancet* 2016;388(10061):2825; *JAMA* 2003;289:959; *NEJM* 1999;340:438.

EMERGENCIES IN THE TRANSPLANT PATIENT

Infectious Complications
- Incidence is 25–80% in 1st year after transplant
- Can be subtle: Immunosuppression can diminish classic sx (eg, fever, localizing sx), radiographic signs, or serology results; maintain high index of suspicion
- Timing of infection after tpx a/w type of infection
  - Nosocomial: Asp PNA, wound infxn, UTI (Foley), donor infxn, line infxn, C, difficile
  - Opportunistic: *PJP, Histoplasma, Coccidioides, Cryptococcus,* HBV, HCV, BK polyoma-virus, CMV, TB, EBV; assess if pt is on ppx (eg, PJP, CMV, fungal ppx)
  - Community: PNA, Influenza, EBV, RSV, Legionella, UTI
- If septic, strongly consider adjunct stress-dose steroids

Infections in Posttransplant pts	
0–1 mo posttransplant	Bacterial > fungal, viral
	Nosocomial > opportunistic, community
1–6 mo posttransplant	Bacterial, fungal, viral
	Opportunistic > nosocomial, community infxn
>6 mo posttransplant	Bacterial, fungal, viral
	Community > opportunistic infxn > nosocomial

Graft Rejection
- Recipient immune-mediated rxn against transplanted organ (esp microcirculation)
- Frequency & sx of rejection vary by organ tpx type
  - 20% kidney; 64% (acute)/23% (late) liver tpx, 30% cardiac (acute), 30% lung (first yr)
- Essential to involve transplant team if considering rejection
- TX: High-dose intravenous steroids; may require additional tx

Signs & sxs of Transplant Rejection	
Renal (20%)	SX: Often asx; fever, malaise, oliguria, graft pain; HTN
	DX: Labs (↑ BUN/Cr, abnml lytes); urine lytes (r/o other dx); Renal US w/ ↑ resistive indices
Liver (60% <6 mo; 25% late)	SX: Fever, malaise, abd pain, organomegaly, ascites
	DX: Labs (↑ LFTs); RUQUS (r/o other dx [eg, thrombosis])
Cardiac (30% <6 mo)	SX: SOB, orthopnea, palpitations, near-syncope, GI sx if R heart predominance (RUQ pain, nausea)
	DX: Labs (↑ Troponin, BNP), ECG w/ ST/Tw chgs, BSUS w/ systolic/diastolic dysfuxn; CXR w/ edema (if L heart)
Lung (30% <1 yr)	SX: SOB, cough, lung exam variable
	DX: Labs (↑ eos), CXR can be nml, Chest CT

Organ-specific Complications
Renal Transplant
- UTI (most common): always cx; consider strongly dual-abx & admx
- Arterial stenosis (10%): HTN, ↓ UOP, edema; U/S w/ flow limitation; tx w/ stent
- Venous thrombosis (4%): Graft pain/erythema, ↓ UOP, N/V; U/S (may need contrast CT); often results in graft failure & need for graft replacement
- Ureteral obstruction (3–6%): ↓ UOP, edema; U/S w/ hydronephrosis; if no correction w/ Foley, may need percutaneous intervention for urinary drainage
- Urinary leakage (2–5%): ↓ UOP, perineal leakage; U/S w/ peritpx fluid collxn; urology c/s
- Lymphocele (5–15%): abd swelling; US w/ hydrocele (CT for definitive dx)

Liver Transplant
- Hepatic artery thrombosis (4–12%): Doppler U/S 90% Se; mortality 80% w/o tx
- Hepatic artery stenosis (14%): Doppler U/S 70% Se; may require angiography for dx
- Pseudoaneurysm: Can cause hemobilia, hemoperitoneum, GIB; dx w/ U/S or CT
- Biliary strictures: May be asx 2/2 denervation; U/S (Se 66%), MRCP (Se 95%); tx stent
- Biliary leaks (2–25%) & bilomas: tx w/ stenting over leak, drain & abx (if biloma)

Cardiac Transplant
- Allograft vasculopathy (30–70%): Chronic & progressive; rapid atherosclerosis in tpx organ; may have s/sx of ischemia, or be asx 2/2 denervation (inc sudden cardiac arrest)
- Bradycardia: 2/2 sinus or AVN trauma; refractory to atropine 2/2 loss of vagal innervation
- Tachyarrhythmias: BB > CCB for Afib/flutter (2/2 med interaction); half-dose adenosine 2/2 sensitivity of transplanted heart

Lung Transplant
- Airway anastomotic stenosis, tracheobronchomalacia (increase in granulation tissue), necrosis; SOB/stridor; CT may help, but bronch is definitive dx; may need stent
- Fistula: Depending on tract, may present w/ PTX, crepitus, hemoptysis
- Pulm artery stenosis: Early & late after tpx; SOB, ↓ O2, LE edema, ↓ BP; dx w/ CTA chest
- Pulm vein thrombosis: Early after tpx; SOB, ↓ O2, LE edema, ↓ BP; dx w/ CTA chest
- Phrenic nerve injury (3–9% lung tpx; 40% heart–lung tpx): SOB; CXR ↑ hemidiaphragm

LEG PAIN AND SWELLING

Approach
- Careful hx: Anatomic distribution, unilateral vs. bilateral, acute vs. chronic, a/w erythema or dermatologic findings; hx of trauma
- Assess for paresthesia, hyperesthesia, or neuropathy
- Complete neurologic & vascular exam, assess for motor weakness

Differential

Pathophysiology	Differential
Cardiac	CHF (edema, venous stasis)
Vascular	DVT (see Ch. 1), PVD, arterial occlusion, vascular ulcers, thrombophlebitis
Infection	Osteomyelitis, necrotizing fasciitis, septic joint, cellulitis/abscess (see Ch. 4)
Musculoskeletal	Fracture, sprain, dislocation, hematoma, compartment syndrome; spinal stenosis (pseudoclaudication)
FEN/GU	Electrolyte abnlties, glomerulonephritis, nephritic syndrome
OB/GYN	Pregnancy, HELLP syndrome
Neurologic	Guillain–Barré, peripheral neuropathy
Environmental	Heat edema
Neoplasm	Sarcoma, SVC syndrome

PERIPHERAL VASCULAR DISEASE

Claudication
History
- Ischemic muscle pain reproducible w/ exertion, improves w/ rest
- Pts often place legs in dependent position to improve flow
- 1–2% have chronic critical limb ischemia: Pain at rest, nonhealing ulcers, dry gangrene

Findings: May have nl exam at rest w/ or w/o ↓ peripheral pulses; shiny, smooth skin
Evaluation
- ABI <0.9 is diagnostic of PVD (sens & spec)
- Careful pulse exam, w/ Doppler if difficult to palpate
- Look for signs of critical ischemia (rest pain, nonhealing ulcers)

Management: If concern for critical ischemia or acute dz, consult vascular surgery
Disposition
- Admit acute dz
- D/C home if chronic w/ vascular surgery f/u, strict return instructions

Acute Extremity Arterial Occlusion
History
- Known PVD +/or RFs (HTN, tobacco, known CAD, AF)
- Abrupt onset of pain w/ distal paresthesias
- Late (concerning findings): poikilothermia, pallor, paresthesia, pulselessness

Findings
- Cold, mottled extremity, ↓ pulse, motor weakness, ± bruit
- Tenderness to palpation out of proportion of exam or ↓ sensation

Evaluation
- Bedside Doppler of all pulses, including unaffected extremities; ABI
- Labs: CBC, BMP, baseline coags, ± lactate
- U/S can demonstrate level of occlusion
- CTA or angiography
- ECG for arrhythmia, may need echo to look for embolic source

Treatment
- Immediate vascular surgery consultation for possible embolectomy
- Anticoagulation (discuss w/ vascular): Heparin 18 U/kg/h IV w/o bolus

Disposition
- Transfer to facility w/ vascular surgery capability if none available

Pearl
- Ischemic tissue D starts by 4 h; sooner in pts w/ chronic arterial insufficiency

	Measurement of Ankle–Brachial Indices (ABIs)
1	W/ pt lying supine, measure SBP at ankle & ipsilateral wrist Place cuff over biceps to measure wrist SBP & over calf to measure ankle SBP Place Doppler U/S over radial pulse for wrist measurement & over posttibialis or DP for ankle measurement Inflate cuff until Doppler pulse no longer heard, record this pressure
2	Divide ankle SBP by wrist SBP nl ABI = 1, <0.9 defines PVD ABI < 1 indicates lower-extremity diminished flow ABI > 1 indicates upper-extremity diminished flow

TRAUMA

Compartment Syndrome

History
- Can occur in any closed fascial space, most commonly in distal lower extremity (calf)
- Hx of trauma (esp crush), burns, rhabdomyolysis, tight cast/dressing, hemorrhage (anticoagulants, coagulopathy), postischemic swelling, snakebites, IVDU

Findings
- Pain out of proportion to exam, pain w/ passive stretch of muscles that run through compartment (see the table below), paresthesias, pallor of the extremity, taut or rigid compartment. LATE: Decreased pulse, sensory/motor deficits.

Evaluation
- Measure compartment pressures: nl <8 mmHg; emergent fasciotomy if >30 mmHg
- Stryker instrument: Enter each compartment perpendicular to the skin
- A-line manometer: Attach 18G needle to A-line manometer; check that the compartment pressure being measured is at the same height as the manometer transducer

Treatment
- Immediate orthopedic/surgical consult for fasciotomy

Disposition
- Admit to ortho for serial manometry & neurovascular checks if compartment pressures <30 mmHg but evolving compartment syndrome suspected

Pearls
- Nl compartment pressure does *not* r/o compartment syndrome; clinical Dx
- 6% incidence w/ open tibia fx; 1% in closed tibia fx; 30% w/ arterial injury; 14% w/ venous

Lower-Extremity Compartments & Associated Muscles	
Deep posterior	Flexor digitorum longus, tibialis posterior, flexor hallucis longus
Superficial posterior	Soleus & gastrocnemius
Lateral	Peroneus longus, peroneus brevis
Anterior	Tibialis anterior, extensor hallucis longus, extensor digitorum longus

LOWER BACK PAIN

Approach
- Careful hx: Anatomic distribution, unilateral vs. bilateral, acute vs. chronic, fever, abd pain, groin pain, syncope hx of trauma; worse at rest or at night; incontinence?

Historical Red Flags for Back Pain	
For fracture	Age >70, any trauma w/ age >50, chronic steroids, osteoporosis, sxs of cancer (eg, weight loss, B sxs)
For malignancy	Elderly, sxs of cancer, worse when supine, >1 mo of sxs
For infection	Fever, IVDU, HIV, immunosuppression, hx of TB
For aortic/vascular	Abd pain, "tearing" pain, syncope, urinary sxs

- Physical exam w/ thorough neurologic exam, straight leg raise, pulses, rectal tone, gait
- Always check urine pregnancy test in females of childbearing age
- X-rays not routinely indicated: Use for red flags above, abnl exam, point tenderness
- Most require only analgesia & f/u but always consider life- & limb-threatening conditions

Differential	
Pathophysiology	**Differential**
GI (see Ch. 3)	Abd aneurysm/dissection, pancreatitis, cholecystitis, ulcer (±perforation)
Trauma	Acute lumbosacral strain, vertebral compression fracture, retroperitoneal bleed (minor/no trauma but on anticoagulant)
Infectious	Spinal epidural abscess, discitis, osteomyelitis, pyelonephritis/perinephric abscess
Neurologic	Cauda equina syndrome, herniated disc, spinal stenosis
Rheumatologic	Rheumatoid arthritis, ankylosing spondylitis, OA
FEN/GU	Nephrolithiasis
Vascular	Spinal hematoma/dissection
Neoplasm	Malignancy (multiple myeloma in elderly), bony metastasis

TRAUMA

Acute Lumbosacral Strain
History
- Usually hx of precipitating event: twisting, lifting, new workout. Acute/subacute onset
- Should have no fever or radicular sxs

Findings: Paravertebral muscle spasm & tenderness, nl neuro exam

Evaluation: No indication for imaging acutely

Treatment
- NSAIDs; if severe, short course opioids or BZD; early activity (no bed rest!)
- Muscle relaxants of no proven value, many side effects (anticholinergic, dependence)

Disposition: D/C home w/ PCP f/u, strict return instructions

Pearl: Lumbar strain is the #1 cause of LBP in ED but a dx of exclusion

Vertebral Compression Fracture
History: Acute-onset LBP usually in elderly pts w/ osteopenia, smoking, on steroids
Findings: Focal tender area on spine, usually no neuro findings
Evaluation: Plain film of affected thoracic, lumbar, or sacral spine

Treatment
- Usually stable fractures; analgesia ± brace for comfort
- Consult ortho or spine for >50% compression or multiple fractures

Disposition: Admit for intractable pain, any neuro findings, >50% compression, multiple fractures

Pearl: Look for neoplastic cause if no other RFs or hx, esp in elderly

NEUROLOGIC

Cauda Equina Syndrome
Definition: Large central disk herniation of distal spinal cord – *neurosurgical emergency*

History
- Severe LBP shooting down 1 or both legs & neuro sxs: Saddle paresthesias, urinary retention w/ overflow incontinence, loss of bowel control or sexual Dysfxn; pts w/ recent trauma or cancer w/ possible mets

Findings: ↓ rectal tone, urinary retention, saddle anesthesia, areflexia, weakness

Evaluation
- MRI is imaging test of choice
- Postvoid residual is the most sens initial finding

Management: Emergent neurosurgery consult, admit

Lumbar Spinal Stenosis
Definition: Narrowing of lumbar spinal canal from degeneration, facet arthritis, or subluxation
History: 40+ y/o, bilateral low back pain, pseudoclaudication (pain w/ walking), age >40, improves w/ rest & flexion of back (walk hunched over to keep back flexed)
Findings: nl exam, nl SLR, pain w/ back extension

Evaluation: Emergent imaging not needed if nl neuro exam; CT, MRI are diagnostic
Treatment: Pain mgmt w/ NSAIDs; hip flexor & abd exercises; surgery if severe
Disposition: Close f/u w/ PCP, spine

Herniated Disc
History
- 30–40 y/o, hx of waxing/waning back pain shooting down leg (past the knee) ± paresthesias
- Exacerbated by leaning forward, coughing, sneezing, & straining (stretches nerve root)

Findings
- See table below (L4–5 is most common)
- SLR test correlates w/ nerve root irritation only if reproduced sxs extend below knee; Ipsilateral is sens, contralateral is spec.

Management
- Neuro intact: Analgesia, DC home. MRI or CT myelogram if no improvement in 4–6 wk.
- Neuro deficits (or acute traumatic herniation): MRI to eval for cord involvement

Disposition: D/C if no cord findings; o/w needs spine consultation
Pearl: Sciatica is lumbar disc herniation impinging on sciatic nerve

Lumbar Nerve Root Compression			
Root	Pain	Sensory Loss	Weakness
L4	Hip, anterior thigh	Anteromedial thigh to medial aspect of foot	Weak quadriceps; ↓ knee jerk
L5	Lateral thigh/calf; dorsal foot, big toe	Lateral calf, dorsal foot, big toe	↓ extensor hallucis longus
S1	Posterolateral thigh, calf, heel	Back of thigh & calf; toes, lateral heel	Gastrocnemius; ↓ ankle jerk
S2–S4	Perineum	Perineum	Bowel/bladder; cremasteric

INFECTIOUS

Spinal Epidural Abscess
History
- Classic triad of fever, local spine tenderness, extremity neurologic deficit
- High-risk population: IV drug abusers, immunocompromised, recent instrumentation, DM

Findings
- Classic sequence: Back pain → root pain/radiculopathy → motor weakness, sensory Δ, bowel/bladder dysfxn → paralysis

Evaluation: MRI w/ IV contrast is test of choice

Treatment
- Cover Staph, Strep, gram-neg. organisms: (nafcillin 2 g OR oxacillin) & (ceftriaxone 2 g OR ciprofloxacin) ± vancomycin, + antipseudomonal abx if instrumentation hx
- Spine surgery consultation; ±steroids; may want biopsy prior to abx

Disposition: Admit, usually to spine surgery; operative washout

Pearl: Avoid LP to prevent introduction of organisms into CSF unless meningitis highly suspected

NEOPLASTIC

Bony Metastasis
History: >50 y/o, 1 mo of sxs, weight loss. Commonly breast, lung, kidney, prostate, thyroid
Findings: Tenderness of lumbar spine to palpation
Evaluation
- Plain film. CT/MRI/bone scan if plain film not definitive
- MRI & spine/oncology consultation if cord syndrome or findings

Treatment
- Pain control, Oncology referral
- If cord compressed, administer dexamethasone 10 mg IV or methylprednisolone 30 mg/kg IV, immediate consult

Disposition: Tx per spine surgery; possible operative decompression

Pearls
- 1° malignancy (esp multiple myeloma) should also be considered, esp in elderly
- Many bony mets missed on x-rays/CT; review films w/ radiologist specifically

JOINT PAIN

Approach
- Careful hx; anatomic distribution, single vs. multiple joints, acute vs. chronic, a/w fevers, skin Δ; hx of trauma
- Eval for systemic sxs in conjunction w/ chief complaint of joint pain
- If considering septic arthritis, evaluate need for arthrocentesis

Differential	
Pathophysiology	**Differential**
Trauma	Fracture, dislocation, hemarthrosis, osteonecrosis, tenosynovitis
Infectious	Non-GC septic arthritis, GC septic arthritis, reactive arthritis, tenosynovitis, Lyme dz (see Ch. 4)
Rheumatologic	Gout, pseudogout, rheumatoid arthritis, OA
Musculoskeletal	Bursitis, tendinitis

Etiology of Common Regional Joint Pains		
Region	**Type**	**Findings**
Shoulder	Rotator cuff injury	Inflammation or tear of rotator cuff tendons from direct trauma or overuse Pain in deltoid area of shoulder, worse w/ moving arm overhead or w/ direct pressure (sleeping) Tenderness to palpation "Empty Can Test": Pain & weakness w/ resisted abduction of arm elevated at 90°, adducted forward 30° Tx w/ NSAIDs, avoidance of aggravating movements, PT, subacromial steroid injections if no improvement
	Frozen shoulder (adhesive capsulitis)	Gradual ↓ ROM (active & passive) of glenohumeral joint due to joint capsule pathology; no known injury Pain at extremes of ROM Tx w/ NSAIDs, PT, 2–4 wk oral corticosteroids
	Acromioclavicular syndrome	Arthritis or injury to AC ligaments Acute or chronic, possible hx of trauma TTP & swelling of AC joint, pain worse w/ ↓ traction or forced passive adduction Acute injury tx w/ sling
Elbow	Lateral epicondylitis (tennis elbow)	Pain along lateral epicondyle at attachment of extensor tendons of forearm ↑ pain w/ resisting wrist dorsiflexion Tx w/ rest, NSAIDs, ±steroid injections
	Medial epicondylitis (golfer elbow)	Less common than tennis elbow Pain along medial epicondyle at insertion of common flexor tendon Resistance to wrist flexion w/ elbow in extension ↑ pain
Hip	Trochanteric bursitis	Most common cause of pain in hip (lateral aspect) Pain ↑ w/ walking, squatting, climbing stairs, ↓ at rest Resisted abduction of hip reproduces pain Tx w/ NSAIDs, corticosteroid injections
Knee	Patellar tendonitis (jumper's knee)	Pain at inferior aspect of patella during repetitive running, jumping, kicking Tx w/ rest, NSAIDs, knee brace, PT, strengthening exercises for quads & hamstrings
Ankle	Achilles tendonitis	Pain, swelling, tenderness, over Achilles tendon from repetitive trauma & microscopic tears from overuse (ballet, distance running, basketball) ↑ pain w/ passive dorsiflexion Tx w/ rest, heat, NSAIDs, shoe modification, heel lift to ↓ tendon stretching, PT, stretching exercises

TENOSYNOVITIS

Definition
- Inflammation of the tendon & tendon sheath. Can result in chronic disability, ↓ ROM, chronic pain, amputation if not treated appropriately.

Types of Tenosynovitis		
Type	**Hx & Findings**	**Management & Disposition**
De Quervain tenosynovitis	Repetitive pinching of thumb & fingers Pain improved w/ rest; no hx of acute trauma Most common in middle-aged women Pain at radial aspect of wrist, worse w/ passive ROM of thumb, ulnar deviation of wrist w/ thumb cupped in closed fist (Finkelstein test)	Rest, NSAIDs Thumb spica Steroid injection Surgery if needed Good prognosis DC home w/ f/u
Stenosing flexor tenosynovitis (trigger finger)	Locking of thumb or ring finger in flexion followed by sudden release, pain radiates to fingers Most common in middle-aged women, diabetics Pain in proximal tendon sheath in distal palm ±Palpable tendon thickening or nodularity May require manipulation to release	NSAIDs Splint 4–6 wk ±Steroid injection Surgical release if injection fails Good prognosis D/C home w/ f/u
Infectious tenosynovitis	Puncture wound, laceration, bite, cracked skin, high-pressure injury; usually *S. aureus*, Strep **Kanavel signs:** 1. Fusiform ("sausage") swelling of finger 2. Flexed position of finger 3. Severe pain w/ passive extension 4. Tenderness along flexor tendon sheath	**Admit** ortho/hand Abx Splint & elevation Fair prognosis even w/ abx, surgery

GOUT

History
- Middle-aged pt w/ abrupt (often recurrent) onset single joint pain, swelling, erythema, warmth; may be precipitated by minor trauma or illness
- RFs: HTN, HLD, DM, obesity. Systemic etiologies: Cancer, hemolysis.
- 75% monoarticular, classically affects 1st MTP joint (aka "podagra")

Findings
- Red, swollen, tender, warm joint (MTP > ankle > torsal area > knee); mimics cellulitis
- Tophi overlying effected joints indicate chronic gouty dz

Evaluation
- Arthrocentesis if: 1st episode (no prior tap), unclear Dx, concern for septic joint
- Joint fluid: Needle-shaped, neg. birefringent crystals; always send for culture
- Serum uric acid level is of no value; 30% will have nl levels
- X-ray findings in chronic gout include bony erosions, punched out lesions, calcified tophi

Treatment
- NSAIDs (no aspirin). Eg, indomethacin 50 mg PO TID for duration of attack (~3–10 d).
- Alternatively: Colchicine (0.5 mg PO q1h up to 8 mg; if nl renal fxn) OR steroids
- Allopurinol for chronic prevention but has no role in acute mgmt of gout attack

Disposition
- D/C home w/ pain control unless intractable pain

Pearl
- Gout is a result of monosodium urate crystal deposition

PSEUDOGOUT

History
- Elderly pt w/ abrupt-onset, single-joint pain, swelling, erythema, warmth; precipitated by minor trauma or illness; usually in large joints (unlike gout)

Findings
• Red, swollen, tender, warm joint (knee > wrist > ankle = elbow)

Evaluation
• If unclear Dx, concern for septic joint, perform arthrocentesis
• Joint fluid: Rhomboid-shaped, positively birefringent crystals
• X-ray findings: Chondrocalcinosis, subchondral sclerosis, radiopaque calcifications

Treatment
• Same as gout

Disposition
• D/C home w/ pain control

Pearls
• Pseudogout is the result of calcium pyrophosphate crystal deposition
• Most common cause of new monoarticular arthritis in pts >60 y/o
• RFs: ↑ Ca, ↓ Mg, ↓ PO_4, hemochromatosis, hemosiderosis, parathyroid dz

BURSITIS

Definition
• Inflammation of bursa, which are flattened sacs lined w/ synovial fluid that helps facilitate movement; bursitis is usually due to overuse, trauma, or OA, but can be septic

History
• Discrete area of pain, swelling, erythema, warmth over a joint
• Less than half of bursitis is septic, but 70% of septic bursitis has preceding trauma
• Most common in joints that are subject to repetitive stresses (elbow, knee), but can be deep (hip) esp in setting of instrumentation (eg, acupuncture, surgery)

Findings
• Warm, swollen, fluid-filled pocket outside the joint ± erythema
• Tenderness, fever, associated cellulitis suggest septic bursitis
• Should have minimal pain w/ passive ROM; o/w consider septic arthritis

Evaluation
• If any concern for septic bursitis, perform bursa aspiration (WBC >5K is suggestive)
• Deep bursae may require aspiration by ortho or IR
• Often clinically difficult to differentiate from septic arthritis; may need arthrocentesis

Treatment
• Rest, ice, elevation, analgesia, ±steroid injection
• If septic bursitis: Abx for *Staph* coverage (ie, dicloxacillin, TMP–SMX, or clindamycin)
• Consult ortho for f/u as these have high outpt failure rate & may need surgical bursal excision or serial aspirations

Disposition
• D/C w/ pain control if no ortho intervention, ±abx
• Admit for fulminant infection, immunocompromised pt, significant surrounding cellulitis

Pearl
• Prepatellar (carpet layer's knee) & olecranon bursitis (student's elbow) are usually due to *Staph* infection from local trauma

INFECTIOUS

Septic Arthritis (Nongonococcal)

History
• Acute onset of painful, swollen, warm, tender joint, often w/ fever
• Hallmark is severe pain w/ any passive ROM
• All joints are at risk but most commonly knee > hip. In peds, hip is most common.
• High-risk groups include IV drug users, immunocompromised

Findings
• Usually single joint involvement; can see multijoint in disseminated GC dz
• Pain w/ minimal passive ROM or axial load; warmth, redness, swelling

Evaluation
• X-ray to identify effusion, FB, fracture, or osteomyelitis
• Arthrocentesis: Gram stain & culture, cell count, protein & glucose, crystal analysis, synovial lactate; positive: WBC >50000 w/ PMN predominance
• Labs: Consider ESR, CRP, blood cx to isolate; UA, CXR for infectious w/u

Management
- Arthrocentesis (hip may need orthopedics or IR), ortho consult, splint in physiologic position
- Supportive care: hydration, antipyretics, pain control
- Abx after arthrocentesis & blood cultures taken; S. aureus is most common
- Adults: Vancomycin & 3rd-generation cephalosporin OR quinolone
- Children <14 yr: Vancomycin & 3rd-generation cephalosporin
- Prosthesis, immunocompromised: Vancomycin & antipseudomonal (piperacillin/tazobactam OR fluoroquinolone)

Disposition: Admit for abx, ortho observation, likely need for operative washout

Pearls
- Septic hips do not present w/ classic signs; can be very subtle
- Presence of crystals in the joint fluid does NOT r/o a septic joint
- Overlying cellulitis is relative CI for arthrocentesis; avoid cellulitic area during tap
- If hardware is present, discuss risk/benefit w/ orthopedics prior to arthrocentesis
- Intra-articular steroid injection for pain relief in septic arthritis is contraindicated

Gonococcal Septic Arthritis
History
- Young, sexually active pt usually c/o single painful, swollen, warm, & tender joint
- May be polyarticular or migratory; smaller joints (elbow, wrist, ankle) commonly involved
- Urethral or vaginal D/C of GC infection may be present

Findings
- Any clinical manifestations of Neisseria GC infection (cervicitis, malodorous, purulent vaginal D/C in female or dysuria & penile D/C in male)
- Swollen, tender, warm, & extremely painful small joint(s), usually slightly flexed at rest, more painful w/ ROM; may have tenosynovitis
- A painless diffuse maculopapular rash w/ necrotic/pustular centers may be present
- RUQ abd pain may indicate Fitz-Hugh–Curtis syndrome

Evaluation
- Same as non-GC septic arthritis + cervical (female) & urethral (male) cultures; blood, pharynx & rectal cultures to ↑ likelihood of definitive dx

Treatment
- Arthrocentesis, ortho consult, splint joint in physiologic position for comfort
- 3rd-generation cephalosporin (ceftriaxone 1 g IV QD) OR quinolone, add doxycycline for chlamydia
- Supportive care: Hydration, antipyretics, pain control

   Disposition: Admit for abx, ortho observation, possible need for operative washout

Pearls
- GC septic arthritis is the only septic arthritis that does not necessarily need operative washout; however, serial arthrocentesis to remove fluid may be indicated
- Gram stain & culture from GC septic arthritis more often neg. than non-GC septic joints
- Intra-articular steroid injection for pain relief in septic arthritis is contraindicated

EAR PAIN

Approach
- Nature of pain, associated sxs, duration, fevers, hearing loss; diabetes

Ear Pain Differential	
Location	**Differential**
Outer ear	OE, malignant OE, trauma, FB, Ramsay Hunt syndrome (herpes zoster oticus)
Middle ear	Acute/chronic OM, trauma
Mastoid air cells	Mastoiditis

Otitis Externa (Swimmer's Ear)
Definition
- Infection (Acute: *Pseudomonas, S. aureus, S. epidermidis;* Chronic: *Aspergillus, Candida*) of the outer ear due to breakdown of natural barriers

History
- Summer, water exposure, cotton swab trauma, hearing aids, pain/itching/drainage

Physical Findings
- Pain w/ movement of tragus/helix, localized LAD, redness/exudate in canal, white/gray debris, ±green d/c/yellow crusting, ±abscess, conductive hearing loss if severe

Treatment
- Remove debris, dry canal w/ suction, drain abscess if present
- Mild infections: Cleanse w/ 2% acetic acid, hydrogen peroxide, OR sterile saline; no good evidence for these. Avoid w/ ruptured TM
- Severe infections: Topical abx (eg, ofloxacin) + steroid × 7 d
  - Use wick (cotton, gauze, or cellulose) 10–12 mm into canal × 2–3 d to allow med delivery
  - If TM rupture, consider oral abx
- No swimming × 48 h, keep ear dry in shower × 1 wk (ear plugs or Vaseline gauze seal)

Disposition
- Home: Diabetics w/ simple OE should get close f/u

Malignant (Necrotizing) Otitis Externa
Definition: Aggressive infection (95% *Pseudomonas*) of the outer ear canal to skull base/bony structures, usually in diabetics/immunocompromised
History: Ear pain extending to TMJ (pain w/ chewing), nocturnal pain, swelling, otorrhea
Physical Findings: Granulation tissue, severe inflammation, may have CN palsy
Evaluation: Consider CT scan to eval extent, underlying osteomyelitis, & intracranial extension

Treatment
- 1st line: IV ciprofloxacin; Increasing rates of resistance; 2nd line: Ceftazidime, imipenem, OR piperacillin/tazobactam
- Consider amphotericin B or voriconazole for aspergillus in HIV/immunocompromised

Disposition: Admission for IV abx ± operative débridement

Pearls
- 10% mortality
- Cx: Cerebral/epidural abscess, osteomyelitis, dural sinus thrombophlebitis, meningitis

Otitis Media
Definition
- Inflammation of the middle ear
- Acute OM: Infection (50% *S. pneumoniae,* 20% *H. influenzae,* 10% *M. catarrhalis,* viral 50–70%) + effusion <3 wk
- Chronic OM: Effusion w/o infection

History: Unilateral ear pain, fever (25%), winter/spring, 2–10 y/o, URI
Physical Findings: Bulging TM, loss of light reflex/TM mobility (most sens), effusion, erythema (not sufficient alone to diagnose OM), purulent drainage

Treatment
- Many improve w/ no abx w/o cx
- Pain control: APAP/ibuprofen, auralgan (topical)
- Nonsevere acute OM: Amoxicillin to start in 2–3 d if sxs do not improve
- Severe (<6 mo, bilateral, bulging TM, otorrhea, fever >39°C, systemically ill) = immediate abx

- Pediatric: Amoxicillin 80–90 mg/kg/d (1st line) 7–10 d, amoxicillin/clavulanate if recent abx or concurrent conjunctivitis *(Pediatrics 2010;125(2):384)*
- Adult: Amoxicillin 500 mg BID (mild to mod), 875 mg BID (severe), Cefpodoxime OR cefuroxime if PCN allergic

Disposition: Home, PCP f/u 2–3 d

Pearls
- Cx (rare): Meningitis, mastoiditis, persistent effusion → hearing loss
- TM perforation does not require any Δ in management

Mastoiditis
Definition: Extension of infection from the middle ear into the mastoid air cells
History: Unilateral ear pain, fever, HA
Physical Findings: Tenderness, erythema, fluctuance over mastoid, outward bulging pinna
Evaluation: CT scan to eval extent/destruction of the septa of the air cells, MRI for intracranial cx, ENT consult

Treatment
- Abx: Nafcillin/cefuroxime/ceftriaxone
- ±Myringotomy/tympanostomy; mastoidectomy (if 50% of air cells involved)

Disposition: Admission, possible operative débridement
Pearl: Cx include meningitis, dural sinus thrombosis, brain abscess, subperiosteal abscess, hearing loss

HEARING LOSS

Approach
- Nature, acuity of onset, unilateral/bilateral, associated pain/systemic sxs

Hearing Loss Differential	
Cause	Differential
Infections	Mumps, measles, influenza, herpes simplex, herpes zoster, cytomegalovirus, mononucleosis, syphilis (sudden onset), viral cochleitis, meningitis
Vascular	SCD, Berger dz, leukemia, polycythemia, fat emboli, hypercoagulability, stroke
Metabolic	Diabetes, pregnancy
Conductive	Cerumen impactions, FB, OM, OE, barotrauma, trauma, TM rupture, cholesteatoma, traumatic ossicle disruption, Ménière's
Medications	AGs, furosemide, salicylates, antineoplastics
Neoplasm	Acoustic neuroma

Cerumen Impaction/Foreign Body
Definition: Buildup of earwax or FB in the external canal
History: Unilateral hearing loss, placement of FB in ear, drainage, pain
Physical Findings: Visualization or cerumen/FB in ear

Treatment
- Irrigate the external canal w/ room temperature NS (cold/hot NS can cause nystagmus/vertigo/nausea), past FB if possible. Do not irrigate batteries
- For live insects, consider liquid lidocaine, isopropyl alcohol, or mineral oil to asphyxiate prior to removal
- For cerumen: Instill colace, cerumenex, or H_2O_2 for 15 min to dissolve, then irrigate
- For FB: Alligator forceps OR cyanoacrylate (glue) to cotton-tipped applicator, hold against object for 60 sec; OR try suction for smooth objects
- Re-examine ear postextraction for TM rupture, canal damage, or residual FB. Consider topical abx if canal damaged

Disposition: D/c

Ruptured Tympanic Membrane
Definition: Rupture of the TM. Etiologies include trauma (open hand slap over ear, lightening), FB (cotton swab, pipe cleaner), barotrauma (high altitude, diving), infection (OM)
History: Pain, hearing loss
Physical Findings: Perforation of TM, ±blood in the canal

Treatment

- Keep ear dry (earplugs during shower, no swimming)
- Abx needed if pre-existing infection; treat as usual OM; consider abx if contaminated water exposure
- Operative repair if >¼ of TM damaged

Disposition

- D/c, ENT f/u 2–4 d for audiogram; perforations usually heal in 2–3 mo
- Admit in acute trauma w/ associated facial nerve injury, incapacitating vertigo

SORE THROAT

Approach

- Nature, acuity of onset, duration, associated sxs (cough, fever, drooling, voice Δ, dysphagia, difficulty breathing)

Sore Throat Differential	
Cause	**Differential**
Infections	Viral (rhinovirus, adenovirus, coronavirus, HSV, influenza, CMV, EBV, varicella, HIV), bacterial (S. pyogenes, gonorrhea, N. meningitides, M. pneumoniae, Chlamydia, S. aureus, H. influenzae, H. parainfluenzae, C. diphtheriae, Legionella, Candida), peritonsillar abscess, retropharyngeal abscess, Ludwig angina, Lemierre syndrome
Systemic	Kawasaki, SJS, thyroiditis
Trauma	Penetrating, FB, laryngeal fx, caustic ingestion, retropharyngeal hematoma
Tumor	Tongue, larynx, thyroid, leukemia

Group A Streptococcus Pharyngitis ("Strep Throat")
Definition: Infection of the oropharynx caused by GABHS
History: Sore throat, odynophagia, myalgias, fever; no cough
Physical Findings: Erythematous oropharynx, tonsillar exudate, cervical LAD

Evaluation

- Centor criteria: Fever >38°C, tonsillar exudate, tender LAD, absence of cough
- Rapid strep: Sens 60–90%, spec 90% (send culture if neg. given low sens)
- GABHS culture: 90% sens
- Consider culture for gonorrhea (if oral sex exposure), or Monospot for EBV

Treatment

- There are multiple conflicting guidelines (NEJM 2011;364:648). One reasonable approach:
  - If 0–1 Centor criteria met: No testing, no tx
  - If 2–3 Centor criteria met: Rapid strep, treat if positive, confirm w/ culture
  - If all Centor criteria met: No testing, yes tx
- Abx
  - Benzathine penicillin 25000 U/kg max 1.2 million U IM ×1 OR penicillin VK, OR amoxicillin OR azithromycin. If refractory: Clindamycin, augmentin
  - Dexamethasone 8 mg ×1 may ↓ time to pain relief (J Emerg Med 2008;35(4):363)

Disposition: D/c
Pearl: Treat w/ abx to prevent scarlet fever, rheumatic fever, abscess, mastoiditis. Poststrep glomerulonephritis is not prevented w/ abx

Croup (Laryngotracheobronchitis)
Definition

- URI in children (6 mo–6 yr) usually by parainfluenza virus causing inflammation/exudate/edema of subglottic mucosa

History: Barky cough, worse at night, low-grade fever, following 2–3 d of URI sxs
Physical Findings: High-pitched inspiratory stridor, barking cough, hoarse voice, tachycardia, tachypnea

Croup Severity Score (Westley Score)	
Inspiratory stridor	None = 0, w/ agitation = 1, at rest = 2
Retractions	None = 0, mild = 1, moderate = 2, severe = 3
Air entry	nl = 0, mildly decreased = 1, severely decreased = 2
Cyanosis	None = 0, w/ agitation = 4, at rest = 5
Level of alertness	nl = 0, altered = 5
Score ≤2 = mild, 3–5 = moderate, >6 = severe	

Evaluation: Neck film is typically of no clinical value → narrowing of subglottic trachea ("steeple sign")

Treatment
- Calm child, monitor pulse oximetry
- Cool mist (no clear benefit)
- Dexamethasone 0.3–0.6 mg/kg (↓ time to improvement) *(Cochrane Syst Rev 2004;(1): CD001955)*
- Moderate–severe or stridor at rest: Nebulized racemic epinephrine 0.5 mL of 2.25%

Disposition
- Admit if no improvement in ED, hypoxic, persistent stridor at rest, <6 mo old, unable to tolerate PO, requiring multiple doses of epinephrine
- Croup severity score ≤4 can usually be D/C, score >6 may require ICU

Pearl: If epinephrine given, should observe for >3–4 h for rebound stridor

Epiglottitis
Definition
- Inflammation of the epiglottis caused by *H. influenzae* >> *Staph/Strep, B. catarrhalis*
- Can lead to rapidly progressing, life-threatening airway obstruction

History
- Sore throat, muffled "hot potato" voice, odynophagia, respiratory distress, fever
- ↓ Pediatric incidence since vaccination, now more common in adult diabetics

Physical Findings: Dysphonia, stridor, drooling, sitting in tripod position

Evaluation
- Lateral neck XR (90% sens): Epiglottis >7 mm ("thumbprint"), loss of vallecular air space
- Adult: If nl x-ray → indirect or fiberoptic laryngoscopy (have surgical airway ready)
- Pediatric: Avoid agitation (↑ risk of acute airway obstruction), do NOT attempt to visualize in the ED. To OR for DL w/ anesthesia & ENT/surgery

Treatment: Abx (ceftriaxone OR ampicillin–sulbactam, add clindamycin or vancomycin if concern for MRSA); no proven benefit w/ steroids
Disposition: ICU admission

Pertussis (Whooping Cough)
Definition: Lower respiratory tract infection by *B. pertussis* (gram-neg. rod)
Presentation
- Commonly a prolonged course (aka "hundred-day cough")
- Stages: (1) *Catarrhal* (most infectious): 2 wk mild URI sxs; (2) *Paroxysmal:* 1–2 wk intense paroxysmal cough ± posttussive emesis, inspiratory "whoop"; (3) *Convalescent:* Several weeks of chronic cough
- ↑ Risk if unvaccinated, but immunity wanes after ~12 yr; ↑ morbidity if <6 mo old

Evaluation
- Rapid PCR may be useful esp during epidemics
- May develop PNA; consider CXR if refractory to abx

Treatment
- Droplet precautions × 7 d, abx (only effective in catarrhal stage)
- Azithromycin or clarithromycin, albuterol prn, treat household contacts
- Low threshold for empiric tx in infants, pregnant, healthcare workers

Disposition: Admit <6 mo–1 y/o or ill appearing

Lemierre Syndrome
Definition
- Suppurative thrombosis of internal jugular vein w/ *F. necrophorum*
- Septic emboli to lung are common (can be confused w/ R-sided endocarditis)

History
- Usually previously healthy young adults w/ high fever, sore throat ± cough
- Typical course is pharyngitis that improves & then followed by severe sepsis

Physical Findings: Unilateral neck swelling, tenderness, induration
Evaluation: Contrast CT of neck
Treatment: Abx: Ampicillin–sulbactam, piperacillin–tazobactam or a carbapenem. Consider adding vancomycin if catheter-associated. Anticoagulation is controversial
Disposition: Admit

SINUSITIS

Acute Sinusitis
Definition
- Inflammation of the paranasal sinuses
- Usually viral or allergic
- Common bacterial etiologies: S. pneumoniae, nontypable H. influenzae, M. catarrhalis
- Pseudomonas is seen in HIV, cystic fibrosis, or after instrumentation
- Mucormycosis is invasive fungal sinusitis (Rhizopus) in diabetics or immunocompromised

Presentation
- Mucopurulent d/c, postnasal drip, cough, sinus pressure, HA, ±fever
- Typically progresses over 7–10 d & resolves spontaneously
- Sxs >7 d, worsening course, or worsening after improving, all suggest bacterial dz
- Consider sinusitis w/ positional HA that is worse when bending forward
- Sphenoid sinusitis is a difficult Dx, often presents late; classically worse w/ head tilt

Evaluation
- Clinical, no routine imaging. CT sens but not spec, can r/o cx
- Cx include orbital cellulitis, osteomyelitis, cavernous sinus thrombosis, cerebral abscess, meningitis, frontal bone abscess (Pott puffy tumor)

Treatment
- Supportive (analgesics, antipyretics, decongestants, antihistamines if allergic)
- Decongestants: Neo-Synephrine nasal spray TID × 3 d, Afrin nasal spray BID × 3 d
- Abx not routinely indicated. Reserve for pts w/ sxs >7 d, worsening sxs, fever, purulent d/c, or high risk for severe infection or cx
  - Amoxicillin–clavulanate 500 mg PO TID × 5–7 d
  - RFs for resistance: high-dose amoxicillin–clavulanate (2000 mg BID)

Disposition
- Vast majority are managed outpt
- Admit if toxic, severe HA, high fever, immunocompromised, poor f/u

Pearl
- Sphenoid/ethmoid sinusitis is less common than maxillary sinusitis but has significant potential cx (eg, orbital cellulites, cavernous sinus thrombosis)

EPISTAXIS

Definition: Bleeding from the nose. 90% of cases are anterior & involve Kiesselbach plexus on the septum. 10% of cases are posterior & arise from a branch of sphenopalatine artery

History
- Etiologies include URI (most common), trauma, nose picking, environmental irritants (dry air), intranasal drug use, neoplasm, FB, polyps, anticoagulation/TCP
- RFs: Alcoholism, diabetes, anticoagulation, HTN, hematologic disorder

Physical Findings
- Evaluate w/ nasal speculum after having pt blow nose to express clots

Evaluation
- Can usually identify anterior source on exam; posterior bleeds are heavy, brisk, can cause airway compromise. If still bleeding after anterior packing, consider posterior source
- Check hematocrit if extensive/prolonged bleeding, INR if on warfarin

Treatment
- If significantly hypertensive, consider antihypertensive to help w/ hemostasis
- Anterior: Start w/ oxymetazoline (Afrin) 3 sprays & hold pressure for 15 min
  - May also insert cotton pledgets soaked in cocaine/lidocaine/epinephrine/phenylephrine
  - Once vasoconstricted, try to identify a focal bleeding site, then use silver nitrate cautery in ring around bleeding (will not work on active bleeding; caution on septum)
  - If bleeding has stopped, observe for 60 min; if recurs, insert a lubricated nasal tampon or vaseline gauze packing
  - If nasal tampon is not successful, pack the contralateral side
- Posterior: Bleeding can cause airway compromise & be life-threatening
  - Commercial double balloon device OR pass Foley catheter through nose into posterior pharynx, fill balloon, hold gentle traction

Disposition
- Anterior: D/c w/ 48 h f/u, typically w/ prophylactic abx for TSS (unproven) (eg, clindamycin, augmentin, or dicloxacillin)
- Posterior: Admit w/ ENT consult

EYE PAIN/REDNESS

Approach
- Ask about FB exposure, chemicals, trauma, contact lens use, freshwater exposure
- *Always* check visual acuity. Use topical anesthetics (tetracaine, proparacaine) for exam
- Complete eye exam: Visual acuity (corrected), visual fields, external inspection, peri-orbital soft tissue & bones, extraocular movement, pupils (including swinging light test for afferent pupillary defect), pressure (tonometry), slit lamp (lids, conjunctiva, sclera, cornea w/ fluorescein, anterior chamber, iris, lens), fundoscopy

Acute Angle-closure Glaucoma
Definition: Increased IOP due to ↓ aqueous outflow. Generally due to reduction in the angle of the anterior chamber in setting of the dilated pupil pushing against trabecular meshwork

History
- Sudden onset of severe unilateral pain, HA, N/V, blurry vision, halos
- May be triggered by dim light, mydriatic drops, stress, sympathomimetics

Physical Findings
- Unilateral perilimbal injection, ↓VA, "steamy" (cloudy) cornea, nonreactive midsize pupil (5–7 mm), shallow anterior chamber, ↑ IOP >22 mmHg, firm globe

Treatment
- *Immediate optho consult; need for urgent laser peripheral iridotomy*
- *Reduce aqueous production:* Timolol 0.5% 1–2 drops q30min (avoid if CI to systemic βB), acetazolamide 500 mg IV, then 250 q6h (avoid in sulfur-allergic pts) or brimonidine 1 drop TID
- *Facilitate aqueous outflow (miotics):* Pilocarpine 2% 1 drop q15min until pupil constricts
- *Decrease vitreous volume (osmotics):* Mannitol 1–2 mg/kg IV over 30–60 min

Disposition
- Per optho recommendations. Admit for intractable vomiting or need for systemic agents

Critical Dx		
Etiology	**Features**	**Management**
Caustic injury (chemical)	Hx: Chemical exposure PE: Corneal burns (esp w/ alkali), pain, blepharospasm	*Immediate optho consult* Immediate copious (2–4 L) irrigation until pH = 7
Acute angle-closure glaucoma	See discussion above	See discussion above
Retrobulbar hematoma	Hx: Often due to trauma, but also spontaneous in coagulopathy or due to tumor PE: Decreased acuity, diplopia, proptosis, afferent pupillary defect ± pale optic disc	IOP >20 = orbital compartment syndrome *Immediate optho consult* Lateral canthotomy if: - Conscious, ↑ IOP, ↓VA - Unconscious, IOP >40 & proptosis - CI: ruptured globe
Penetrating trauma/ scleral penetration	Hx: Blunt (blow to orbit or globe) or penetrating PE: ↓ acuity, afferent papillary defect, classically teardrop-shaped pupil, Seidel sign (aqueous leak on fluorescein)	Apply eye shield *Immediate optho consult* IV abx Tetanus prophylaxis CT scan to assess for FB
Corneal ulcer/ keratitis	Hx: Pain, FB sensation, photophobia, tearing, blurry vision. Recent contact lens use, UV light exposure, Bell palsy or abrasion PE: Fluorescein: Corneal infiltrate (white spots/haze) around sharply demarcated "scooped out" epithelial defect - Herpes: Dendritic - UV keratitis: Many punctate ulcers (snowflake pattern)	*Immediate optho consult* May need to débride or culture prior to abx - Ciprofloxacin - Cycloplegics - Acyclovir if possibly HSV

Etiology	Features	Management
Orbital cellulitis (vs. preseptal cellulitis)	Orbital cellulitis: Posterior to orbital septum, drains into cavernous sinus *Both orbital & preseptal:* - May have fever, leukocytosis - Lid swelling, erythema, warmth - Eye tenderness - ±Conjunctivitis, chemosis *Suspect orbital cellulitis if:* - Ill appearance, high fever - Pain w/ EOM movement - Ophthalmoplegia/diplopia - Visual impairment - Proptosis - Increased IOP	*Immediate optho consult for orbital cellulitis* IOP > 20: Optho emergency CT orbit to r/o FB, abscess Obtain blood cx Start IV abx (vancomycin + ceftriaxone or ampicillin/sulbactam) In diabetics, consider mucormycosis *Admit all orbital cellulitis* If preseptal cellulitis, outpt abx w/ amoxicillin/clavulanate & optho recheck in 1 d Cx: vision loss, cavernous sinus thrombosis, CNS involvement, abscess, osteomyelitis
Emergent Diagnoses		
Hyphema	Hx: Pain, ↓ visual acuity, usually after blunt trauma PE: Gross or microscopic blood layering in anterior chamber, ±fixed & dilated pupil	First r/o open globe *Discuss w/ optho-"eight ball" hyphema requires urgent f/u* IOP > 30: Treat as glaucoma IOP > 20: Use cycloplegic to prevent iris motion Elevate HOB 45 degrees Screen for FH of sickle cell Most can be D/C home w/ 1–2 d recheck Return for ↑ pain or ↓ vision
Corneal abrasion/FB	Hx: Pain worse w/ blinking, photophobia, FB sensation PE: Conjunctival injection. Evert lids to look for FB. Use fluorescein to eval -Rust ring = metallic FB -Seidel test to r/o corneal penetration	If high velocity: XR or CT to r/o ocular penetration If embedded FB, remove w/ 25 g needle tip under magnification, or burr Give tetanus prophylaxis Abx (erythromycin), use quinolone if contact use or freshwater exposure DC home w/ optho f/u in 1–2 d for recheck, rust ring removal if needed. No contacts until resolved
Anterior uveitis/iritis	Def: Inflammatory process involving anterior chamber, iris, ciliary body, or choroid Hx: Usually due to trauma, autoimmune dz, or infection (HSV, Lyme). Unilateral painful red eye, "deep" pain, blurred vision, photophobia Physical Findings: Perilimbal injection, photophobia (consensual suggests iritis), ± ↓ visual acuity, slit lamp shows anterior chamber cell & flare	• Traumatic iritis: Cycloplegic for comfort, *optho f/u in 1–2 d* • Inflammatory: Cycloplegics, *consult optho for possible steroids*
Other Causes of Red Eye		
Conjunctivitis (allergic, viral > bacterial)	Def: Inflammation of mucus membranes that line sclera/lids. Usually viral Hx: Drainage, irritation, pruritus, crusting, concurrent URI PE: Injection/edema, usually sparing limbus nl exam o/w Gonorrhea = copious, green exudate	Culture if neonate or concern for *Chlamydia, gonorrhea* Warm soaks, artificial tears Antihistamine if allergic Abx if concern for bacterial: - Erythromycin, Polytrim - Quinolone if contact lens or freshwater exposure D/c home, optho f/u in 2 d if not improving *Consult optho if gonorrhea suspected*

Etiology	Features	Management
Lid disorders (blepharitis, chalazion, dacrocystitis, hordeolum/stye)	*Blepharitis:* Inflamed eyelid margins *Chalazion:* Inflamed meibomian gland (subcutaneous lid nodule) *Dacrocystitis:* Inflamed lower eye lid w/ redness, tenderness *Hordeolum (stye):* Abscess in eyelash follicle or lid margin (can be external or internal)	*Blepharitis:* Warm compresses *Chalazion:* Warm compresses, gentle massage *Dacrocystitis:* R/o periorbital or orbital cellulitis. If mild, d/c w/ clindamycin & warm compresses. Admit if systemically ill *Hordeolum:* - External: Warm compresses ± abx ointment for *Staph* - Internal = PO abx for *Staph*

VISION CHANGE & VISION LOSS

Approach
- Complete eye exam: Visual acuity (corrected), visual fields, external inspection, periorbital soft tissue & bones, extraocular movement, pupils (including swinging light test for afferent pupillary defect), pressure (tonometry), slit lamp (lids, conjunctiva, sclera, cornea w/ fluorescein, anterior chamber, iris, lens), fundoscopy, & full neurologic exam

Differential of Vision Δ & Loss	
	Differential
Painful	Trauma, glaucoma, uveitis, corneal ulcer, temporal arteritis, optic neuritis
Painless	Amaurosis fugax/TIA, central retinal artery/vein occlusion (CRAO/CRVO), vitreous hemorrhage, retinal detachment, lens dislocation, hypertensive encephalopathy, pituitary tumors, macular disorders, toxic ingestions (toxic alcohols, heavy metals)

Differential of Diplopia	
	Differential
Monocular	Astigmatism, cataracts, lens dislocation
Binocular	Entrapment, CN palsy, intracranial mass effect, thyroid dz, microvascular dz

Central Retinal Artery Occlusion
Definition: Retinal artery occlusion, most commonly embolic

History
- Sudden painless, monocular vision loss (or visual field cut if branch of retinal artery), may have transient loss prior to complete loss (amaurosis fugax)
- RFs: HTN, DM, CVA, AF, carotid dz, hypercoagulable, vasculitis, endocarditis, sickle cell anemia

Physical Findings
- Afferent pupillary defect, funduscopic exam shows cherry-red spot at fovea (spared), pale disc (late finding)
- May have carotid bruit, irregular HR, murmur; r/o temporal arteritis

Evaluation
- CBC, ESR
- For embolic w/u: Neuroimaging (CT/CTA or MRI/MRA), carotid imaging, echo, EKG

Treatment
- Initiate immediately (>2 h = irreversible vision loss)
- *Immediate ophthalmologic consult*
- Intermittent globe massage (to try to dislodge embolus & move it further downstream)
- Reduce IOP as in glaucoma (eg, acetazolamide, mannitol, timolol)
- Anterior chamber paracentesis
- Surgical decompression, anticoagulation, intra-arterial thrombolysis, hyperbaric O_2

Disposition: Admit

Pearl: Cardiac embolus most common in >40 y/o, coagulopathies most common in <30 y/o

Central Retinal Vein Occlusion
Definition: Retinal vein occlusion, usually thrombotic

History
- Sudden painless monocular vision loss (may be gradual onset)
- RFs: CAD, HTN, glaucoma, venous stasis, hypercoagulable, DM, vascular dz

Physical Findings: Afferent pupillary defect, funduscopic exam w/ retinal hemorrhages/ disk edema ("blood & thunder"), cotton wool spots
Management: *Immediate optho consult.* Start ASA, outpt hypercoagulability w/u
Disposition: Home

Temporal Arteritis (Giant Cell Arteritis)
Definition: Granulomatous inflammatory vasculitis of medium/large arteries

History
- Unilateral HA, jaw/tongue claudication, malaise, low-grade fevers, visual impairment
- Usually >50 y/o (90% >60 y/o), F > M, hx of PMR (50% of pts)

Physical Findings: Tenderness over temporal artery, decreased visual acuity, afferent pupillary defect
Evaluation: ↑ ESR, ↑ CRP, temporal artery biopsy

Management
- If visual deficits: IV methylprednisolone 1g daily × 3 days
- No visual deficits: Prednisone 60 mg/d (do not withhold pending biopsy results) & biopsy w/i 2 wk. Consult rheumatology, ophthalmology

Disposition: Admit only for visual deficits

Pearls
- Failure to diagnose & treat may result in permanent blindness
- 75% of pt w/ visual deficits in one eye will develop contralateral deficits w/i 3 wk
- 20× higher risk of thoracic aortic aneurysm

Optic Neuritis
Definition
- Inflammation of the optic nerve usually due to focal demyelination
- A/w MS (⅓ pts will be diagnosed w/ MS), but also sarcoidosis, SLE, leukemia, alcoholism, syphilis, idiopathic, postviral

History: Vision loss (minimal → complete), ↓ color perception, pain w/ eye movement

Physical Findings
- ↓Visual acuity, afferent pupillary defect, central scotoma, funduscopic exam
- Disk swelling/pallor

Evaluation: MRI shows inflammation of optic nerve, 20% have other demyelinating lesions
Treatment: Immediate ophthalmology/neurology consult, steroids
Disposition: Admit

Retinal Detachment
History
- Painless, classically "curtain-like" visual field deficit, "coal dust" or "spider webs," floaters, photopsia (scintilla)
- RFs include myopia, trauma, surgical hx (cataract removal), DM, HTN, malignancy (breast CA, melanoma, leukemia), SCD, eclampsia, prematurity

Physical Findings: Visual field cut, "billowing" retina, may see pigmented vitreous or visible line demarcating detachment (usually by indirect ophthalmoscopy)
Evaluation: Bedside ED ocular U/S highly sens for detachment

Management
- Immediate optho consult if suspected
- If macula still attached, surgical repair indicated w/i 24–48 h
- Most inflammatory retinal detachments are treated medically (NSAIDs, steroids), but sometimes require emergent surgery depending on etiology, size, location

Disposition: Admit if acute

TOOTHACHE

Toothache Differential	
Trauma	Dental fractures, tooth subluxation, tooth avulsion
Atraumatic	Dental caries, periapical/periodontal abscess (see Ch. 4), acute necrotizing ulcerative gingivitis, alveolar osteitis

Tooth Numbering	
Upper right 1, 2, 3, 4, 5, 6, 7, 8 (midline)	Upper left (midline) 9, 10, 11, 12, 13, 14, 15, 16
Lower right 32, 31, 30, 29, 28, 27, 26, 25 (midline)	Lower left (midline) 24, 23, 22, 21, 20, 19, 18, 17

Dental Fractures
Definition
- Ellis I: Enamel; Ellis II: Enamel + dentin; Ellis III: Involves pulp (+ bleeding)

Evaluation: Consider CXR in trauma pt for aspirated fragments
Management
- Dental blocks & oral analgesia
- Ellis I: Smooth sharp edges if needed, dental f/u in 2–3 d
- Ellis II: Cover w/ calcium hydroxide paste, zinc oxide paste, glass ionomer composites (pulp necrosis 1–7%), *dental f/u in 24 h*
- Ellis III: Cover w/ calcium hydroxide paste, zinc oxide paste, glass ionomer composites (pulp necrosis 10–30%), dental consult or urgent referral for pulpotomy/ pulpectomy
- High risk infection. Rx abx
- Need urgent (<24 h) dental f/u
- If bleeding → gauze soaked in epinephrine, inject lidocaine w/ epinephrine into pulp

Tooth Subluxation & Avulsion
Definition: Loose teeth or loss of teeth due to trauma
Evaluation: X-ray if mobility suggests alveolar fracture

Management
- Dental blocks & oral analgesia
- Minimal mobility: Soft diet 1–2 wk, dental f/u in 2–3 d
- Grossly mobile: Stabilize w/ periodontal paste or splint, *dental f/u in 24 h*
- Avulsion: Only permanent teeth. Transport tooth in Hank's solution or milk (preserves up to 8 h), do not clean tooth, replace tooth to socket w/ stabilization if w/i <60 min. 1% loss of tooth survival for every minute out. *Immediate dental consult w/ f/u in 24 h*

Dental Caries
Definition: Bacterial infection of hard tooth structure (enamel, dentin, & cementum)
Presentation: Tooth pain, poor dentition
Management: Dental block & oral analgesia, dental f/u in 1–2 d

Periapical Abscess
Definition: Bacterial infection of alveolar space
Presentation: Severe tooth pain, often fluctuant abscess
Management: Dental block. I&D if fluctuant. Abx (penicillin V or clindamycin), warm saline rinses, dental f/u in 1–2 d.

Acute Necrotizing Ulcerative Gingivitis (Trench Mouth)
Definition
- Polymicrobial infection of gums causing bleeding, deep ulcers, & necrotic gums
- RFs: Poor oral hygiene, local trauma, smoking, immunodeficiencies

Presentation
- Rapid onset diffuse mouth pain, halitosis, fever, gum bleeding
- Gingival erythema/edema, interdental papillae ulceration, gray pseudomembrane

Management: Oral anesthetic solution (viscous lidocaine), dilute hydrogen peroxide rinses QID or chlorhexidine, abx if extensive or systemic (penicillin, clindamycin), *dental flu in 1–2 d*

Pearl: Cx: Vincent angina–spread to pharynx & tonsils

Alveolar Osteitis (Dry Socket)

Definition: Irritation of bone exposed to the oral cavity after premature disintegration of blood clot 3–5 d after tooth extraction

History: Sudden onset, severe pain after dental extraction, foul odor/taste

Management: Dental block, oral analgesia, irrigate socket, pack w/ iodoform gauze soaked in medicated dental paste or eugenol. Abx (penicillin, clindamycin). *Dental flu in 1–2 d.*

RESUSCITATION

Broselow Tape (equipment size & drug doses based on child length), Handtevy method

Airway: RSI (See 17-1)
- Pretreatment: Atropine (0.02 mg/kg, max 1 mg) prn bradycardia; lidocaine (1.5 mg/kg) prn if ↑ ICP
- Sedation: Etomidate (0.3 mg/kg); thiopental (3–5 mg/kg); ketamine (1–2 mg/kg)
- Paralysis: Succinylcholine (1–2 mg/kg); rocuronium (0.6–1.2 mg/kg)
- ETT size: 3 mm cuffed (newborns); (age/4 + 4) – 0.5 mm cuffed (>1 mo); depth (cm) = ETT size × 3
- Laryngoscope size: 0 (<2.5 kg); 1 (<3 yr); 2 (3–12 yr); 3 (12 yr to adult)

Shock
- nl SBP (mmHg) = 70 + (age in years × 2) b/w 1 & 10 yr
- Start w/ 20 cc/kg NS, up to 3 boluses
- Dopamine (2–20 μg/kg/min); epinephrine (0.05–1 μg/kg/min) for cold shock; norepinephrine (0.05–1 μg/kg/min) for warm shock; dobutamine (2–20 μg/kg/min) for cardiogenic shock
- Consider hydrocortisone if at risk for adrenal insufficiency
- In trauma, start w/ 20–40 mL/kg NS; then add 10–20 mL/kg PRBCs

ABDOMINAL PAIN

Approach
- Nature of pain: Location, constant or intermittent, relation to eating, associated sxs
- PMH: Previous abd surgeries, prematurity
- Exam: Always perform genital exam to r/o testicular torsion
- Labs: CBC, CRP, BMP, UA, LFTs, lipase if in the upper abdomen

Abd Pain Differential		
Location	**Infancy**	**Childhood/Adolescence**
Mechanical	Malrotation w/ midgut volvulus, intussusception, hernia, Meckel diverticulum, Hirschsprung	Constipation, hernia, Meckel diverticulum, bowel obstruction (3a)
Inflammatory/ infectious	NEC	Gastroenteritis, appendicitis, HSP, pancreatitis, gastritis, biliary tract dz (3a), colitis (3a), pancreatitis
GU	UTI (14bb)	UTI (14bb), renal colic (6b), pregnancy/ectopic (7), PID (7), testicular/ovarian torsion (7)
Other	Colic, trauma (abuse)	DKA (14r), trauma, sickle cell (14aa), toxic ingestions, PNA, strep pharyngitis

APPENDICITIS

Definition
- Inflammation of the appendix

History
- Diffuse/periumbilical pain → localizing to RLQ, anorexia, N/V, irritability (may be the only sx in age <2), fever

Physical Findings
- RLQ tenderness, rebound/guarding, Rovsing sign (RLQ pain w/ palpation in LLQ), psoas sign (RLQ pain w/ hip extension), obturator sign (RLQ pain w/ leg flexion + internal hip rotation)

Evaluation
- Labs: CBC, UA (sterile pyuria/mild hematuria), hCG
- Imaging: U/S (90% sens: Much lower if perforated/large habitus/operator dependent), abd plain films (fecalith 10%), CT scan (95% sens/spec)

Treatment
- Surgical consult for operative management, abx (ampicillin 50 mg/kg, gentamicin 1 mg/kg + metronidazole 15 mg/kg or cefoxitin 20–40 mg/kg)

Disposition
- Admit

Pearls
- 90% of children <2 y/o have perforation at presentation (thinner walled/looser omentum → ↑ perforation)
- Young children may not have anorexia

INTUSSUSCEPTION

Definition
- Invagination of bowel into another, most commonly ileocolic (most frequent cause of SBO in <6 y/o)

History
- Age 3 mo–3 yr (peak 5–9 mo), M > F, lethargy, vomiting, intermittent fussiness/crying/inconsolability w/ drawing legs to chest, cramping abd pain

Physical Findings
- Not tender b/w episodes, abd tenderness, RUQ sausage-like mass, heme + stool, "currant jelly" stool (late finding in <1/3 of pts)

Evaluation
- Upright plain abd film to r/o free air, crescent sign, U/S (95% sens/spec): Target, bull's eye, doughnut, pseudokidney sign; barium/air/water enema: Diagnostic/therapeutic (90% successful)

Treatment
- Barium/air/water enema, NGT, surgical consult for operative management in case barium enema fails, hydration (severe dehydration is common), NPO

Disposition
- Admission for 24 h observation

Pearls
- <3 y/o likely idiopathic
- Barium enema is contraindicated if peritoneal signs
  - If >2 y/o, consider abnl lead point (tumor, Meckel's, polyp)

MALROTATION WITH MIDGUT VOLVULUS

Definition
- Malrotation & weak fixation of the duodenum & colon during embryologic development → twisting of the mesentery causing duodenal obstruction/SMA compression → necrosis

History
- Neonate (3 y/o) acute abd pain, bilious vomiting, ±distension, irritability/lethargy, FTT, mostly occur w/i 1st year of life

Physical Findings
- Ill appearing/dehydration, heme + stool/grossly bloody, abd tenderness, often peritoneal

Evaluation
- Upright plain films: "Double bubble" (dilated stomach & duodenum)/pneumatosis/SBO; U/S: "Whirlpool sign"; upper GI series (diagnostic): "Corkscrew sign," coiled-spring appearance of jejunum

Treatment
- Immediate surgical consult for operative management, NGT, NPO, abx, fluids

Disposition
- Admission

INCARCERATED/STRANGULATED HERNIA

Definition
- Defects in the abd wall that allow protrusion of abd contents through the inguinal canal

History
- More commonly male, abd/groin/testicular pain, inguinal fullness w/ prolonged standing/coughing, vomiting, irritability in infants

Physical Findings
- Intestine/BS in scrotal sac

Evaluation
- Scrotal/abd U/S if physical exam is unclear, x-ray can be used to r/o free air

Treatment
- Reduction: Place in Trendelenburg → gentle pressure ± ice analgesic/BZD; >12 h concern for perforation/gangrene → surgical management

Disposition
- Admission if operative management required

MECKEL DIVERTICULUM

Definition
- Omphalomesenteric duct remnant w/ 60% containing heterotopic gastric (80%) or pancreatic tissue

History
- Any age (sxs usually begin <2 y/o), ±LLQ pain, melanotic stool (acid secretion → ulceration/erosion of mucosa), vomiting, sx of SBO, intussusception

Physical Findings
- LLQ mass, heme + stool/brisk bleeding, abd distension

Evaluation
- Technetium scan (Meckel scan): Identifies heterotopic gastric tissue (90% sens)

Treatment
- Type & cross/transfuse for brisk bleeding, surgical consult for Meckel diverticulectomy

Disposition
- Admit

Meckel's Rule of 2s
2% of the population
Only 2% of those w/ Meckel are symptomatic
2 in long
2 ft proximal from ileocecal valve
Presents in the 1st 2 yr of life
2 types of epithelium: Gastric & pancreatic

NECROTIZING ENTEROCOLITIS (NEC)

Definition
- Inflammatory condition of intestinal wall due to bacterial overgrowth w/ translocation

History
- Preterm neonate (90%), age < 1 mo (usually first days of life), bilious vomiting, abd distension, bloody stool, feeding intolerance

Physical Findings
- Ill appearing, hypotension, lethargic, abd tenderness, heme + stools, diarrhea

Evaluation
- Abd x-ray: Pneumatosis intestinalis (75%), portal venous air; barium enema if x-ray is ambiguous

Treatment
- NPO, hydration/transfusion, NGT, abx (ampicillin/gentamicin/metronidazole), surgical consult

Disposition
- Admit

Pearls
- Bell stages: I. Vomiting/ileus, II. Intestinal dilation/pneumatosis on x-ray, III. Shock/perforation
- Cx: DIC, strictures, obstruction, fistulas, short gut syndrome

HIRSCHSPRUNG DISEASE

Definition
- Absence of ganglion cells in the myenteric plexus of the colon → constant contraction & proximal dilation → constipation, obstruction (4:1 male predominance)

History
- Chronic constipation, delayed 1st meconium, FTT, abd distension, vomiting

Physical Findings
- Sx in 1st days to weeks of life, palpable stool in abdomen, tight sphincter, fecal mass in LLQ, no stool in rectal vault, "squirt" – explosive release of stool when finger is withdrawn

Evaluation
- Abd plain film: Dilated colon/fecal impaction/air fluid levels; barium enema; Dx → biopsy (aganglionosis) or anal manometry

Treatment
- Outpt surgical eval

Disposition
- D/c unless cx: Toxic mega colon, perforation, enterocolitis

CYANOSIS

Approach
- Differentiate cyanosis that is central (mucous membranes, tongue, trunk, 2/2 right-to-left shunt) vs. peripheral (feet, hands, lips, 2/2 peripheral vasoconstriction)

Definition
- Acrocyanosis: Blueness in hands/feet only seen in newborns, 2° perfusion of the extremities → nl & resolves w/i 1st few days of life
- Breath-holding spell: Prolonged period w/o attempt to breathe a/w intense crying from pain, anger, fright → benign, but Dx of exclusion

Cyanosis Differential	
Pathophysiology	**Differential**
Hypoventilation	Apnea, breath-holding spell, sz
Respiratory	Upper airway obstruction, 1° lung dz, bronchiolitis/asthma
Cardiovascular	Cyanotic congenital cardiac dz
Other	Sepsis, hypothermia, methemoglobinemia, CN^-, acrocyanosis of the newborn

History
- Age of onset, central or peripheral, med ingestion, recent illness, environmental exposures
- Δ w/ crying: Improvement → respiratory etiology (↑ alveolar recruitment); exacerbation → cardiac etiology (↑ CO)

Findings
- Appearance (ill or well), VS, respiratory distress, heart murmur

Evaluation
- Provide O_2, obtain CXR, ECG
- Hyperoxygenation test: Compare ABG on RA on 100% O_2 for 10 min, P_{O_2} of >250 excludes hypoxia 2/2 congenital heart dz
- Improvement in O_2 sat w/ O_2, lack of murmur, nl ECG → pulmonary process
- No Δ in O_2 sat w/ O_2, murmur, abnl ECG → cardiac cause → obtain echo (see 14-19)

Treatment
- O_2, identify then tx underlying condition
- Consider PGE_1 for pts <2 wk of age in circulatory failure

Disposition
- Admit any pt who is ill appearing, low O_2 sat or PaO_2
- Consult cardiology for any pt w/ suspected congenital cardiac dz

PEDIATRIC FEVER

Approach
- Fever (38°C or 100.4°F) management is different in pediatric population compared to adults
- ABCs, check O_2 saturation, rectal temperature
- Need for abx & hospitalization depends on age, tox, exposures, immune status, identified source, seriousness of source

- Introduction of *H. influenzae* & pneumococcal vaccines have changed the incidence & etiology of febrile illness in pediatric populations

Fever Differential	
Pathophysiology	**Differential**
Pulmonary	Bronchiolitis, croup, pertussis, pharyngitis, PNA
GI	Appendicitis, gastroenteritis, rotavirus
GU	UTI, pyelonephritis
Noninfectious	SCD, Kawasaki's Dz, rheumatologic & oncologic etiologies
Misc infections	Cellulitis, HIV, sepsis, varicella, epiglottitis, measles, meningitis, mumps, OM, omphalitis, roseola, rubella, scarlet fever, osteomyelitis, HSV, enterovirus, bacterial conjunctivitis, nonsp viral syndromes

FEBRILE INFANT 0–90 D OLD

History
- Difficult to obtain localizing hx; standardized w/u to Dx serious bacterial illnesses, high-risk 2/2 immature immune sz
- Exposures (travel, ill family members) & immunizations are helpful

Findings
- Fever >38°C or 100.4°F rectal considered standard; fussy, irritable, poor feeding
- Assess frequency & # of wet diapers, cap refill, fontanelles, tears, to estimate dehydration
- Ask about any rashes (viral exanthems, meningococcus)

Evaluation
- Sepsis w/u: See table

Treatment
- Less than 1 mo: Cefotaxime 50 mg/kg IV q12h + ampicillin 25–50 mg/kg IV q8h
- 1–3 mo: Ceftriaxone 50 mg/kg IV q24h, consider IM ceftriaxone 50 mg/kg if being D/C
- Higher doses for suspected meningitis, consider adding acyclovir 20 mg/kg IV (see 14-16)
- Treat other identified bacterial source appropriately
- If LP was not performed, consider withholding abx in well-appearing infant w/ nl WBC

Disposition
- If <30 d or <90 d & toxic appearing, admit & follow cx even if all labs nl
- Can d/c 30–90 d w/ neg. sepsis w/u & well appearing/feeding w/ f/u in 24 h. Consider 1 dose ceftriaxone prior to d/c

Pearl
- Due to inability to localize source of infection, relative immaturity of immune systems, & prevalence of occult bacteremia, all pts receive extensive sepsis w/u

FEBRILE CHILD 3–36 MO

History
- Vulnerable immune system, esp to encapsulated organisms' exposures
- Exposures (travel, ill family members) & immunizations helpful

Findings
- Irritable, poor feeding; elicit hydration status via # of wet diapers, tears, fontanelle, cap refill
- Ask about any rashes (viral exanthems, meningococcus)

Evaluation
- See table

Treatment
- If ill appearing w/ fever, 1 dose ceftriaxone (50 mg/kg IV & 24-h admission for cx)
- Treat identified bacterial source appropriately

Disposition
- If well appearing w/ neg. w/u & fully immunized, d/c home w/ close f/u
- If well appearing w/neg. w/u & incomplete immunization:
  - WBC >15K (ANC >9000), give empiric abx (ceftriaxone IV or IM) &24 h f/u or admit if f/u uncertain
  - WBC <15K (ANC <9000), d/c w/o abx, but close f/u in 24–48 h

- Prevalence of occult bacteremia in well-appearing children <36 mo is now 0.25–0.4%
  (Acad Emerg Med 2009;16(3):220; Arch Dis Child 2009;94(2):144)

EVAL of Pediatric Fever by Age			
Age	Temp	Appearance	Eval
0–90 d	>38°C	Any	Straight cath urine & culture CBC w/ differential, blood culture, CRP CXR if ↑ RR, respiratory sxs CSF culture, cell count, glucose/protein, ±HSV/ enterovirus PCR Stool culture if diarrhea is present
3–36 mo	<39°C	Any	UA & Ucx CXR if ↑ RR, resp sxs
	>39°C	Well	UA & Ucx CBC w/ differential, blood culture, CRP CXR if ↑ RR, resp sxs
		Ill	UA & Ucx CBC w/ differential, blood culture, CRP If neg., LP CXR if ↑ RR, resp sxs

JAUNDICE

Definition
- Yellowish discoloration of the skin/tissue/body fluids caused by ↑ bilirubin production or ↓ excretion

Approach
- Bilirubin: Formed from degradation of hemoglobin → bound to albumin in blood (unconjugated/indirect) → conjugated in liver by glucuronyl transferase (conjugated/direct) → excreted in bile

History
- Differential depends on age (neonates ≤4 wk), gestational age, breast-feeding status
- Time of onset of sx: Yellowing of skin, dark urine

Physical Findings
- Scleral icterus, jaundice

Labs
- Total/fractionated bilirubin (visible >5 mg/dL in neonates), LFTs, CBC (hemolysis/anemia → Coombs test, smear, ABO/Rh type), reticulocyte count, serum haptoglobin
- Neonates → unconjugated (can be physiologic, treat to prevent kernicterus)/conjugated (always pathologic)

Differential Dx of Unconjugated Hyperbilirubinemia in Children	
Hemolytic disorders	ABO incompatibility
	G6PD deficiency
	Sickle cell anemias
	Thalassemias
	Hereditary spherocytosis
	HUS
Enterohepatic recirculation	Hirschsprung dz, pyloric stenosis, GI obstructions
Other	Cephalohematoma, birth trauma, hypothyroidism, Down syndrome, polycythemia, Gilbert syndrome, Crigler–Najjar syndrome (deficiencies in glucuronyl transferase)

PHYSIOLOGIC JAUNDICE

Definition
- Elevated unconjugated bilirubin in the 1st wk of life, 60% newborns will be jaundiced (peaks 2–5 d), due to low activity of glucuronyl transferase, increased production, & increased enterohepatic circulation

Evaluation
- Total/fractionated bilirubin, CBC (hemolysis/anemia → Coombs test, smear, ABO/Rh type), total bilirubin usually <6 mg/dL, up to 12 mg/dL in premature infants

Treatment
- No tx necessary

Disposition
- Home

Pearls
- Pathologic: In the 1st 24 h of life, peak >17 mg/dL in breast-fed/>15 mg/dL in formula-fed infants, persists beyond 1st wk of life, ↑ bilirubin >5 mg/dL/d
- Cx of severe hyperbilirubinemia: kernicterus (bilirubin deposition in basal ganglia → neurodevelopmental deficits)
- Sepsis can rarely present as jaundice

BREAST-FEEDING JAUNDICE

Definition
- ↑ unconjugated bilirubinemia in breast-fed infants possibly due to hormonal mediators or altered intestinal secretion/absorption of bile, early onset after birth
  - May be related to caloric deprivation or insufficient frequency of feeding

Evaluation
- Total/fractionated bilirubin, CBC

Treatment
- No tx necessary if bilirubin <17 mg/dL, encourage breast feeding, phototherapy

Disposition
- Home

BREAST MILK JAUNDICE

Definition
- Due to substances in breast milk that prevent conjugation & excretion of bilirubin. Occurs after 3–5 d of life, persists for weeks.

Evaluation
- Total/fractionated bilirubin, CBC

Treatment
- If bilirubin <17 mg/dL, continue breast feeding, phototherapy
- If >17 mg/dL, stop breast feeding, will not recur when resumed

Disposition
- Home

ABO AND RH INCOMPATIBILITY/HEMOLYTIC DISEASE

Definition
- Hemolytic dz caused by maternal antibodies against fetal A or B type proteins or maternal Rh antibodies (sensitized from previous pregnancy) against Rh-positive fetus (Rh incompatibility)

History
- Yellowing of skin w/i 1st 24 h of life, dark urine, lethargy

Physical Findings
- Severe jaundice, scleral icterus, ill appearing

Evaluation
- Total/fractionated bilirubin, CBC (hemolysis/anemia → Coombs test, smear, ABO/Rh type)

Treatment
- Phototherapy, exchange transfusion (see table)

Disposition
- Admit

Indications for Therapy in Unconjugated Hyperbilirubinemia				
Age	Consider Phototherapy (mg/dL)	Phototherapy (mg/dL)	Consider Exchange Transfusion if Phototherapy Fails (mg/dL)	Exchange Transfusion (mg/dL)
≤24 h	—	—	—	—
25–48 h	≥12	≥15	≥20	≥25
49–72 h	≥15	≥18	≥25	≥30
≥72 h	≥17	≥20	≥30	≥30

CONJUGATED HYPERBILIRUBINEMIA

Definition
- Pathologic increase in direct bilirubin leading to jaundice (conjugated bilirubin >20% of total, or >2 mg/dL)

History
- Yellowing of skin, dark urine, lethargy, ±genetic syndrome/metabolic syndromes/ sepsis

Physical Findings
- Severe jaundice, scleral icterus, ill appearing

Evaluation
- Total/fractionated bilirubin, CBC, blood cultures, blood smear, LFTs, blood type, KUB if signs of obstruction, U/S: Biliary obstruction, UA, Ucx

Treatment
- Hydration, tx based on cause (see below)

Disposition
- Admit

Differential Dx of Conjugated Hyperbilirubinemia in Children	
Biliary obstruction	Biliary atresia
	Choledochal cyst
	1° sclerosing cholangitis
	Gallstone (usually pigmented stone from hemolysis in sickle cell/ thalassemia)
Infections	TORCH infection (toxoplasmosis, rubella, CMV, & herpes virus)
	Bacterial sepsis
	UTI
	Viral hepatitis
Metabolic	Cystic fibrosis
	Galactosemia
	α1-antitrypsin deficiency
	Wilson dz
Drugs	Aspirin
	APAP
	Iron
	Sulfa
Miscellaneous	Reye syndrome
	Neonatal lupus
	Neonatal hepatitis, autoimmune hepatitis

LIMP

Approach
- Examine abdomen, genitalia, spine, hips, long bones, knees, ankle, feet; observe gait
- Careful hx from pt & care giver: Acute vs. chronic, fevers, skin Δ; trauma
- Obtain x-rays although pain is often referred (classically, knee pain referred from hip)
- Consider systemic sxs in conjunction w/ chief complaint of joint pain

Limp Differential	
Pathophysiology	**Differential**
Trauma	Fracture, dislocation, sprains, hemarthrosis, back pain
Hematologic	Sickle cell anemia (14aa), hemophilia
Neuromuscular	Peripheral neuropathy, muscular dystrophy, myositis
Infectious	Septic arthritis, toxic synovitis, osteomyelitis, PID, diskitis, epidural abscess
Rheumatologic	Juvenile rheumatoid arthritis, gout, pseudogout, lupus, rheumatic fever
GI/GU	Psoas abscess, testicular torsion, orchitis, appendicitis
Musculoskeletal	Legg–Calvé–Perthes dz, SCFE, Osgood–Schlatter dz
Neoplastic	Leukemia, Ewing sarcoma, osteosarcoma, osteochondroma

INFECTIOUS

Septic Arthritis of the Hip
History
- Most commonly in children <3 y/o, but can occur at any age
- Limp or refuse to walk, hx of fever & irritability (sxs may be far more subtle in infants)

Findings
- Febrile & toxic appearing
- Flexed, externally rotated, abducted hip; antalgic gait (if walking)
- Significant pain w/ ROM but not necessarily warm, swollen or erythematous

Evaluation
- ↑ WBC, ↑ CRP, ↑ ESR; arthrocentesis shows ↑ WBC, +Gram stain & culture
- X-rays & U/S may show effusion

Treatment
- Orthopedic consultation for drainage & washout in the OR
- Abx: β-lactamase–resistant PCN (IV nafcillin or oxacillin 50–100 mg/kg/d QID) & 3rd-generation cephalosporin (cefotaxime or ceftriaxone 50 mg/kg); consider vancomycin
- Pain control

Disposition
- Admit for surgical wash-out

Pearl
- Hip > knee > elbow likely to be septic in children

Toxic (Transient) Synovitis
History
- 3–6 y/o, M:F 2:1, acute or chronic unilateral hip, thigh, or knee pain
- May be mildly febrile, possibly recent URI

Findings
- Nontoxic appearing
- Limited hip ROM 2/2 pain; mild restriction of passive ROM to internal rotation & extension; most sens to log roll
- Antalgic gait, painful to palpation

Evaluation
- X-ray of hip nl; may show effusion
- WBC & ESR nl or slightly ↑; afebrile children w/ nl labs can avoid arthrocentesis
- U/S can diagnose effusion, but cannot differentiate type

Treatment
- Pain control w/ NSAIDs, heat, & massage

Disposition
- Orthopedic f/u, crutches to keep weight off hip until pain resolves

Pearls
- Most common cause of acute hip pain in children from 3–10 yr; arthralgia & arthritis secondary to transient inflammation of the synovium of the hip
- Recurrence rate <20%, most develop w/i 6 mo, no ↑ risk for juvenile chronic arthritis, may go on to develop Legg–Calvé–Perthes dx

Predicted Probability of Septic Arthritis (%)		
No. of Factors	Modified Kocher Criteria (J Bone Joint Surg Am 2006;88(6):1251)	Kocher Criteria (J Bone Joint Surg Am 1999;81(12):1662)
0	16.9	0.2
1	36.7	3
2	62.4	40
3	82.6	93.1
4	93.1	99.6
5	97.5	

Factors: Temp >38.5°C, WBC >12, ESR >40, refusal to bear weight ± CRP >20 (if using modified Kocher criteria)

MUSCULOSKELETAL

Legg–Calvé–Perthes Disease (Avascular Necrosis of Femoral Head)
History
- Most commonly in 5–7 y/o w/ limp & pain in groin, thigh, or knee; worse w/ ↑ activity
- No fever or irritability, no hx of trauma

Findings
- Nontoxic appearing, antalgic gait
- ↓ Hip ROM secondary to pain w/ possible thigh atrophy, ↑ w/ internal rotation & abduction

Evaluation
- WBC & ESR nl
- X-rays often nl initially; frog-leg views helpful
  - Widening of cartilage space, diminished ossific nucleus
  - Subchondral stress fx of femoral head; linear lucency in femoral head epiphysis
  - Femoral head opacification & flattening known as coxa plana
  - Subluxation & protrusion of femoral head from acetabulum

Treatment
- Goal is to avoid severe degenerative arthritis, maintain ROM, relieve weight bearing
- Orthopedic eval; bone scan & MRI more rapidly diagnostic than x-rays

Disposition
- Orthopedic f/u, crutches to keep weight off hip until pain resolves

Pearls
- Idiopathic osteonecrosis of capital epiphysis of femoral head; 15–20% bilateral
- Caused by interruption of blood supply to capital femoral head → bone infarction
- Better prognosis at younger onset; proportional to degree of radiologic involvement

Slipped Capital Femoral Epiphysis (SCFE)
History
- 12–15-y/o boy or 10–13-y/o girl, c/o limp & groin, thigh, or knee pain
- If sxs >3 wk, considered chronic
- If unable to bear weight, considered unstable (higher cx rate)

Findings
- Affected leg externally rotated, shortened w/ pain when flexing hip; antalgic gain

Evaluation
- nl temp, WBC, ESR
- X-ray: Femoral head is displaced posteriorly & inferiorly in relation to femoral neck w/i confines of acetabulum; AP & frog-leg views best

Treatment
- Orthopedic consult for operative internal fixation; goal to prevent AVN of femoral head

Disposition
- Admission for orthopedic surgery

Pearls
- Obesity is the RF; genetics play role; bilaterality more common in younger pts who also tend to have metabolic/endocrine disorders
- If traumatic hip injury w/ obvious external rotation & shortening of the leg, do not force ROM as this can worsen epiphyseal displacement

Osgood–Schlatter Disease

Definition
- Microtrauma to the tibial tubercle tuberosity apophysis occurring during use

History
- Preteen boy w/ knee pain, worse w/ activity & better w/ rest

Findings
- Edema & pain of tibial tubercle; enlarged & indurated tibial tuberosity
- Tender over anterior knee, esp over thickened patellar tendon
- Pain reproduced by extending knee against resistance, stressing quads or squatting w/ knee in full flexion, running, jumping, kneeling, squatting, stairs

Evaluation
- Clinical dx. X-ray may show swelling over tuberosity & patellar tendon; no effusion

Treatment
- Guided by severity: Range from decreasing activity in mild cases to rest in severe cases
- NSAIDs for pain control, ice, ±crutches

Disposition
- D/c home w/ pain control

Pearls
- One of the most common causes of knee pain in adolescent; benign & self-limited
- Bilateral in 25% of cases; 50% give hx of precipitating trauma

PEDIATRIC SEIZURE

Definition
- Abn, paroxysmal d/c of CNS neurons leading to abn neurologic fxn

Approach
- ABCs, check O_2 saturation, temperature, determine if still seizing
- Immediate bedside glucose fingerstick & tx, consider administering empiric glucose
- If actively seizing, quickly administer suppression medications
- Careful hx: Description of events before & after sz, associated sxs (HA, photophobia, vomiting, visual Δ, ocular pain), focal neurologic sxs
- Assess for head or neck trauma, meningismus, skin finding (petechiae, café-au-lait spots, port-wine stain, ash leaf spots), ↑ICP (bulging fontanelle)
- Thorough neurologic exam; Todd paralysis: Transient paralysis after a sz
- CBC, CMP, tox screen, UA, CXR: Tox screen, anticonvulsant levels, infectious w/u
- Consider CT if persistent AMS, neurologic deficit, or trauma
- Consider LP after head CT if persistently AMS, fever, & therapeutic med levels
- 1st-time sz w/u: Consider head CT, ECG, CBC, CMP, tox screen, LP
- EEG days to weeks after sz unless concern for nonconvulsant status epilepticus
- Status epilepticus is recurrent or continuous sz activity lasting >30 min w/o return to baseline MS
  - Can result in cerebral hypoxia, lactic & respiratory acidosis, hypercarbia, hypoglycemia
- Disposition: Admission for abnl neuro exam, others w/ neurology f/u

Sz Differential	
Pathophysiology	**Differential**
Neurologic	1° sz, status epilepticus, febrile, sz degenerative CNS dz (neurofibromatosis, tuberous sclerosis, Sturge–Weber syndrome), epilepsy, cerebral palsy
Head injury	IPH, SAH, SDH, epidural (19b)
Infection	Meningitis (5d, 14i), encephalitis (5d), brain abscess, toxoplasmosis, tetanus, neurocysticercosis
Metabolic	Hypoglycemia, hyperglycemia, hyponatremia, hypernatremia, hypocalcemia, hypomagnesemia, alkalosis (5e), pyridoxine deficiency

Pathophysiology	Differential
Toxic	Lead, PCP, amphetamine, cocaine, aspirin, CO, organophosphates, theophylline, lidocaine, lindane, drug withdrawal (anticonvulsants), s/p DPT immunization
Neoplasm	Brain tumor
Pediatric	Reye syndrome, CMV, congenital syphilis, maternal rubella, PKU
Vascular	Embolism, infarction, HTN encephalopathy, malformations
Other	Psychological, hyperventilation, breath-hold spells, inadequate drug level, neurocutaneous syndromes, inborn errors of metabolism

Primary Seizures

History
- Presence/absence of aura, abrupt onset & termination of sz activity, stereotyped purposeless behavior, fecal or urinary incontinence, postictal confusion or lethargy

Findings
- Depends on type of sz, LOC secondary to simultaneous activation of entire cerebral cortex

Evaluation
- As above

Treatment
- Acute vs. chronic meds, airway mgmt often w/ only nasal trumpet, supplemental O_2
- **Abortive tx**
  - BZD are 1st line (lorazepam 0.1 mg/kg up to 4 mg IV)
  - BZD: Diazepam ($t_{1/2}$ 15–20 min), lorazepam ($t_{1/2}$ 12–24 h), midazolam ($t_{1/2}$ <12 h)
  - 2nd-line: fosphenytoin (20 PE/kg IV)
  - Phenobarbital (20 mg/kg IV load), 1st line in neonates, watch for hypotension & bradypnea
  - If refractory szs, give pyridoxine 100 mg IV; consider thiamine 100 mg IV in adolescents
- **Long-term Anticonvulsant Medications**
  - If known sz disorder & subtherapeutic levels, load w/ chronic med
  - Long-term anticonvulsants not routinely indicated in 1st unprovoked sz

Disposition
- Explicit instructions to not drive, operate hazardous machinery, or perform tasks where recurrent sz may cause harm; some states have mandatory reporting to department of motor vehicles

Pearls
- Keep differential broad even if known sz d/o, esp if tx med levels
- If meningitis suspected, give abx pre-emptively while awaiting confirmation
- Pseudosz is Dx of exclusion
- Tx EtOH withdrawal sz w/ BZD, almost never responsive to antiepileptic meds
- Consider Neurology consult if starting new long-term med in 1st-time sz (will need close f/u)

Pediatric Sz Suppression Steps		
Tx of Sz		
Step	**Antiepileptic**	**Dose**
1	Lorazepam (slower)	0.1 mg/kg IV or prn, repeat 0.05 mg/kg q5min
2 (>30 min)	Phenobarbital (consider intubating)	20 mg/kg (<20 kg) or 10 mg/kg (>20 kg) IV
	Phenytoin Fosphenytoin	20 mg/kg IV at 1 mg/kg/min 20 mg PE/kg at 3 mg PE/kg/min
	Levetiracetam	20 mg/kg IV
3 (>1 h)	Pentobarbital, midazolam, valproic acid, propofol infusions, general anesthesia	

Epilepsy

History
- Typical sz recurrence, may be a/w lip biting, incontinence of bowel or bladder followed by lethargy/combativeness & confusion (postictal period)

Findings
- Depends on type of sz, LOC secondary to simultaneous activation of entire cerebral cortex

Evaluation
• As above

Treatment
• Acute vs. chronic meds, airway mgmt often w/ only nasal trumpet, supplemental O_2

Disposition
• Neurology f/u for medication adjustment if indicated

Pearls
• Keep differential broad even if known sz d/o, esp if tx med levels
• Systemic illness such as URI or fever can lower sz threshold

Cerebral Palsy
History
• Nonprogressive lesion sustained during brain development → motor, speech, & learning disabilities, high risk (50%) for szs. Prematurity is the biggest RF

Findings
• Depends on type of CP:
  • I. Quadriplegia: Hypotonic trunk & spastic extremities
  • II. Diplegia: Spastic lower extremities, ↑ DTRs, clonus, & "scissoring"
  • III. Hemiplegia: Unilateral spasticity, usually UE > LE
  • IV. Athetoid: Writhing, involuntary movements of extremities
  • V. Ataxic: Unsteady, uncoordinated movements
  • VI. Hypotonic: Lacking muscle tone

Evaluation
• Head CT if new onset sz or recent trauma
• Outpt EEG if new onset sz or Δ in sz pattern or frequency

Treatment
• Standard sz tx

Disposition
• Neurology f/u for medication adjustment if indicated

Pearls
• Pts w/ CP often have breakthrough sz & low sz thresholds, look for underlying illness (URI, PNA, UTI, etc.), adjust outpt meds w/ 1° neurologist
• CP pts also commonly present to the ED w/ chronic aspiration, PNA, feeding difficulties, G-tube malfunction, UTIs

Pediatric Sz Types	
Sz Type	Findings
Generalized absence	Staring spell w/ loss or motor/speech activity, w/ brief LOC
Generalized tonic–clonic	Contracted posture followed by rhythmic jerking movements of extremities in pts w/ impaired consciousness
Myoclonic	Repetitive, rhythmic muscular contractions
Simple partial	Unilateral tonic–clonic movements, nl consciousness
Complex partial	Unilateral tonic–clonic movements w/ impaired consciousness, both cerebral hemispheres involved
Somatosensory	Numbness, tingling, paresthesias, or visual Δ
Autonomic	Δ in HR, pupil size, sweating, aphasia
Psychomotor	Repetitive behaviors such as clapping, verbalizations, chewing, swallowing, not remembered after sz

Febrile Seizures
History
• T ≥38.3°C (101°F) in child b/w 6 mo & 5 yr of age
• No hx of sz; 1 generalized sz lasting <15 min a/w rapidly ↑ temp

Findings
• Generalized sz activity, usually lasts <15 min; high fever, postictal period
• Complex febrile sz: Last >15 min, >1× in 24-h period, or focal component

Evaluation
• Evaluate for underlying (infectious) cause: CXR, UA, labs, bedside glucose, ±LP

Treatment
• Antipyretic, observation until pt back to baseline, parental reassurance
• Anticonvulsants like BZD & phenobarbital are not indicated

Disposition
- 1st febrile sz, nonfocal exam, neg. ED w/u can be D/C w/ neuro f/u

Pearls
- Focal sz do not present as simple febrile sz
  - Consider meningitis/encephalitis in unvaccinated children
- Febrile sz not a/w an epilepsy or brain damage
- Incidence of another febrile sz is 35%
- >2 febrile sz/yr or >3 total febrile sz must be evaluated for other etiologies

NAUSEA AND VOMITING

Approach
- Common sxs of many dz processes (eg, intra-abd causes, metabolic derangements, toxic ingestions, neurologic causes)

History
- Relation to eating, bilious (require eval for obstruction), ability to tolerate POs, urine output (making wet diapers), presence of bloody stools, HA, AMS

Labs
- BMP, serum glucose (↑ risk of hypoglycemia)

Treatment
- Treat under lying cause, antiemetics, hydration (PO or IV)

Nausea & Vomiting Differential		
Location	Infancy	Childhood/Adolescence
Mechanical	GERD, malrotation w/ midgut volvulus (14a), intussusception (14a), pyloric stenosis	Constipation, hernia (14a), Meckel diverticulum (14a), bowel obstruction (3a)
Inflammatory/ infectious	NEC (14a), gastroenteritis, sepsis (14j), meningitis (14i), PNA, OM	Gastroenteritis, OM, appendicitis (14a), pancreatitis (14a), HSP (14a), biliary dz (3a)
GU	UTI (14bb)	UTI (14bb), renal colic (6b), pregnancy/ectopic (7), PID (7), testicular/ovarian torsion (7)
CNS (persistent vomiting w/o systemic/GI sxs)	Hydrocephalus, intracranial injury/tumor (18b)	Hydrocephalus, intracranial injury/tumor (18b), migraine (5d)
Metabolic	DKA (14r), urea cycle defects, fatty acid oxidation disorders, amino acidopathies, organic aciduria	DKA (14r), urea cycle defects, fatty acid oxidation disorders, RTA, adrenal insuf
Other	Toxic ingestions, trauma, Reye syndrome	Trauma, sickle cell (14aa), toxic ingestions

PYLORIC STENOSIS

Definition
- Hypertrophy of the antrum of the stomach, 5:1 male-to-female ratio

History
- 2–5 wk of age (rare after 3 mo), nl feeding after birth → nonbilious/±blood streaked projectile vomiting after feeding, weight loss, lethargy

Physical Findings
- RUQ olive-size mass, dehydration (loose skin, sunken eyes, dry mucous membranes)

Evaluation
- BMP (hyperchloremic metabolic alkalosis), U/S (+ pylorus >4 mm thick, >16 mm long, 95% sens, study of choice), upper GI series: "String sign," abd x-ray: Dilated stomach

Treatment
- Hydration, surgical consult for pyloromyotomy

Disposition
- Admit

GASTROESOPHAGEAL REFLUX DISEASE

Definition
- Loose esophageal sphincter → retrograde passage of food into esophagus

History
- <2 y/o, nonbilious vomiting/spitting during/after eating, type of formula (cow vs. soy)

Physical Findings
- Sandifer syndrome: Startled/jerky movements after eating, often confused for sz

Evaluation
- Outpt w/u: 24 pH probe (most sens), nuclear milk scan, barium swallow, heme + stools (if esophagitis present), bloody diarrhea can indicate formula allergy

Treatment
- Small feeding volumes w/ burp breaks, keep semiupright for 30–40 min after eating, thicken feeds by adding cereal
- Acid-reducing agents: Ranitidine 2–4 mg/kg/d divided q8h, PPI, metoclopramide 0.1–0.2 mg/kg q12h

Disposition
- Home

Pearls
- Cx: FTT, apnea, laryngospasm, esophagitis, PNA
- Usually resolves by 1 yr

GASTROENTERITIS

Definition
- Vomiting & diarrhea caused by infectious source

History
- Vomiting, diarrhea, sick contacts, recent abx, travel

Physical Findings
- Lethargy, dehydration (skin turgor, cap refill, mucus membranes, tears, VS)

Evaluation
- BMP (if severely dehydrated), stool culture/ova/parasites (protracted/bloody diarrhea)

Treatment
- Electrolyte correction, hydration (PO preferred, IV prn), most self-resolve, avoid anti-motility agents (↑ pain/cramping/prolonged sxs)
- Ondansetron prn; zinc supplementation (10–20 mg/d × 10–14 d) reduces severity, duration, & incidence of diarrheal illnesses in children <5 yr of age (*WHO: Treatment of Diarrhea: A Manual for Physicians & Other Healthcare Providers.* 4th rev ed. 2005)

Disposition
- Home or admit (severe dehydration, bicarb <16 mEq/L, inability to tolerate POs)

Etiology-sp Sxs & tx of Gastroenteritis			
Agents	**Classic Hx & Findings**	**ED Intervention**	**Clinical Pearls**
Viral			
Rotavirus	Watery diarrhea, in fall (Southwest)/ winter (Northeast) months; common among children attending daycare or preschool	Hydration	~70% of children under age 2 yr admitted for diarrhea dehydration are infected w/ rotavirus; very infectious
Adenovirus	Watery diarrhea w/ concurrent respiratory illness usually in spring or early summer	Hydration	
Norwalk virus	Watery diarrhea w/ fever, HA, & myalgia	Hydration	Major cause of diarrhea epidemics

Agents	Classic Hx & Findings	ED Intervention	Clinical Pearls
Bacterial			
C. jejuni	Watery or bloody diarrhea w/ fever & crampy abd pain	Hydration & azithromycin, erythromycin, or ciprofloxacin	Contracted through contaminated food or water
Shigella	Diarrhea possibly w/ blood/mucus/pus a/w fever, HA, & abd pain	Hydration; fluoroquinolones, Bactrim, ampicillin, or azithromycin	Contracted through contaminated food or water; increasing abx resistance
Salmonella	Bloody diarrhea w/ fever	Hydration; ciprofloxacin, azithromycin, ampicillin, or Bactrim	Abx can induce a carrier state Treat only if risk of invasive dz (<3 mo of age, sickle cell, immunosuppression)
E. coli	Watery diarrhea	Hydration; fluoroquinolones, azithromycin, or Bactrim	Tx w/ abx may trigger HUS in pts w/ E. coli 0157 (controversial)
V. cholerae	Watery diarrhea	Hydration; tetracycline or erythromycin	
V. parahaemolyticus	Rice-water diarrhea in pt who ingested inadequately cooked seafood	Bactrim 10 mg (TMP)/kg/24 h BID for 7–10 d in severe cases	
Y. enterocolitica	Diarrhea possibly w/ blood/mucus/pus a/w fever, vomiting, & RLQ pain	Hydration	Mimics appendicitis
C. difficile	Diarrhea a/w recent abx use	Metronidazole 15–30 mg/kg/24 h PO TID or vancomycin 40 mg/kg/24 h PO q6h	Toxic megacolon very rare in children, but possible
S. aureus	Foodborne toxin mediated w/ abrupt, dramatic onset of sxs w/i 2–6 h of ingestion	Hydration, supportive care	
Parasitic			
G. lamblia	Watery diarrhea & excessive, particularly malodorous, flatulence in pt exposed to children in daycare or mountain streams	Hydration & supportive care; metronidazole 15–30 mg/kg/24 h PO TID for 5 d	
E. histolytica	Diarrhea w/ blood & mucus	Hydration; metronidazole 15–30 mg/kg/ 24 h TID	A/w hepatic abscesses Consider paromomycin to treat intraluminal infection

QID, 4 times daily; BID, twice daily; q6h, every 6 h; CBC, complete blood count; BUN, serum urea nitrogen; Cr, creatinine; RLQ, right lower quadrant; TMP, trimvibrio colethoprim; PO, by mouth; TID, 3 times daily.

PEDIATRIC MENINGITIS (SEE 5D)

History
- HA, fever, neck stiffness, lethargy (AMS), N/V, rash, irritability, sz, somnolence

Findings
- Meningismus (stiff neck) occurs <15% of the time in children <18 mo old, petechial rash, irritability/lethargy, hemodynamic instability, fever, sz

Evaluation
- If bacterial etiology suspected, abx should be given immediately, then LP (see 4d)

Treatment
- Dexamethasone 0.15 mg/kg IV before 1st dose of abx (↓ ICP, risk of hearing loss 2/2 H. influenzae)
- Abx
  - <1 mo: Ampicillin (100 mg/kg) + gentamicin (2.5 mg/kg) OR cefotaxime (50 mg/kg)
  - 1–2 mo: Ampicillin + ceftriaxone (100 mg/kg) OR cefotaxime
  - >2 mo: Vancomycin (15 mg/kg) + ceftriaxone OR cefotaxime
- Consider adding acyclovir 20 mg/kg IV

Clinical Pearl
- Ampicillin necessary to cover *Listeria* in infants

NEONATAL COMPLAINTS

Approach
- Differentiate nervous parents from a child w/ true dz

Common Neonatal Presentations	
Pathophysiology	**Complaint**
GI	Poor feeding, reflux/regurgitation, vomiting, diarrhea, constipation, jaundice
Infectious dz	Fever
Other	Crying/colic, ALTE, sudden infant death syndrome (SIDS)
Respiratory	Stridor, apnea, cyanosis

History
- Events during pregnancy, delivery, gestational age & weight @ birth, alertness, diet, frequency of diaper Δ, crying patterns, color Δ; FH

Findings
- Weight, VS, color; undress baby → full exam

Pearl
- Many signs/sxs are nonsp: Abnl tone, weak suck, decrease PO intake, jaundice, abnl breathing, peripheral cyanosis, vomiting

POOR FEEDING

Approach
- Check for appropriate weight gain (5–7% wt loss during 1st week nl, then gain 1 oz/d for 1st 3 mo), take a careful hx/physical exam to identify any other abnlty

Treatment
- If weight gain is appropriate & pt has no other issues, attempt feeding trial

Disposition
- Pts w/ appropriate wt gain who tolerate POs in ED may be D/C home w/ parental reassurance & outpt f/u; all other pts require further eval (see w/u for inconsolability below)

CONSTIPATION

Approach
- Differentiate functional (no underlying condition) from pathologic constipation

Constipation Differential	
Pathophysiology	Differential
Obstruction	Bowel obstruction, anal atresia, meconium ileus, viral illness w/ ileus
Metabolic	Hypothyroid, hypercalcemia, heavy metal poisoning
Neuro	Cerebral palsy, Down syndrome, spina bifida occulta, neuromusc dz
Other	Dehydration, rectal prolapse, anal fissure, botulism, Hirschsprung dz

History
- Sx time course, Δ in stool consistency, baseline stooling patterns, 1st meconium passage after birth (>24–48 h = abnl), recent illness, V/D, fever, ingestion of honey

Findings
- Abd (distension), rectal exam (patency, stool @ vault), neuro exam (CNs, muscular tone)

Evaluation
- KUB (if obstruction is suspected); consider Chem 7, TSH, Ca, heavy metal screen

Treatment
- For functional constipation: Glycerin suppository, disimpaction, increased water b/w feedings, consider bisacodyl, lactulose, enemas, high fiber diet in older children
  - Fleets enemas may cause hypocalcemia, avoid in young infants

Disposition
- Functional constipation → d/c w/ PCP f/u: Pathologic causes warrant further w/u & may require admission

CRYING AND COLIC

Definition
- Colic: Recurrent pattern of inconsolable crying & irritability lasting >3 h/d on >3 d/wk, 3 wk–3 mo of life. Benign GI colic is Dx of exclusion.

Approach
- Excessive crying/colic are nonsp complaints that can be the presenting signs of benign GI distress or life-threatening dz

Colic Differential	
System	Differential
CNS	Meningitis/encephalitis, ICH
HEENT	FB in eye, corneal abrasion, OM, pharyngitis
Cardiac	CHF, SVT
GI	Gastroenteritis, intussusception, appendicitis, anal fissure, GERD, incarcerated hernia, benign GI colic, constipation, milk allergy
GU	Testicular torsion, UTI
Other	Hair tourniquet (finger, toe, penis), trauma, child abuse, extremity fracture, septic arthritis, drug ingestion, electrolyte disturbance, vaccine rxn

History
- Timing of crying, trauma, fever, medication ingestion, feeding hx, complete ROS & PMH

Findings
- Observe behavior, thorough physical exam

Evaluation
- UA; consider further testing (eg, abd U/S, x-ray, LP, tox screen) to r/o spec etiologies

Treatment
- Treat the underlying d/o

Disposition
- Home: If etiology is thought to be benign & pt has cry-free period in ED
- Admit: Any pt w/o clear etiology identified & no cry-free period in ED

APPARENT LIFE-THREATENING EVENT (ALTE) (Emerg Med J 2002;19:11)

Definition
- Observed episode frightening to the observer & characterized by ≥1 of the following: Apnea, color Δ, Δ in muscle tone, choking, &/or gagging
- Separate clinical entity from SIDS & represents a wide spectrum of etiologies

ALTE Differential	
Pathophysiology	**Differential**
Cardiac	Arrhythmia, myocarditis, hemorrhage
GI	GERD
Infectious	UTI, sepsis
Metabolic	Hypoglycemia, inborn error of metabolism
Neuro	Sz, head trauma, hydrocephalus, meningitis/encephalitis
Other	Toxins/drugs, child abuse, nl periodic breathing, Munchausen by proxy
Respiratory	Respiratory tract infection, airway obstruction, breath-holding spell

History
- Obtain 1st-hand account of event when possible, appearance of child (central vs. peripheral cyanosis, pallor, etc.), preceding sxs, prior episodes, presence of apnea or gagging, muscle tone, sz-like activity, spontaneous or facilitated recovery

Findings
- Through physical exam

Evaluation
- No standard diagnostic strategy exists. Testing should be guided by hx & physical exam. Consider: CBC, Chem 7, Ca, UA, urine/blood cx, ECG, RSV swab; CT head/LP (based on clinical suspicion); also consider ABG, serum/urine tox, pertussis screen, EEG

Disposition
- Observe in the ED; pts w/o true ALTE (eg, breath-holding spell) can be D/C w/ f/u in 24 h
- Infant w/ hx of apnea, pallor, cyanosis, limp, unresponsive req stimulation or CPR or have inadequate f/u require admission for observation & further revaluation

Pearl
- Definitive etiology of the ALTE is found in only ~50% of pts

---

SIDS

Definition
- D of child <12 mo of age that is unexplained after careful investigation, autopsy, exam of the D scene, & hx; most common @ 2–5 mo

Approach
- Approach parents of SIDS pts w/ sympathy, as child abuse rare in SIDS (<1–5%)

Risk Factors for SIDS	
Category	**fro**
Infant	Male, preterm or multiple birth, low birth weight, low Apgar scores, ICU tx, congenital dz, neonatal respiratory abnlty, recent viral illness, previous ALTE, sibling w/ SIDS, prone sleeping position, heavy layers
Maternal	Age <20 y/o, unmarried, low socioeconomic status, low educational level, inadequate prenatal care, illness during pregnancy, smoking during pregnancy, use of illicit drugs, bed sharing

Prevention
- Remind parents to lay their children in the supine position, avoid smoking, head covering, soft sleeping surfaces, & multiple layers to reduce risk

CONGENITAL HEART DISEASE

Approach
- Consider Dx in pts w/ sudden onset cyanosis, hypoxemia, &/or shock, typically in the 1st 1–2 wk of life, though some pts present weeks to years later
- Differentiate cyanotic vs. noncyanotic & ductal vs. nonductal dependent congenital heart dz
- Hyperoxia test: Compare ABG on room air & on 100% O_2 for 10 min, P_{O_2} of >250 makes hypoxia 2/2 congenital heart dz unlikely
- Give PGE_1 to any pt w/ suspected ductal-dependent lesion & circulatory compromise

Definition
- Cyanotic lesions: Congenital cardiac dz w/ right-to-left shunt
- Ductal dependent lesions: Congenital cardiac dz in which fetal life depends on a PDA, either from impaired systemic or pulmonary blood flow

Congenital Heart Dz Differential	
Type of Lesion	**Differential**
Cyanotic	Tetralogy of Fallot, *transposition of the great vessels, truncus arteriosus, *pulmonary atresia, *critical PS, *tricuspid atresia/ Ebstein anomaly, total anomalous pulmonary veins, *hypoplastic left heart, *interrupted aortic arch
Noncyanotic	PDA, ASD, VSD, AS, *aortic coarctation, PS

*Ductal dependent.

History
- Cyanosis, fussy baby, poor feeding

Findings
- ↓ O_2 sat, cyanosis, ↓ BP, cardiac murmur, hepatomegaly, check 4-extremity BPs

Evaluation
- ABG, response to O_2, CXR, ECG, echo

Treatment
- O_2, consider PGE_1 (alprostadil): 0.05–0.1 µg/kg/min (max 0.4 µg/kg/min) if ductal-dependent lesion suspected, side effects: bradycardia, hyperthermia, hypotension, & apnea
- Inotropic support w/ milrinone, dopamine, or dobutamine & intubation prn

Disposition
- Cardiology consult, ±cardiac surgery consult, admit

Pearls
- Pts w/ ductal-dependent lesions p/w circulatory failure, usually during 1–2 wk of life
- Acyanotic lesions may p/w CHF

TETRALOGY OF FALLOT

Approach
- Recognize/tx Tet spells

Definition
- PA stenosis, VSD, RV hypertrophy, & deviation of aortic origin to the right (overriding); degree of severity dictated by degree of RV outflow tract obstruction

History
- Presentation usually w/i 1st few years of life, though occasionally into adulthood
- Cyanosis (often during feeds), ↓ PO intake, agitation, ↑ RR; ↑ sxs w/ exercise, szs, CVA
- **"Tet" spell:** Infundibulum spasm → ↑ RV outflow obstruction → cyanosis, respiratory distress

Findings
- ↓ O_2 sat, systolic ejection murmur, cyanosis, squatting pt

Evaluation
- See above, ECG (RAD, RVH, RAE, RBBB), CXR (boot-shaped heart), CBC, VBG

Treatment
- See above, 100% O_2, calm child, bring knees to chest; consider morphine & IV fluid bolus, correct hypoglycemia, consider propranolol, phenylephrine, intubation

Disposition
- Cardiology, cardiac surgery consult, admit

Pearl
- Onset determined by slowly ↑ infundibulum hypertrophy → ↑ RV outflow tract obstruction → ↑ RV hypertrophy → ↑ right-to-left shunt; thus presentations at later age have poorer long-term outcomes

RESPIRATORY COMPLAINTS

PNEUMONIA

History
- Fever, cough; quality of sputum usually unascertainable (children often swallow secretions); recent URI, malaise, lethargy, N/V, SOB, nasal flaring & grunting
- Older children: Abd pain, neck stiffness
- Infants/neonates: Difficulty feeding, tachypnea, restlessness, or lethargy
- RFs: Lack of immunizations/incomplete immunizations, travel, daycare

Bacterial (10–40%)
- Abrupt, follows URI, appearing ill, usually <5 yr

Atypical
- Fever, malaise, & myalgia, HA, photophobia, sore throat, & gradually worsening nonproductive cough

Viral
- Nontoxic, associated upper airway sxs (runny nose, nasal congestion)

Physical Exam
- Fever, tachypnea (most sens), O₂ saturation; full pulmonary exam (rales, rhonchi, decreased breath sounds)

Evaluation
- **Labs:** Chem 7 (severe dehydration), CBC (elevated WBC), blood cultures (if seriously ill); consider viral panel (including RSV)
- **Imaging:** CXR

Treatment
- Supportive: IVFs (if dehydrated), O₂ monitoring & therapy
- Viral: Supportive
- Abx (duration is 14 d for neonates, o/w 7–10 d), add vancomycin if critically ill
  - *Neonate* – ampicillin + gentamicin inpt
  - *1–3 mo* – 3rd-generation cephalosporin + macrolide inpt
  - *3 mo–5 yr* – 3rd-generation cephalosporin + macrolide (inpt) or high-dose amoxicillin (outpt)
  - *5–18 yr* – 3rd-generation cephalosporin + macrolide (inpt) or macrolide alone (outpt)

Disposition
- Home: Immunizations up to date, HD stable, on room air, >3 mo
- Admit: <3 mo, temp >38.5°C, tachypnea (>70 breaths in <12 mo & >50 breaths in older children), retractions in infants, respiratory distress, nasal flaring, cyanosis or hypoxemia (O₂ <92%), intermittent apnea, grunting, poor POs, signs of dehydration, social concerns, inadequate f/u, sepsis, immunosuppressed, comorbidities, cx, virulent pathogens *(Thorax 2002;57(suppl 1))*

ASTHMA AND BRONCHIOLITIS

History
Asthma
- Cough (usually early), dyspnea & wheezing (generally worse at night). Consider frequency, severity, duration, home txs, required past txs, baseline peak flow, number of ED visits, hospitalizations, ICU admissions, intubations
- Triggers: Exercise, infection, cold air, allergens, any respiratory irritant

Bronchiolitis (usually <2 yr of age)
- Fever (usually ≤38.3°C), cough, wheezing, mild respiratory distress; etiology from viral exposure (usually RSV, but also parainfluenza, adenovirus, influenza, rhinovirus). Often preceded by a 1–3-d hx of nasal congestion & mild cough
- RFs for severity: Prematurity, low birth weight, <12 wk old, congenital dz, immunodeficiency, neurologic dz

Physical
Asthma
- Tachypnea, tachycardia, inspiratory/expiratory wheezes, decreased or no air movement, use of accessory muscles, anxious/agitated, signs of dehydration

Bronchiolitis
* Same as asthma; may hear crackles & have signs of other infections such as OM

Evaluation
* **Pulse ox:** Continuous, unless very mild sxs
* **Labs:** Usually not necessary, consider RSV testing (bronchiolitis) if admission
* **Imaging:** CXR only if concomitant PNA suspected or 1st-time wheezer
* **Peak flow** (asthma): In children >6 yr (compare to predicted based on height)

Treatment
* Supportive: ABCs, O_2 therapy (O_2 sat >90%)

Asthma
* Mild/moderate:
  * **Albuterol:** 0.15 mg/kg (max 5 mg) q20–30min × 3 doses (short acting β-agonist)
  * **Ipratropium bromide:** 250 µg/dose (<20 kg) OR 500 µg/dose (>20 kg) q20–30min × 3 doses may decrease need for hospitalization
  * **Steroids:** Prednisolone/prednisone 2 mg/kg PO (max 60 mg) OR methylprednisolone 1–2 mg/kg IV (max 125 mg) OR dexamethasone 0.6 mg/kg PO (max 16 mg)
* Severe (add):
  * **Albuterol:** As above but may be used continuously
  * **Magnesium:** 75 mg/kg IV (max 2.5 g) over 20 min (optimal dose unknown)
  * **Heliox:** 80% helium/20% O_2. Use only if O_2 saturation can be maintained above 90%
  * **Terbutaline or epinephrine:** Terbutaline 0.01 mg/kg SC (max 0.4 mg) q20min × 2 doses &/or epinephrine 0.01 mg/kg SC (max 0.4 mg) q20min × 3 doses then repeated q4–6h
* Ventilation:
  * **Noninvasive (BiPAP):** May reduce respiratory fatigue & improve oxygenation/ventilation
  * **Intubation:** For impending respiratory failure; use large ETT; consider permissive hypercapnia (increased expiratory time & low VTs to prevent barotraumas). Consider ketamine for induction (bronchodilating properties)

Bronchiolitis
* Supportive tx is the mainstay including humidified O_2, suctioning, oral hydration
* Trial of albuterol, can continue only after documented response
* Nebulized hypertonic saline not a/w decreased hospital LOS after controlling for heterogeneity (*JAMA Pediatr* 2016;170(6):577)
* Racemic epinephrine may be helpful
  * <2 yr: 0.25 mL of 2.25% solution via nebulizer diluted in 3 mL NS
  * ≥2 yr: 0.5 mL of 2.25% solution via nebulizer diluted in 3 mL NS
* Consider ribavirin if documented RSV bronchiolitis w/ severe dz or immunosuppression &/or HD unstable

Disposition
Asthma
* Reassess pt in 3 h (more frequent if sxs more severe) after nebulizers, steroids, O_2 therapy
* Home: Improved peak flow (to >70% predicted), significant improvement in RR/O_2 saturation; d/c w/ inhaled β-agonist, steroid burst × 5 d (see *Adult Asthma Table for further home management*) w/ close f/u
* Admission:
  * Floor: Persistent wheezing w/ nasal flaring, tachypnea, hypoxia, & unable to tolerate POs
  * ICU: If pt maintains severe wheezing/poor air movement w/ peak flow <50% & worsening tachypnea or possible impending respiratory fatigue, PCO_2 >42 mmHg, intubated, requiring continuous nebs, heliox, or terbutaline

Bronchiolitis
* Home: Age >2 mo, no hx of intubation, eczema, RR <45, no/mild retractions, O_2 sat >93%, tolerating PO, fewer albuterol/epinephrine txs in 1st hour (*Pediatrics* 2008;121(4):680)
* Admission: Age <6 wk, hypoxia, persistent respiratory distress, significant comorbidities, or immunosuppression

---

BRONCHOPULMONARY DYSPLASIA

Definition
* Chronic lung dz in preterm neonates w/ hx of ICU, malnutrition, exposure to high O_2 concentrations, inflammation, infection (sepsis, chorioamnionitis, funisitis, post-natal infections), & PPV → impaired alveolar/pulmonary vascular development

Dz Severity	
Severity of BPD	O$_2$ Supplement >36 wk Postmenstrual Age
Mild	None
Moderate	<30% O$_2$
Severe	>30% O$_2$ &/or positive pressure

History
• Preterm birth, hx of ICU stay w/ mechanical ventilation, recent respiratory infection, poor feeding, increased O$_2$ requirement

Physical Exam
• Abnl VS, nasal flaring, retractions, grunting, wheezes, rales, decreased breath sounds

Evaluation
• CXR – hyperinflation, cystic areas, scarring; RSV testing will identify those who require hospitalization

Treatment
• Supportive; O$_2$, consider inhaled & systemic corticosteroids, abx (see *Pediatric Pneumonia*), bronchodilators (see *Pediatric Asthma*), furosemide (1 mg/kg q6–12h, titrate to effect)

Disposition
• Admission: If increased respiratory distress, hypoxia, hypercarbia, new pulmonary infiltrates, inability to maintain oral hydration, RSV infection

UPPER AIRWAY EMERGENCIES

Definition
• Actual or impending obstruction of the upper airway

Approach to the Patient
History
• Agitation or fidgeting, cyanosis, AMS, choking, SOB, increased work of breathing, panic, unconscious, unusual breathing noises
• ROS **(fever, drooling)**, PMH/MEDS **(see differential chart)**

Diagnostics
• CXR or neck films, esp if abnl O$_2$ sat & temp

Treatment
• O$_2$, calm the child, head tilt, chin lift, "position of comfort" (upright while leaning forward)

Disposition
• Largely will depend on hemodynamic stability & airway issues

UAE Differential	
Pathophysiology	Differential
Structural	Tracheomalacia, laryngomalacia, tumors, macroglossia
Infectious	Peritonsillar abscess, epiglottitis, retropharyngeal abscess, bacterial tracheitis, croup
Other	Allergic rxn, chemical burns, FB aspiration, trauma

FOREIGN BODY/UPPER AIRWAY OBSTRUCTION
(SEE ADULT RESPIRATORY SECTION)

Croup (Laryngotracheobronchitis)
Definition
• Viral infection primarily of the larynx & trachea (often parainfluenza), age 6 mo–6 yr

History
• Hoarseness, barking cough, & inspiratory stridor w/ variable degree of respiratory distress; preceded by nonsp respiratory sxs (rhinorrhea, sore throat, cough); fever is usually low grade

Physical Exam
• Inspiratory stridor, retractions, decreased air entry

Evaluation
- Labs: None
- Imaging: not routinely indicated
- CXR: PA view may show steeple sign, (subglottic narrowing), lateral view may reveal a distended hypopharynx (ballooning) during inspiration

Treatment
- Supportive: Humidified air, O_2, keep child as comfortable as possible
- Steroids: Dexamethasone (0.6 mg/kg ×1, max of 10 mg)
- Racemic epinephrine: Below dosing mixed w/ 3 cc NS (may repeat q20–30min), for children w/ stridor at rest, requires 2–3 h observation for "rebound stridor"
  - <20 kg: 0.25 mL
  - 20–40 kg: 0.5 mL
  - >40 kg: 0.75 mL

Disposition
- Home: If maintaining O_2 saturation; advise symptomatic tx w/ Tylenol & humidified air
- Admit: If hypoxia, depressed sensorium, moderate to severe respiratory distress, stridor at rest, poor oral intake, dehydration

Epiglottitis
Definition
- Pharyngeal infection classically due to H. influenzae; incidence in children has declined since introduction of H. influenzae vaccine, most common organisms now include S. pyogenes, S. aureus, S. pneumoniae, Moraxella

History
- Fever is usually 1st sx w/ abrupt onset sore throat, stridor, labored breathing, drooling muffled/hoarse voice, age 2–7 yr, lack of cough

Physical Exam
- Toxic, irritable, anxious, sitting in tripod or sniffing position (chin hyperextended & leaning forward), drooling, retractions, adenopathy; may visualize edematous epiglottis on oral exam

Evaluation
- **Labs:** Postpone IV & labs until airway secured; CBC, blood cultures, Chem 7
- **Imaging:** Lateral neck x-ray: Swollen epiglottis (ie, thumbprint sign), thickened aryepiglottic folds, obliteration of the vallecula, & dilation of the hypopharynx

Treatment
- Supportive: O_2 therapy, keep child as comfortable as possible; place child & mom in a quiet & controlled for complete eval/tx
- Airway: Preferable secured in OR under controlled environments but if not available, consider partial sedation & fiberoptic intubation. Cricothyrotomy kit at bedside for emergent surgical airway; tracheostomy.
- Abx: Ceftriaxone 100 mg/kg IV q12h (max 2 g/d) + Vancomycin OR clindamycin if concern for MRSA
- Consult: ENT or anesthesia for STAT OR airway

Disposition
- Admit: All to the ICU

Pearls
- Avoid procedures which may cause distress to the pt & further thereby compromise airway
- Give child or parent Yankauer suction to maintain secretions & alleviate associated anxiety

Bacterial Tracheitis
Definition
- Infection of subglottic region causing edema, pseudomembrane formation; polymicrobial (S. aureus, S. pneumoniae, H. influenzae, Pseudomonas, Moraxella), average age 3 yr

History
- Preceding URI infection w/ rapid deterioration, high fevers, age 3 mo–5 yr

Physical Exam
- Stridor, retractions, tachypnea, barking cough, wheezing, high fevers, toxic appearing

Evaluation
- Labs: None
- Imaging: X-ray shows subglottic & tracheal narrowing, irregular tracheal margins, PNA

Treatment
- Supportive: O_2, frequent suctioning, use one size smaller ETT
- Broad spectrum abx (3rd-generation cephalosporin, vancomycin)

Disposition
- ICU

DIABETIC KETOACIDOSIS

History
- Fatigue & malaise, N/V, abd pain, polydipsia, polyuria, polyphagia, weight loss, AMS/HA (may be signs of cerebral edema), fever/sxs of infection (cough, URI sxs, dysuria, rash); toddlers may not present w/ classic sxs
- RFs: Infection, poor compliance w/ insulin, puberty, inadequate caregiver

Physical Exam
- AMS, tachycardia, tachypnea, Kussmaul respirations, normo- or hypotensive, delayed capillary refill, mottled, lethargy/weakness, fever, N/V, acetone on breath (metabolic acidosis)

Evaluation
- Labs: FSG, Chem 10 (elevated anion gap acidosis, pseudohyponatremia, total body K generally depleted despite lab value, ↓ phosphorus, ↓ Mg), urine/serum ketones, β-hydroxybutyrate, UA, CBC, lactate, lipase, LFTs, urine hCG, VBG; ABG if HD unstable or comatose; blood & Ucxs if febrile
  - Corrected Na = measured Na + [1.6 × (measured glucose − 100)/100]
  - Definition: Glucose >200, venous pH <7.3 or bicarb <15, ketonemia & ketonuria
- ECG: T wave Δ (hyper/hypokalemia)
- Imaging: If concern for focal infection

Treatment
- Supportive: Continuous cardiac monitoring, O_2 sat monitoring, 2 large-bore IVs, intubate if necessary, evaluate & treat sources of infection
- Electrolyte monitoring: Glucose fingerstick q1h (goal = 150); Chem 7, Ca, Mg, phosphorus q2h

Acute Tx	
Medication	**Dose/Frequency**
IV hydration	Slow NS bolus 10–20 cc/kg over 1–2 h + maintenance (weight based) (adjust for dehydration) Add dextrose once serum glucose <250 mg/dL
Insulin	0.1 U/kg/h *Persistent anion gap:* Continue drip *Resolution of anion gap:* Δ to SC insulin (overlap IV w/ SC by 2–3 h)
Electrolyte repletion	*Potassium:* Add 20–30 mEq/L IVFs (K+: 3.5–5) OR 40 mEq/L IVFs (K+ <3.5) as insulin promotes K+ entry into cells *HCO3:* ↑ risk of cerebral edema. Avoid use *Phosphate:* Replete if <2, monitor for hypocalcemia
Mannitol or hypertonic saline (signs of cerebral edema)	*Mannitol:* 0.25–1 g/kg IV over 20 min (may repeat in 2 h if no improvement) *Hypertonic saline:* 5–10 cc/kg over 30 min × 1

Disposition
- Admit: All pts; HD unstable, pts w/ cerebral edema/AMS or newly diagnosed diabetes pts should go to the ICU

Pearl
- Children more likely than adults to develop cerebral edema; carry a 25% mortality rate; avoid insulin bolus & large-volume isotonic fluid boluses

HYPOGLYCEMIA

Definition
- Glucose <50 in children; glucose <40 w/ age 3–24 h; glucose <45 in infants >24 h of age

Hypoglycemia Differential	
Pathophysiology	Differential
Congenital	Glycogen storage disorders, disorders of gluconeogenesis, disorders of fatty acid or amino acid metabolism
Autoimmune/ endocrine/ neoplasm	Hypothyroidism, insulinoma, hypopituitarism, adrenal insufficiency, glucagon deficiency, GH deficiency
GI	Liver pathology, Reye syndrome
Other/meds	Oral hypoglycemics, pentamidine, alcohol ingestion, βB, salicylates, INH, sepsis, burns, cardiogenic shock

Approach to the Patient
History
- Irritability, sweating, jitteriness, feeding problems, lethargy, cyanosis, tachypnea, &/or hypothermia. May be a/w sepsis, congenital heart dz, ventricular hemorrhage, tox, & respiratory distress syndrome, PMH/meds (see chart)

Physical Exam
- Hypotonia, lethargy, cyanotic, hypothermic, apneic, tachycardic, pallor, vomiting, tremulousness, ataxia, sz, diplopia, signs of CVA

Evaluation
- **Labs:** FSG, Chem 7, LFTs, serum insulin, UA (ketones), C-peptide (low in exogenous insulin, high in insulinoma or sulfonylureas); growth hormone, cortisol, glucagon levels; tox screen if indicated

Treatment
- Glucose replacement
  - PO: Glucose paste, fruit juice (preferred)
  - Infants: IV bolus: 10% dextrose: 2 mL/kg followed by infusion at 6–9 mg/kg/min
  - Children: IV bolus: 10% dextrose at 5 mL/kg followed by infusion at 6–9 mg/kg/min
  - IM: Glucagon 0.03–0.1 mg/kg/dose SC q20min prn; not to exceed 1 mg/dose

Disposition
- Home: Obvious cause treated, sx reversed, after high-carbohydrate meal
- Admit: No obvious cause, toxic ingestion w/ oral hypoglycemic, long acting insulin, persistent sxs

FLUID AND ELECTROLYTE ABNORMALITIES

Definition
- See *Adult Metabolic Abnormalities* for etiologies

History
- Hyponatremia: Fatigue, weakness, lethargy, agitation, szs; ask re: renal dz or GI distress
- Hypernatremia: Irritability, lethargy, szs, fever, over or lack of urination
- Hypokalemia: Weakness, smooth muscle dysfxn, lethargy, confusion, decreased GI motility, respiratory insufficiency, rhabdomyolysis, polyuria
- Hyperkalemia: Asymptomatic to generalized weakness, paralysis, paresthesias
- Hypocalcemia: Tetany, weakness, fatigue, paresthesias, laryngospasm, sz, irritability
- Hypercalcemia: Weakness, respiratory distress, apnea, HA, sz, abd pain, lethargy, anorexia, constipation, bone pain, signs of kidney stones, pancreatitis, N/V, psychosis
- Hypomagnesemia: Anorexia, nausea, weakness, nonsp psychiatric sxs
- Hypermagnesemia: Lethargy, confusion, respiratory distress

Physical Exam

- Hyponatremia: May appear euvolemic, dehydrated or hypervolemic; severe hyponatremia = lethargy, hyporeflexia, Cheyne–Stokes respiration
- Hypernatremia: Poor skin turgor, increased muscle tone, altered sensorium; severe hypernatremia = spasticity, lethargy, hyperreflexia, respiratory paralysis
- Hypokalemia: Skeletal muscle weakness, hyporeflexia, lethargy, confusion
- Hyperkalemia: Paralysis, hyporeflexia, confusion
- Hypocalcemia: Tetany, wheezing/inspiratory stridor, Chvostek/Trousseau
- Hypercalcemia: Respiratory distress, apnea, hyporeflexia, epigastric tenderness, ↑ BP
- Hypomagnesemia: Anorexia, nausea, weakness, clonus, tetany, Chvostek/Trousseau
- Hypermagnesemia: Lethargy, hyporeflexia, hypotension, respiratory failure

Evaluation

- Labs: R/o spurious lab draws, hemolysis (hyperkalemia); CBC, Chem 7, Ca/Mg/phosphorus, urine electrolytes; ABG if acidotic & respiratory decline, UA, lipase
- ECG: U wave (hypokalemia), peaked T/widened QRS/ventricular tachycardia (hyperkalemia), prolonged QT (hypocalcemia), shortened QT (hypercalcemia), ventricular arrhythmia/torsades de pointe (hypomagnesemia)

Treatment

- Supportive: Continuous cardiac monitoring, O_2 sat monitoring, 2 large-bore IVs
- Electrolyte monitoring: Chem 7, Ca, Mg, phosphorus q4h
- Electrolyte correction:
  - Hyponatremia: See *Adult Metabolic section*; determine volume status; children should not be corrected >10 mEq/L/d in hypovolemia; acute onset <48 h hyponatremia can be corrected more quickly over 24 h; 3% NS 3–5 mL/kg for severe neuro sx (ie, szs); consider loop diuretics; tx underlying cause
  - Hypernatremia: See *Adult Metabolic section* for Na correction (goal Na reduction rate of 0.5–1 mEq/L/h); consider vasopressin/DDAVP for DI
  - Hypokalemia: Correct alkalosis, hypomagnesemia
    - IV: 0.5–1 mEq/kg/h IV (max 40 mEq/dose) over 1–2 h. Goal ↑ potassium by 0.3–0.5 mEq/L (require ECG monitoring)
    - PO: 1–4 mEq/kg/d PO in divided doses (max 20 mEq/dose)
  - Hyperkalemia:
    - Calcium gluconate: 50–100 mg/kg/dose IV, up to adult dose
    - Calcium chloride (code situation): 10–20 mg/kg/dose IV, up to adult dose over 2–5 min
    - Glucose + insulin: 1 g/kg IV of $D_{25}W$ + 0.25 U/kg IV insulin
    - Sodium bicarbonate: 1–2 mEq/kg/dose IV over 5–10 min
    - Albuterol: 2.5–5 mg nebulized
    - Furosemide: 1–2 mg/kg IV/PO; hydrochlorothiazide 1 mg/kg PO up to 200 mg
    - Kayexalate: 1 g/kg PO
    - Dialysis
  - Hypocalcemia: Send ionized calcium
    - Symptomatic:
      - Calcium gluconate 10%: 50–100 mg/kg IV slowly over 5–10 min to control szs; IV infusion at 50–75 mg/kg/d over 24 h; use calcium chloride (dose as in hyperkalemia) in code situation
    - Asymptomatic:
      - Calcium carbonate: Neonates: 30–150 mg/kg/d PO divided QID; children: 20–65 mg/kg/d PO divided BID/QID
  - Hypercalcemia: Send ionized calcium
    - NS: (Weight-based bolus + 1.5 times maintenance); furosemide
    - Consider bisphosphonates, calcitonin
    - Dialysis: In extreme hypercalcemia & renal failure
  - Hypomagnesemia:
    - PO: Magnesium gluconate 10–20 mg/kg TID/QID
    - IV: Magnesium sulfate 25–50 mg/kg IV over 2–4 h
  - Hypermagnesemia:
    - NS infusion, furosemide 1 mg/kg/dose q6–12h; titrate to effect
    - Calcium gluconate/calcium chloride (same dose as hyperkalemia)
    - Dialysis: Severe renal failure, cardiac or neuromuscular Dysfxn

- Home: Mild, asymptomatic electrolyte abnlty may be D/C home w/ PCP f/u in 1–2 d for repeat labs
- Admit: All pts w/ symptomatic electrolyte abnlty should be admitted & monitored; consider ICU level care for HD unstable or those w/ severe cardiac or neurologic disturbances

PEDIATRIC EXANTHEMS

ERYSIPELAS

Definition
- Infection caused most commonly by group A Strep

History
- Any age but > in children <3 yr

Physical Findings
- Red/hot tender area of skin, purulent d/c at entry site, ±fevers

Treatment
- Penicillin G, dicloxacillin

Disposition
- Home

VIRAL EXANTHEM

Definition
- Diffuse rash caused by nonpolio enteroviruses (coxsackievirus, echovirus, enterovirus) & respiratory viruses (adenovirus, parainfluenza virus, influenza, RSV)

History
- Any age, recent viral illness

Physical Findings
- Diffuse blanchable erythematous macules on trunk & extremities

Treatment
- Supportive

Disposition
- Home

HAND-FOOT-AND-MOUTH DISEASE

Definition
- Caused by coxsackievirus B

History
- Summer/fall, 1–4 y/o

Physical Findings
- Ulcerative oral lesions on soft palate, macular → pustular → crusted lesions on palms/soles, resolves in 5–6 d

Treatment
- Supportive

Disposition
- Home

IMPETIGO

Definition
- Secondary infection in pts w/ underlying dermatoses caused by S. aureus & group A Strep

History
- Warm humid summer months, any age

Physical Findings
- Papule/vesicle → golden crusted lesions commonly around mouth & on cheeks

Treatment
- Topical abx (2% mupirocin, dicloxacillin, 1st-generation cephalosporins)

Disposition
- Home

KAWASAKI DISEASE

Definition
- Systemic vasculitis of microvessels of unknown etiology, often self-limited

History
- Febrile illness, peak onset 18–24 mo, usually in children <5 yr of age

Physical Findings
- To make the Dx, requires unexplained fever × 5 d + 4 of the following:
  - Edema/desquamation of extremities
  - Bulbar conjunctivitis
  - Polymorphous rash
  - Cervical LAD
  - Mucous membrane Δ (ie, strawberry tongue)

Evaluation
- CBC (↑ WBC, ↑ PLT), ↑ LFTs, ↑ ESR, ↑ CRP, sterile pyuria, ECG, echocardiography, RUQ U/S

Treatment
- High-dose ASA 100 mg/kg/d divided QID
- IVIG 2 g/kg infused over 8–12 h single dose (reduces risk of coronary artery aneurysms)

Disposition
- Admit

Complications
- #1 cause of acquired heart dz in children
- Cx: coronary artery aneurysm, CHF, MI, dysrhythmias, valvular insufficiency, gallbladder hydrops, uveitis

SERUM SICKNESS

Definition
- Immune-complex–mediated type III hypersensitivity rxn

History
- Any age but > in children <3 yr, fever, arthralgias, rash, possible etiologies include blood products, antitoxins (ie, spider or snake envenomations), clostridial infections, meds

Physical Findings
- Fever, rash (urticarial, serpiginous)

Treatment
- Supportive as dz is self-limited, resolves in 2–3 wk, discontinue offending agent
- Short course of corticosteroids can be used for severe arthralgias

Disposition
- Home

HENOCH–SCHÖNLEIN PURPURA

Definition
- Small-vessel vasculitis

History
- Age 2–11 yr; preceding respiratory infection (Group A β-hemolytic Strep); fever, arthralgia, abd pain, bloody stools, hematuria

Physical Findings
- Palpable purpura in dependent regions, fever, joint swelling, guaiac positive, scrotal edema

Diagnosis
- Clinical; CBC (↑ WBC, ↑ PLT, anemia), ↑ ESR, antistreptolysin antibodies (+ in 50%), UA (hematuria, proteinuria, pyuria), abd U/S (intussusception), scrotal U/S

Treatment
* Majority is self-limiting w/ resolution in a few weeks; supportive, NSAIDs, treat underlying infection
* Corticosteroids does not prevent recurrences, which occur in 50%; but can be used for severe arthritis, renal involvement, GI, scrotal or CNS cx

Disposition
* Home unless cx: HTN, oliguria, obstruction, intussusception, GIB

Complications
* Bowel obstruction, perforation, intussusception, renal failure, hypertensive encephalopathy, acute scrotum (mimics torsion), pancreatitis, CNS cx (sz, coma, neuro deficits)

URINARY TRACT INFECTION

(*Pediatrics* 2011;128;595)

History
* Adolescents: Dysuria, urgency, frequency, hematuria; fever; flank pain, abd pain
* Younger children: Enuresis, foul-smelling urine, abd pain, N/V
* Infants: Fever, irritability, poor feeding, vomiting, jaundice, FTT

Physical Exam
* Fever, suprapubic tenderness, bladder fullness; CVA tenderness; GU exam to assess for vaginitis

Evaluation
* **Labs:** UA/Ucx (may require straight cath for clean specimen); Chem 7 (dehydration), CBC/blood cultures (if considering sepsis)
* Renal U/S in febrile infant or young child b/w 2 mo & 2 yr w/ 1st UTI
* VCUG for recurrent infections, poor urinary stream, palpable kidneys, unusual organism, HTN, bacteremia or sepsis that fails to respond to abx, unusual presentation, or hydronephrosis/scarring seen on renal U/S

Treatment
* Supportive: Oral rehydration if child able to tolerate o/w establish IV for hydration
* Abx (usually *E. coli*):
  * IV: Cefotaxime, ceftriaxone, gentamicin
  * PO: Augmentin, Bactrim, cefixime, cefpodoxime

Disposition
* Home: Stable, tolerating POs, nontoxic appearing; PCP f/u in 2–3 d
* Admit: <2 mo old, toxic appearing, unable to tolerate POs, signs of urinary obstruction, suspected sepsis, underlying comorbidities, ↑ Cr

PSYCHIATRIC PATIENT

Approach
- Always consider medical disorders → esp if no previous psych hx
- Anticipate need for psychiatry consult & restraints (meds, physical) early to assure safety

Definition
- Medical clearance: An ambiguous term suggesting no "organic" cause for pt's psych complaint; however, pts can have medical condition that exacerbates their psychiatric presentation (ie, drug abuse, infection)
- Focused medical assessment: The process of excluding medical illnesses that require acute care to determine who is medically stable (Ann Emerg Med 2006;47:79)

"Organic" Disorders That Mimic Psychiatric Dz	
Pathophysiology	Differential
Neurologic	Brain tumor, head trauma, encephalopathy, epilepsy, dementia, hydrocephalus, CVA, ICH, migraine, vasculitides
Other	Porphyria
Infections	Meningitis, encephalitis, UTI, PNA
Medications	Polypharmacy, benzos, anticholinergics, SSRIs, opioids, Dig, furosemide, warfarin, hydrochlorothiazide
Toxicologic	EtOH, substance abuse, overdoses, withdrawal
Metabolic/endocrine	Hypo/hyperglycemia, hypoxia, thyroid, parathyroid dz, electrolyte abnlty, hyper/hypocortisolism

Depression/Suicidality (Emerg Med Clin North Am 2015;33:765)
History
- Ask open-ended questions about thoughts, feelings, personal relationships; drug use; prior hospitalizations/psych hx; psych medications; physical/sexual abuse
- Sxs (SIG E CAPS): Sleep, Interest, Guilt, Energy level decreased, Concentration, Appetite, Psychomotor activity, Suicidal ideation
- SI/HI: Access to weapons, plan, prior SI/HI or attempt; command hallucinations
- Risk of suicide (SAD PERSONS): Sex (male), Age (<19, >45), Depression, Previous attempt, EtOH abuse, Rational thinking loss, Social support lacking, Organized plan, No spouse, Sickness

Findings
- Abnl VS; appearance, mental status exam
- Head-to-toe exam: E/O trauma, pupils, nystagmus, thyroid, pulm/cardiac/abdomen, skin
- Neuro: CNs, DTRs, motor, sensory, cerebellar, asterixis, gait, catatonia

Evaluation
- There is no data to support routine use of lab testing in psych pts whose H&P exclude significant medical illness
- βhCG (all women reproductive age), consider ECG & psych med levels (ie, Li)
- Tox: If concern for unreported drug abuse or ingestion (ie, APAP)
- Psychiatry consult: If needed for hospitalization, suicide/homicide attempt, uncertain at risk of danger to self/others
- Other labs: If concern for "organic" d/o or required for psych hospital: CBC, Chem 7, LFTs, UA, TSH, ammonia, CXR
- More thorough w/u is necessary for new onset psych Dx: Consider RPR, CT head, LP, EEG

Treatment
- Treat any underlying medical illness
- Typically antidepressants are not initiated by the ED physician

Anxiety/Panic Disorder
History
- Associated physical sxs (CP, SOB), substance use, prior similar episodes, current life stressors
- SI/HI (see above)

Findings
- Look for clues for underlying medical conditions: abnl VS (tachycardia, hypoxia), trauma, thyroid, nystagmus, cardiopulmonary exam

Evaluation
- Consider EKG, CXR or other cardiopulmonary testing

Treatment
- Treat any underlying medical illness
- BZD may help in acute setting but are a/w possible abuse & rebound

Psychosis (Emerg Med Clin North AM 2015;33:739.)

History
- Often challenging if pt is unable to interact appropriately
- Hallucinations? Delusions? Disorganized thoughts or speech?

Findings
- Look for clues for underlying medical conditions: abnl VS, trauma, nystagmus, thyroid, asterixis, focal neurologic deficits, fluctuating sxs, nonauditory hallucinations

Evaluation
- There is no data to support routine use of lab testing in psych pts whose H&P exclude significant medical illness
- βhCG (all women reproductive age), consider ECG & psych med levels (ie, Li)
- Tox: If concern for unreported drug abuse or ingestion (ie, APAP)
- Psychiatry consult: If needed for hospitalization, suicide/homicide attempt, uncertain at risk of danger to self/others
- Other labs: If concern for "organic" d/o or required for psych hospital: CBC, Chem 7, LFTs, UA, TSH, ammonia, CXR
- More thorough w/u is necessary for new onset psych Dx: Consider RPR, CT head, LP, EEG

Treatment
- Nonpharmacologic strategies: creating a safe environment, seclusion, verbal de-escalation
- Medications:
  - Haldol (IM/IV), ziprasidone (IM), olanzapine (PO/SL/IM); side effects ↑QT, akathisia, dystonia
  - Lorazepam/diazepam (PO/IV/IM): preferred for drug-related agitation; avoid in the elderly
- Physical restratints: Soft/leather (1–4 point), posy, mitts. Use as temporizing measure in conjunction w/ pharmacologic tx & sitter.
- Should attempt to use least restrictive strategies for the shortest time possible

Pearls
- Signs suggestive of "organic disorder": Age >40 w/ no prior psychiatric hx, abnl VS, recent memory loss, clouded consciousness
- Engage family members/friends/partners for collateral whenever possible

Approach
- (1) ABCs, resuscitate/stabilize → (2) decontaminate (GI tract, skin, eyes)/enhance elimination (charcoal, dialysis) → (3) treat w/ antidote, if available & indicated
- Consider empiric naloxone, dextrose, thiamine in pts w/ depressed MS. Use flumazenil w/ caution as it may precipitate sz
- Call Poison Control Center: 1 (800) 222-1222

Common Toxidromes	
Drug Class	**Toxidrome**
Anticholinergics	↑ Temp, ↑ HR, dry skin, mydriasis, dry MM, AMS, urinary retention, sz, coma
Sympathomimetics	↑ Temp, ↑ HR, diaphoresis, mydriasis, agitation, dysrhythmia, sz, coma
Sympatholytic	↓ HR, ↓ BP, miosis, ↓ peristalsis
Opioids	AMS, ↓ RR, miosis
Anticholinesterases	DUMBELS* + muscle weakness, AMS, sz, coma
Sedative-hypnotics	↓ BP, ↓ RR, AMS, ↓ temp, slurred speech, ataxia
Alpha-adrenergic	↑ BP, ↓ RR, mydriasis, moist skin

*Defecation, urination, miosis, bronchorrhea, bronchospasm, bradycardia, emesis, lacrimation, salivation

History
- Always consider Drug, Dose, & Pt: timing, quantity of ingestion/exposure, access to household chemicals/other meds, coingestions, enteric-coated/extended-release substances

Physical Exam
- VS, pupils, skin, neuro findings (AMS, nystagmus, myoclonus, tremor), peristalsis, smell

Evaluation
- ECG, FSG, CBC, BMP, LFTs, UA, ABG, hCG, osmolar/anion gap
- Drug levels
  - Exposures for which drug level is useful: APAP, salicylates, theophylline, lithium, Dig, EtOH, carboxyhemoglobin, methemoglobin, iron, methanol, ethylene glycol, lead, mercury, arsenic, organophosphate, anticonvulsants

Treatment

GI Decontamination			
Tx	**Indications**	**Dose**	**Relative CIs**
Activated charcoal	Given ideally w/i 1 h from ingestion	50 g (adults) 25 g (children) Give w/ antiemetics	Concern for bowel perforation, obstruction, aspiration, acid/alkali ions, EtOH, lithium, iron poorly adsorbed, AMS
Whole bowel irrigation	Significant ingestion not absorbed by charcoal or bags of illicit drugs	PEG via NGT 2 L/h (children 500 mL/h) until clear rectal effluent	Low-risk ingestion, risk of aspiration, toxin absorbed by charcoal, ileus or obstruction, obtundation

Dermal Decontamination
- Irrigation w/ copious volumes of H_2O (unless metallic Na, K, or phosphorus)

Ocular Decontamination
- Irrigation w/ copious volumes of H_2O, check pH after irrigation

Enhanced Elimination
- Urinary alkalinization w/ $NaHCO_3$ (eg, salicylates, phenobarbital, formic acid)
- HD (eg, ethylene glycol, methanol, lithium, salicylates, severe acidosis)

Common Toxicology Tx	
Tx	**Toxicologic Agent**
Antivenom	Snake, black widow spider, brown recluse spider, scorpion envenomation
Botulinum antitoxin	*Clostridium botulinum*
Calcium	CCB, ↑ K, ↑ Mg, ↓ Ca, hydrofluoric acid
Edetate calcium disodium	Lead

Tx	Toxicologic Agent
Cyanide kit (amyl nitrite, sodium nitrite, thiosulfate); Cyanocobalamin	Cyanide, smoke inhalation
Deferoxamine	Iron
Dig antibody fragments	Dig
Dimercaprol	Arsenic, lead, mercury
EtOH	Ethylene glycol, methanol
Flumazenil	Benzos
Fomepizole	Ethylene glycol, methanol
Glucagon	βB, CCB
Hyperinsulinemia–euglycemia therapy	βB, CCB
N-acetylcysteine	APAP
Naloxone	Opioids
Octreotide	Sulfonylureas
Physostigmine	Anticholinergics
Pralidoxime	Organophosphates
Protamine	Heparin
Sodium bicarbonate	TCAs
Succimer	Arsenic, lead, mercury
Vitamin K	Coumadin

Disposition

- Admit for any significant ingestion/exposure; consider transfer for complex presentations & inadequate hospital resources

Pearl

- Hospital tox screens vary → know your hospital's screen to guide your practice

ANTICHOLINERGIC INGESTION

Definition

- Antagonists @ **muscarinic** cholinergic receptor → inhibit parasymp system

Medications w/ Significant Anticholinergic Activity	
Class	**Medication**
Belladonna alkaloids	Atropine, scopolamine, ipratropium
Antiparkinsonian agents	Benztropine
Antihistamines	Diphenhydramine (Benadryl), meclizine (Antivert), promethazine (Phenergan), hydroxyzine (Atarax), dimenhydrinate (Dramamine)
Cyclics	Cyclobenzaprine (Flexeril)
Psychopharmacologics	TCA, phenothiazines

History

- AMS w/ medication exposure, ingestion hx, teas, supplements, or polypharmacy

Differential

- Sympathomimetic OD, EtOH/benzo withdrawal, thyroid storm, sepsis, meningitis, hypoglycemia

Findings

- ↑ HR, ↑ temp, dilated pupils, dry MM/skin, ↓ bowel sounds, urinary retention, myotonic activity, choreoathetosis, confusion/delirium, sz; "blind as a bat, dry as a bone, hot as a hare, mad as a hatter, red as a beet, bloated as a toad"

Evaluation

- ECG (↑ **QRS, QT**$_c$ → **TCAs, neuroleptics**); electrolytes; total CK (rhabdomyolysis); tox screen → r/o other ingestions; pulse ox; tele

Treatment
- **Supportive:** IV hydration, external cooling
- **Decontamination/elimination:** Activated charcoal (1 dose, w/i 1 h), HD
- **BZD** (IV): For agitation, szs
- **Physostigmine** (IV): Reverses anticholinergic effects via acetylcholinesterase inhibition
  - NOT for routine use due to risk of intractable szs, AV block, asystole
  - Half-life of physostigmine often shorter than toxidrome!

Disposition
- Admit; ICU for pts w/ cardiac instability or szs

Pearl
- Rarely fatal unless significant hyperthermia is present

PSYCHOPHARMACOLOGIC INGESTION

Selective Serotonin Reuptake Inhibitors and Serotonin Syndrome
Approach
- Spectrum for serotonin intoxication ranges from mild lethargy to serotonin syndrome
- Consider serotonin syndrome for anyone on meds w/ serotonin activity, esp ≥2 agents
- Greatest risk w/i minutes to hours after starting new med or increasing dose of old med

Definition
- SSRI: Selective serotonin reuptake inhibitors; SRIs: Serotonin reuptake inhibitors (also exhibit activity on epinephrine, norepinephrine, dopamine)

Common Drugs That Inhibit Serotonin Reuptake	
SSRIs	**SRIs**
Fluoxetine, paroxetine, sertraline, citalopram	Venlafaxine, duloxetine, mirtazapine, bupropion

Drugs w/ Serotonin Activity		
Antidepressants	**Illicit Drugs**	**Other**
SSRIs, SRIs, MAOIs, lithium	Amphetamines, cocaine, LSD, MDMA	Buspirone, levodopa, carbidopa, triptans, tramadol, dextromethorphan, trazodone, mirtazapine

Differential for Serotonin Intoxication	
Pathophysiology	**Differential**
Toxic ingestion	Sympathomimetics (16f), MAOIs, lithium, salicylates (16g), anticholinergics (16b), NMS
Chemical withdrawal	EtOH (16e), sedative-hypnotics (16d)
Infection	CNS (4c), SIRS (1f)
Other	Thyrotoxicosis (9d), tetanus (4i), malignant hyperthermia (10k)

History
- Akathisia, AMS, szs

Findings
- ↑ HR, ↑ temp, ↑ reflexes, diaphoresis, mydriasis, ↑ ↓ BP, **tremor, clonus,** neuromuscular rigidity, ataxia

Evaluation
- VS, CBC, BMP, CK (rhabdo), ECG (↑ QRS, ↑ QT_c, torsades), pulse ox, Tele

Treatment
Acute Overdose
- Activated charcoal, admit for monitoring

Serotonin Syndrome
- Supportive: IV fluids, electrolyte correction, external cooling (may require sedation/ paralysis for severe hyperthermia)
- Benzos (IV): For agitation, rigidity, szs
- (Controversial) Consider cyproheptadine (12 mg initially, 4 mg PO q1h), chlorpromazine 25–50 mg IV for severe sxs

Characteristics of Serotonin Syndrome vs. Neuroleptic Malignant Syndrome		
Signs & Sxs	Serotonin Syndrome	NMS
Onset	Sudden	Often over days to weeks
Resolution	w/i 24 h	Over ~1 wk
Hyperthermia	Common	VERY common
AMS	Common	VERY common
Autonomic dysfxn	Common	VERY common
Muscle rigidity	Common	VERY common
↑ Total CK	Uncommon	VERY common
Metabolic acidosis	Uncommon	VERY common
↑ Reflexes	VERY common	Uncommon
Myoclonus	VERY common	Uncommon

NEUROLEPTICS, NEUROLEPTIC MALIGNANT SYNDROME

Definition
- Characterized by D_2 antagonism ± **serotonin receptor antagonism**

Common Neuroleptics		
Typical Neuroleptics	Atypical Neuroleptics	Antiemetics
Chlorpromazine, haloperidol	Aripiprazole, clozapine, olanzapine, quetiapine, risperidone, ziprasidone	Promethazine, prochlorperazine, droperidol

History
- Slurred speech, sedation, anticholinergic toxidrome, extrapyramidal sxs (dystonia, akathisia, parkinsonism, tardive dyskinesia)
- **NMS:** ↑ HR, rigidity, AMS, szs, autonomic instability, metabolic acidosis, rhabdomyolysis

Evaluation
- CBC, BMP, CK (rhabdo), ECG (↑QT$_c$, torsades, dysrhythmia), UA (myoglobin)

Treatment
- Dystonia/akathisia: Diphenhydramine, benztropine, BZD
- **NMS:** External/Internal cooling, IV fluids, benzos, nondepolarizing neuromuscular blockade, dantrolene, bromocriptine, amantadine

LITHIUM

Clinical Effects			
System	Side Effects	Acute Overdose	Chronic Toxicity
GI	N/V, diarrhea, abd pain	N/V, diarrhea	N/V
Neurologic	Tremor, weakness	Tremor, rigidity, clonus, ↑ reflexes, lethargy, sz, coma	Tremor, rigidity, pseudotumor cerebri, tinnitus, ataxia, blurred vision, sz, coma
CV	Sinus node dysfxn	↓ BP	↓ BP, ↓ T-wave, ↓ ST seg, sinus node dysfxn, ↑ QTc
Renal	Polyuria	—	Nephrogenic DI (↑Na), interstitial nephritis, renal acidosis
Endocrine	Goiter, ↓ thyroid	—	Goiter, ↑ or ↓ thyroid, ↑ Ca

History
- Acute tox: GI sxs initially; neurologic findings may develop later
- Chronic tox: Neurologic sxs

Severity of Lithium Toxicity		
Grading of Toxicity		**Tx**
1	N/V, tremor, ataxia, muscle weakness, ataxia	IV fluids, Kayexalate
2	Rigidity, hypertonia, ↓ BP, stupor	IV fluids, Kayexalate, ± dialysis
3	Coma, sz → D	Dialysis

Evaluation
- VS, ECG, CBC, BMP, Ca, Mg, PO4, TSH, free T4, UA
- Lithium level: Not useful in acute ingestion (development of neurologic sx is better reflection of tox); in chronic tox, level >1.5 mEq is significant
- Assess for causes of decreased lithium clearance (eg, dehydration, renal failure)

Treatment
- IV fluids: Decreases tox & promotes Li excretion, NS bolus then ½ NS
- GI decontamination: Activated charcoal ineffective, whole bowel irrigation may be useful
- Sodium polystyrene sulfonate (Kayexalate), consider thiazides, indomethacin, or amiloride for nephrogenic DI
- BZD for szs (avoid phenytoin, which ↓ **Li renal excretion**)
- HD: For pts w/ severe neurologic sxs &/or clinical deterioration, Li level >3.5

Disposition
- Admit all pts w/ sustained release ingestions, Li level >1.5 mEq, or new neurologic signs; lesser ingestions can be treated & observed 4–6 h → re√ level ± psychiatry eval

Pearl
- Li has very narrow therapeutic window; consider Li tox in pts w/ ARF/↓ UOP

TRICYCLIC ANTIDEPRESSANTS

Approach
- Sxs of overdose almost always occur **w/i 6 h** of ingestion

Physiologic Mechanism of Toxicity	
Receptor	**Clinical Manifestations**
Histamine antagonist	Sedation, coma
ACh (muscarinic) antagonist	↑ HR, ↑ BP, mydriasis, dry skin, ileus, urinary retention
α1-adrenergic antagonist	Sedation, orthostatic ↓ BP, miosis (can counteract muscarinic mydriasis)
Amine reuptake inhibition	↑ HR, myoclonus, ↑ reflexes
Na channel inhibition	↑ PR/QRS intervals, RAD, ↓ cardiac contractility, heart block
K channel antagonist	↑ QT interval → torsades de pointes
GABA-A antagonist	Szs

Severity of TCA Toxicity	
Degree of Toxicity	**Clinical Manifestations**
Mild to mod	Drowsiness, confusion, slurred speech, ataxia, dry MM, ST, urinary retention, myoclonus, ↑ reflexes
Severe	SVT, ↑ QRS, ↑ PR, ↑ QT, VT, ↓ BP, sz, coma

Evaluation
- **ECG,** CBC, BMP, Ca/Mg/PO4, CK, UA tox screen, pulse ox, Tele

Treatment
- Supportive: IV fluids
- GI decontamination/elimination: Activated charcoal ± **gastric lavage**, intralipid for clomipramine
- **Sodium bicarbonate:** 1–2 mEq/kg boluses titrated to pH 7.45–7.55
- **Indications:** QRS >100, new RAD, ↓ BP, &/or ventricular dysrhythmia
- BZD: For szs
- Lidocaine: For ventricular dysrhythmias refractory to NaHCO3, avoid procainamide or other type Ia or Ic antiarrhythmics
- Lipid emulsion: Case reports only, 1.5 mg/kg bolus followed by 400 mL infusion over 30 min

Disposition
- Admit all pts w/ e/o cardiotoxicity or sz; d/c pts w/o sxs at 6 h after ingestion

Pearl
- Antimuscarinic effects are absent in many cases of TCA overdose

ALCOHOLS

Definition
- Ingestions of toxic alcohols

Approach
- Hx
- Type of alcohol ingested, time of ingestion, coingestants
- PE: Monitor for airway protection, occult trauma (head injury)
- Labs: FSG (may be all that's needed), consider BAL (declines ~20 mg/dL/h), anion gap, serum/urine tox (if coingestants suspected), osmolar gap for alcohols other than EtOH
- Osmol calc = $2 \times Na + BUN/2.8 + glucose/18 + EtOH/4.6$
- Osmol gap = Osmol measured − osmol calc
- Tx: Charcoal doesn't bind alcohol, ±thiamine/folate

Alcohol Ingestion Differential		
Alcohol	**Toxic Metabolites**	**Anion Gap Acidosis**
EtOH	Acetaldehyde	No (unless alcoholic ketoacidosis)
Methanol	Formic acid	Yes
Ethylene glycol	Oxalic acid	Yes
Isopropyl alcohol	Acetone	No

ETHANOL

History
- EtOH ingestion, found down, lethargy, N/V, ± associated trauma, ± aspiration, gastritis

Physical Findings
- CNS, respiratory depression, slurred speech, ataxia, nystagmus

Evaluation
- FSG (hypoglycemia common in alcoholics), ± BAL (if ingestion uncertain), ± CBC/BMP/LFTs/lipase, ± ECG (if pulse if irregular), ± magnesium level

Treatment
- Maintain airway, serial exams, ± IVF/thiamine/folate (given but may not be necessary)

Disposition
- Ambulating w/o ataxia + speaking clearly → d/c

Pearls
- R/o head trauma, CNS infection, Wernicke encephalopathy, alcoholic ketoacidosis, hypoglycemia, alcohol withdrawal/DT, coingestions, SI/HI
- Known EtOH ingestion/intoxication in pt w/ hx of same does not require lab & can be observed until clinically sober

METHANOL

Definition
- Ingestion of methanol (peak levels 30–60 min, 24–30 h ½ life, hepatic metabolism)

History
- Drinking: Paint solvents/antifreeze/windshield-washing fluid/canned fuels/gasoline additives, shellac/copy machine fluid/home heating fuels

Physical Findings
- CNS depression, vomiting, papilledema/hyperemia, visual Δ/loss, gastritis

Evaluation
- ↑ Methanol level, ↑ Osmol gap, ↑ anion gap (profound), BMP, ABG

Treatment
- Based presumptive Dx if levels delayed, maintain airway

- Fomepizole: Loading dose (15 mg/kg in 100 mL D_5S over 30 min) → maintenance (10 mg/kg q12h × 4 doses → 15 mg/kg q12 to methanol concentration <20/dL)
- Folate 50 mg IV q4h until resolution of acidemia (cofactor to convert formic acid → $CO_2 + H_2O$)
- Dialysis: Absolute indications → visual impairment + detectible methanol level or >50 mL/dL, osmol gap >10, ingestion >1 mg/kg, severe acidosis, renal failure

Disposition
- Admit

ETHYLENE GLYCOL

Definition
- Ingestion of ethylene glycol (peak levels 30–180 min, 3–7 h ½ life, 70% hepatic metabolism)

History
- Drinking: Antifreeze, coolants, paint, polishes, detergents, fire extinguishers

Physical Findings
- 3 phases: <12 h → ↓ CNS (like EtOH), gastritis; 12–24 h → ↑ HR/RR/BP/SOB; >12 h → ATN (oxalate crystal deposition)

Evaluation
- Ethylene glycol level, ↑ osmol gap, ↑ AG, calcium oxalate crystals in urine, beta-hydroxybutyrate (used to distinguish from alcoholic ketoacidosis)

Treatment
- Based presumptive Dx if levels delayed, maintain airway
- Fomepizole: Loading dose (15 mg/kg in 100 mL D_5W over 30 min) → maintenance (10 mg/kg q12h × 4 doses → 15 mg/kg q12h to ethylene glycol concentration <20/dL)
- Folate/thiamine 100 mg IV q6h/pyridoxine 50 mg IV q6h until resolution of acidemia (cofactors in oxalic acid metabolism)
- HD: Severe acidosis (pH <7.25) + osmol gap >10, renal failure (Cr >1.2 mg/dL), ethylene glycol level >50 mg/dL, deterioration despite supportive care

Disposition
- Admit

Clinical Pearl
- Urine/gastric contents fluoresce w/ Wood lamp due to antifreeze additives (early)

ISOPROPYL ALCOHOL

Definition
- Ingestion of isopropyl alcohol (peak levels 30–180 min, 3–7 h ½ life, 80% hepatic metabolism, lethal dose 2–4 mL/kg)

History
- Drinking: Rubbing alcohol, paint thinner, solvents, skin/hair products, nail polish remover

Physical Findings
- Profound ↓ CNS (2–4 × EtOH), fruity odor on breath, respiratory depression, ↓ BP, gastritis

Evaluation
- BMP, UA, FSG, isopropyl level, nl AG, ↑ osmol gap, falsely ↑ Cr (from acetone)

Treatment
- Based presumptive Dx if levels delayed
- Supportive (rarely lethal)
- Dialysis: Refractory hypotension, levels >500 mg/dL

Disposition
- Admit if severe toxicity, may D/C 2 h after resolution of sxs if no coingestions or SI

ALCOHOL WITHDRAWAL

Definition
- Abrupt cessation or significant reduction in alcohol intake (begins 6–24 h/peaks 48–72 h after last drink)

History
- Heavy alcohol use w/ cessation, insomnia, anorexia, N/V, restlessness, diaphoresis, sz

Physical Findings
- Tremulousness, szs (25% of pts at 6–48 h), delirium, hallucinations (visual > auditory), autonomic hyperactivity (tachycardia, HTN, irritability, hyperreflexia), delirium tremens (rare/serious, 24 h–5 d after last drink): Tremor/autonomic hyperactivity/confusion/hallucinations/low-grade fever

Evaluation
- FSG, CBC, BMP, LFTs/coags (if liver dysfxn suspected), BAL

Treatment
- Glucose (if hypoglycemic), thiamine, lorazepam 2 mg IV for sz, IV/IM/PO long-acting BZD (ie, lorazepam 1–4 mg IV q10–30min to sedation, diazepam 5–10 mg IV q5–20min to sedation, chlordiazepoxide 25–100 mg PO q1h), phenobarbital as 2nd-line

Disposition
- Admit if requiring IV medication/DTs ± ICU

Clinical Pearls
- Rarely fatal (increased w/ aspiration due to sz) when treated appropriately
- May require very large doses of IV BZD to control/treat

DRUGS OF ABUSE

Focused Differential		
Class	**Drugs**	**Effects**
Sedative-hypnotics	BZD, barbiturates, gamma-hydroxybutyrate (GHB), opioids	Sedation, ataxia, slurred speech, apnea, hypotension, hypothermia, dysrhythmias
Stimulants/ sympathomimetics	Cocaine, amphetamine, methamphetamine, MDMA, caffeine, ephedrine, dextromethorphan, LSD, bath salts	HTN, tachycardia, agitation, vasospasm/ischemia (CVA/ACS), AMS, anxiety, mania, psychosis, szs, rhabdomyolysis, muscle rigidity, hyperthermia

BENZODIAZEPINES

Definition
- GABA agonists

History
- Usually suicidal gesture or abuse, hypnotic/sleep agents (zaleplon, zolpidem, eszopiclone) have similar effects as BZD in overdose

Physical Findings
- CNS, respiratory depression, slurred speech, ataxia, hyporeflexia, midpoint/small pupils, hypothermia, hypotension

Evaluation
- FSG, consider ABG, Serum/urine tox, ETCO$_2$ monitor, Tele, pulse ox if severe toxicity

Treatment
- Supportive (airway protection if needed), Flumazenil 0.1–0.2 mg, repeat up to 3 mg → may precipitate szs, indications are rare, use only to reverse when known benzo is overadministered as part of procedural sedation & must be reversed for life-threatening sxs, monitor for resedation after 1–2 h, may require repeat dose
- Decontamination: Activated charcoal if ingestion occurred w/i 30 min

Disposition
- Home (rarely require admission) if resolution of sxs after monitoring & if no SI

Pearls
- Monitor for withdrawal, which is similar in presentation (agitation, szs) & tx to EtOH withdrawal
- Isolated benzo OD rarely life-threatening although usually presents as polysubstance OD

GAMMA-HYDROXYBUTYRATE (GHB)

Definition
- GABA & GHB receptor agonist

Physical Findings
- Initial euphoria, AMS/obtundation, hypothermia, bradycardia, hypotension, sz, respiratory depression, myoclonus, aspiration, rarely pulmonary edema & sz

Evaluation
- FSG, ± Serum/urine tox screen (rapidly metabolized → GHB levels not readily available)

Treatment
- Supportive, maintain airway, recovery w/i 2–4 h, resolution w/i 8 h

Disposition
- Home

OPIOIDS

Definition
- Opioid receptor agonist

History
- Witnessed or reported use of opioids (heroin, methadone, morphine, hydromorphone, fentanyl, oxycodone)

Physical Findings
- ↓ CNS, ↓ RR/BP, apnea, ± miosis, track marks, aspiration, noncardiogenic pulmonary edema

Evaluation
- Glucose, serum/urine tox screen (for coingestants), end-tidal CO_2 monitor, Tele, pulse ox

Treatment
- Maintain airway
- Naloxone (titrate to effect) 0.2–0.4 mg IV → 1 mg IV → 2 mg IV → IV drip (duration 1–2 h)
- Activated charcoal (recent ingestion), whole bowel irrigation (long-acting opioid)

Disposition
- May require ICU admission for long-acting opioid toxicity on naloxone drip

Pearls
- Pts die from untreated apnea, often in prehospital setting
- Pts w/ hypoxia/cyanosis have risk of aspiration/ARDS
- Pts w/ recurrent apnea after naloxone likely have longer-acting opioid

Opioid Withdrawal

Definition
- Cessation or rapid reduction of opioid use in a dependent individual

History
- Chronic opioid use, anxiety, N/V, abd pain, diarrhea, myalgias

Physical Findings
- Yawning, rhinorrhea, mydriasis, piloerection, tachycardia

Treatment
- Clonidine 0.1 mg PO q30–60min (central α-agonist) → ↓ duration, methadone (not indicated in the ED), IVF

Disposition
- Home or detox

Pearl
- Not life-threatening, do not require admission, may be precipitated by administration of naloxone & caution should be used before treating w/ additional opioids

COCAINE

Definition
- Snorting, injecting, smoking, ingesting (body packing vs. stuffing) cocaine (peak 5–15 min, duration 1–4 h, releases norepinephrine/blocks reuptake)

History
- Cocaine use, anxiety, CP, focal weakness (CVA/ICH), sz, psychosis

Physical Findings
- ↑ HR, ↑ BP, hyperthermia, diaphoresis, agitation, nasal septal perforation, mydriasis

Evaluation
- Serum/urine tox screen, cardiac markers (if CP present), ECG (↑ QRS, ischemia), Cr (renal failure), CK (rhabdomyolysis), head CT (if ICH suspected), consider aortic dissection, intestinal infarction, stroke

Treatment
- Supportive care, BZD for anxiety/agitation/CP, treat hyperthermia (ice packs, cooling blankets, cooling mist), avoid βBs (unopposed α-adrenergic stimulation)
- Activated charcoal (recent ingestion), whole bowel irrigation (packers/stuffers)

Disposition
- Varies depending on severity & mechanism of toxicity

Pearl
- Cocaine wash-out syndrome: After cocaine binging, MS (lethargy, obtundation), lasts up to 24 h

METHAMPHETAMINE ("METH")

Definition
- Norepinephrine release, dopaminergic (causes addiction)

History
- Ingestion, snorting, smoking, injection, rectal insertion of methamphetamines & derivatives (LSD, bath salts), ADHD, & narcolepsy medications

Physical Findings
- ↑ HR, ↑ BP, hyperthermia, diaphoresis, agitation, poor dentition ("meth mouth"), poor hygiene, compulsive scratching lesions ("meth mites"), tremors, sz

Evaluation
- Serum/urine tox screen, ECG, consider CT head (ICH), UA, CK (rhabdomyolysis), BMP, cardiac enzymes (CP), Tele

Treatment
- Supportive care, BZD for anxiety/agitation/CP, cool hyperthermic pts (ice packs, cooling blankets, cooling mist)
- Activated charcoal (recent ingestion), whole bowel irrigation (packers/stuffers)

METHYLENEDIOXYMETHAMPHETAMINE (MDMA, "ECSTASY"), LYSERGIC ACID DIETHYLAMIDE (LSD)

Definition
- Serotonergic

History
- Ingestion of MDMA, LSD, other hallucinogens

Physical Findings
- ↑ HR, ↑ BP, hyperthermia, anxiety, mydriasis, hallucinations, sz, diaphoresis, bruxism

Evaluation
- Serum/urine tox screen, BMP (↓ Na due to excessive water ingestion), ECG, consider CT head (ICH), INR, UA, CK (rhabdomyolysis), cardiac enzymes (CP), Tele

Treatment
- Supportive care, BZD & haloperidol for agitation, cool hyperthermic pts (ice packs, cooling blankets, cooling mist)
- ± Activated charcoal (recent ingestion)

ANALGESIC OVERDOSE

ACETAMINOPHEN (APAP) POISONING

History
- Witnessed or reported ingestion of any APAP-containing meds (many Rx & OTC drugs)
- Often coingestions w/ other substances

Findings
- 4 stages of APAP poisoning
  - I. Asymptomatic (0–24 h)
  - II. GI upset, N/V, abd pain (24–72 h)

- III. Jaundice, fulminant liver failure, encephalopathy (3–5 d)
- IV. Recovery (1 wk after) if survive phase III or multisystem organ failure

Evaluation
- APAP level 4 h after ingestion, serum/urine tox for coingestants, baseline LFTs & coags, BMP for calculation of anion gap, preop labs if potential for need for transplant, ECG

Treatment
- N-acetylcysteine (NAC) is glutathione substitute used as antidote
- Cardiac monitor, 2 large-bore IVs, ± NGT for anticipated NAC tx (PO NAC noxious), antiemetics
- Begin NAC if (acute ingestion, APAP level >140 μg/mL), (chronic ingestion of >200 mg/kg, 150 mg/kg, 100 mg/kg over 1, 2, 3 d, or ↑ LFTs, detectable serum APAP, or high risk)
- NAC 140 mg/kg per NGT × 1, then 70 mg/kg PNGT or 150 mg/kg IV × 1, then 50 mg/kg IV q4h × 5 doses, prolong therapy past initial 20 h if persistent serum APAP detected or ↑ LFTs until improvement in LFTs
- Activated charcoal (recent ingestion), HD (APAP >1,000 mg/L + coma/hypotension)

Disposition
- Admission to hospital vs. ICU based on clinical picture; transfer to transplant facility
- Consider Psych eval

Pearls
- Maximal safe APAP dose 15 mg/kg (up to 1000 mg) QID, max daily dose 3–4 g/24 h
- APAP metabolism produces NAPQI (toxic metabolite) → direct hepatocyte damage
- When coupled to glutathione, NAPQI made inert & is excreted in urine; APAP tox results from overwhelmed/depleted glutathione stores
- Many unintentional APAP OD from confusion b/w pediatric vs. infant APAP preparations
- Infant: 80 mg/0.8 mL = 100 mg/mL; children: 160 mg/5 mL (5 mL = 1 tsp) = 32 mg/mL

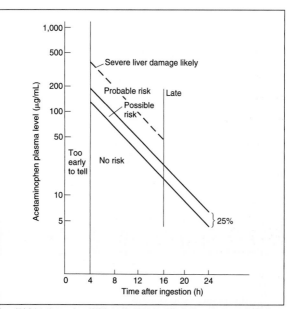

Figure 16.1 Relation between plasma APAP level and hepatotoxicity correlated with time after ingestion. Reprinted with permission from Helms RA, Quan DJ. *Textbook of Therapeutics: Drug and Disease Management.* Philadelphia, PA: Lippincott Williams & Wilkins; 2006.

SALICYLATE POISONING (ASA)

History
- Witnessed or reported ingestion of ASA or ASA-containing meds
- Often coingestions w/ other substances, occasionally inadvertent (elderly)
- Suspect ASA poisoning in any pt who reports tinnitus

Findings
- 1st 8–12 h: Fever, hyperventilation (respiratory alkalosis + metabolic acidosis), hyperpnea, tachycardia, hypotension, diaphoresis, dysrhythmias, N/V, epigastric pain, confusion
- By 24 h: Coma, cerebral edema, szs, noncardiogenic pulmonary edema, DIC

Evaluation
- Serum tox screen for ASA level & coingestants, BMP for anion gap, CBC, baseline coags, ABG, CXR, ECG
- Check ASA level q4h to ensure that levels are not rising due to bezoar formation or enteric-coated formulation delayed metabolism
- Bedside ferric chloride test (sens but not spec), serum quantitative assay preferred
- Add 2–4 drops 10% ferric chloride to 2 mL urine: Bluish purple color indicates + ASA; acetone & phenylpyruvic acid cause false + (pt w/ DM, ketoacidosis alcoholics)
- Ferric chloride testing will be + if as little as 2 ASA tablets ingested 24 h prior to test; takes 2 h from time of ingestion for ASA to be renally cleared

Treatment
- Airway protection if pt tires, hyperventilate & maintain respiratory alkalosis w/ vent
- Cardiac monitor, 2 large-bore IVs, Foley to monitor UOP & pH, dextrose for hypoglycemia
- Alkalinize urine to enhance ASA excretion
- 3 amps $NaHCO_3$ to 1 L D_5W or 2 amps $NaHCO_3$ to 1 L ½ NS, bolus over 30 min
- Continue $NaHCO_3$ IV fluid to maintain serum pH >7.45, <7.55, UOP 1.5 mL/kg/h
- Add 20–40 mEq K^+ to replete K^+ exchanged into cells for H^+ ions; hypokalemia prevents effective alkaline diuresis
- Activated charcoal (recent acute ingestion), consider whole bowel irrigation
- Arrange for HD for symptomatic pt, if chronic ASA poisoning w/ ASA >60 mg/dL or acute ASA poisoning w/ ASA >90 mg/dL w/ severe acidosis

Disposition
- Admission to floor vs. ICU (if symptomatic), observe for at least 6 h (asymptomatic, nonenteric-coated, smaller ingestions), screen for SI/psych eval if indicated

Pearls
- ASA uncouples oxidative phosphorylation, causes a 1° metabolic acidosis & 1° (centrally mediated) respiratory alkalosis
- Methyl salicylate (found in BenGay, Icy Hot muscle balm, oil of wintergreen food flavoring) produces ASA tox in very small amounts (1 tsp of oil of wintergreen contains 7 g of ASA)
- Done nomogram created for ASA in the same way as the APAP-tox nomogram; considered to be inaccurate & of no clinical value due to the wide metabolic swings that occur w/ salicylate tox; is **no longer** used

Potential Severity of Single ASA Ingestion	
Amount Ingested	**Effect**
<150 mg/kg	None → mild tox
150–300 mg/kg	Mild → mod tox
301–500 mg/kg	Serious tox
>500 mg/kg	Potentially lethal tox

CARDIAC MEDICATION OVERDOSE

β-BLOCKER (βB) OVERDOSE

History
- Witnessed or reported overingestion of βB
- Children who have been at homes of older relatives taking prescribed medications

Findings
- Symptomatic bradycardia, hypotension, AMS, weakness, bronchospasm
- Lipid-soluble βB (propranolol) – sz; sotalol – ↑ QTc, torsades de pointes
- May have hypoglycemia, N/V, hyperkalemia

Evaluation
- ECG shows bradycardia, AV or intraventricular block, asystole
- Check cardiac enzymes, BMP; drug levels not available

Treatment
- Continuous Tele, 2 large-bore IVs, place transcutaneous pacer pads on pt
- Place a cordis in the R IJ or L subclavian vein if transvenous pacing indicated
- For symptomatic or refractory βB OD, administer:
  - Atropine 0.5–1 mg IV (ACLS protocol) for severe bradycardia &/or hypotension
  - Glucagon 5–10 mg IV bolus followed by infusion of 1–5 mg/h if hypotensive
  - Pressors if indicated (epinephrine), cardiac pacing prn
  - Sodium bicarbonate 1–2 mEq/kg for wide-complex conduction defects
  - Consider hyperinsulinemia–euglycemia therapy &/or IV lipid emulsion (benefit in animals & case reports)
- No role for activated charcoal or whole bowel irrigation unless massive recent OD
- HD only useful for βB w/ low volume of distribution (acebutolol, atenolol, nadolol, timolol, sotalol) if unresponsive to medical intervention, or if pressors/glucagon necessary to maintain BP

Disposition
- Admission to floor vs. ICU (if symptomatic)
- Clinically significant βB OD develop sxs w/i 6 h; if remain asymptomatic, can be D/C unless ingested sustained release formulation (24 h observation)

CALCIUM CHANNEL BLOCKER (CCB) OVERDOSE

History
- Witnessed or reported overingestion of CCB
- Children who have been at homes of older relatives taking prescribed medications

Findings
- Symptomatic bradycardia, hypotension, AMS, N/V, weakness
- Transient hyperglycemia; sz rare

Evaluation
- ECG shows bradycardia, ventricular escape rhythm, 2nd- or 3rd-degree AV block; usually nl QRS complex (vs. βB OD)
- Check cardiac enzymes, BMP; drug levels not available

Treatment
- Continuous Tele, 2 large-bore IVs, place transcutaneous pacer pads on pt
- Place a cordis in the R IJ or L subclavian vein if transvenous pacing indicated
- Continue supportive therapy including volume resuscitation & pressors for hypotension & depressed inotropy
- For either symptomatic βB or CCB OD, administer:
  - Atropine 0.5–1 mg IV (ACLS protocol)
  - Glucagon 5–10 mg IV bolus followed by infusion of 1–5 mg/h if hypotensive
  - Calcium gluconate 3 g slow IV push or calcium chloride 1 g IV q5–10min prn
    - Can reverse depression of cardiac contractility; no effect on sinus node depression or peripheral vasodilation; variable effect on AV node conduction
  - Pressors if indicated (dopamine, norepinephrine, amrinone)
- For CCB OD, hyperinsulinemia–euglycemia therapy can provide fuel for enhanced myocardial contractility
- If glucose <200 mg/dL, give dextrose 0.25 g/kg D25 up to 1 amp D50
- If K+ <2.5 mEq/dL, administer 40 mEq IV; monitor & replete K+ prn
- Administer regular insulin 0.5–1 U/kg IV bolus, followed by infusion of 0.5–1 U/kg/h
- Start D10 ½ NS at 80% maintenance rate
- Recheck glucose q20min × 1 h, then qh; titrate insulin infusion to maintain glucose b/w 100 & 200
- Consider IV lipid emulsion (promising in animal studies & case reports), glucagon
- No role for activated charcoal or whole bowel irrigation unless massive recent OD of extended-release formulation; then use multidose charcoal
- HD not useful for CCB OD due to extensive protein binding

Disposition
- Admission to floor vs. ICU (if symptomatic)
- CCB should be monitored for 6 h or 24 h for sustained release formulations

---

DIGOXIN OVERDOSE

History
- Usually in pts on chronic Dig, occasional acute intentional OD occurs
- Weakness, fatigue, palpitations, syncope, AMS, N/V, diarrhea, HA, paresthesias
- Yellow-green vision or other vision disturbances pathognomonic in chronic OD (not always present)
- Recent worsening renal fxn, dehydration, electrolyte abn, recent addition of new med

Findings
- GI sxs (common), generalized neuro sxs, visual Δ w/ few objective findings
- Hemodynamic instability related to dysrhythmias or acute CHF

Evaluation
- ECG may show a number of cardiac dysrhythmias (see table)
- Dig level, cardiac enzymes, BMP (↑ K in acute OD, nl or ↓ K, ↓ Mg in chronic OD)

Treatment
- Continuous Tele, trend Dig & serum K levels w/ ECG & clinical picture
- Correct electrolyte abnl
- Acute overdose
  - ↑ K is bad prognostic sign; treat immediately w/ calcium, glucose/insulin & bicarb (the notion that calcium is contraindicated in Dig overdose is based on very weak evidence from animal models)
  - Magnesium, lidocaine, antiarrhythmic until Digibind available
  - Dig spec Ab (antidote) if level >6, K >5, high-deg AV block, ventricular arrhythmias, AMS, hemodynamic compromise
  - Each vial of Dig spec Ab binds 0.5 mg of Dig
  - # of Dig spec Ab = (serum Dig [ng/mL] × TBW [kg])/100
  - For unknown amount/level, empirically treat w/ 10 vials, repeat once prn for acute ingestion, 6 vials for chronic ingestion
  - Phenytoin & lidocaine safe to control tachydysrhythmias
  - Activated charcoal (if recent ingestion), dialysis ineffective due to large Vd
- Chronic tox
  - Stop Dig
  - Verify need for Dig spec Ab, check Cr, electrolytes

Disposition
- Admission to floor vs. ICU (if hemodynamic instability, refractory dysrhythmia)
- If asymptomatic, no cardiac dysrhythmias, nl K & dig level, can d/c after 6 h

Pearl
- Many drug interactions (BZD, βB, CCB, diuretics, succinylcholine, some abx)

Dysrhythmias Suggestive of Dig Toxicity
PVCs (most common); bigeminy or trigeminy
Slow AF w/ regularized ventricular rate (AV dissociation)
NPJT (rate 70–130)
AT w/ block
Bidirectional ventricular tachycardia
Asystole or ventricular fibrillation

CAUSTIC INGESTIONS

Background
- Cause tissue injury by acidic or alkaline chemical rxn
- pH <2 is considered strong acid, pH >12 considered strong base
- Severity of tissue injury determined by duration of contact, pH, concentration, type of substance (liquid vs. solid)

Approach
- Careful hx: Spec agent, amount, duration, pH, & timing of ingestion, coingestions
- Often a suicidal gesture; assess mental state as well as physical

- Rapid physical exam: Look for respiratory compromise, stridor, hoarseness, oropharyngeal burns, drooling, subcutaneous air, acute peritonitis (signs of perforation), hematemesis
- Do NOT induce emesis; re-exposure could worsen injury
- Do NOT attempt to neutralize ingestions due to possible exothermic rxn

ACID/ALKALINE INGESTIONS

History
- Alkaline: Ingestion of ammonia, cleaning agents: drain, oven, swimming pool, dishwasher detergents, bleach, cement, hair relaxers
- Acid: Ingestion of battery liquid, toilet bowl cleaners, rust or metal cleaning products, drain cleaners, cement cleaning products

Findings
- Alkaline: Liquefactive necrosis – severe injury starts rapidly after ingestion, w/i min of contact, tissues that 1st contact alkali are most severely injured (oropharynx, hypopharynx, esophagus). Tissue edema occurs immediately, may persist for 48 h, progress → airway obstruction. Over 2–4 wk get scar tissue thickening → strictures (depends on depth of burn).
- Acid: Coagulation necrosis → desiccation → eschar formation; stomach most commonly affected, small bowel exposure possible. Eschar sloughs in 3–4 d, then granulation tissue development. Perforation after 3–4 d as eschar sloughs; gastric outlet obstruction if scar tissue contracts over 2–4 wk. Pyloric sphincter spasm may delay gastric emptying & ↑ contact time to 90 min.
- In hydrofluoric acid (HF) ingestion, ↓ Ca may lead to arrhythmias, sudden cardiac arrest
- Both may cause esophageal perforation

Evaluation
- pH of product & of saliva, CBC, BMP, ABG, baseline LFTs, UA, preop labs, tox screen; cardiac monitoring, ECG; x-rays, consider CT for extraluminal air
- Endoscopy if symptomatic, small child, AMS but not if e/o perforation or airway edema

Treatment
- Airway protection, large-bore IV access; surgical/GI consultation, antiemetics
- Gastric lavage controversial
- Activated charcoal not helpful due to poor adsorption
- Dilution w/ small amts of water/milk may be beneficial if done w/i 30 min after ingestion
- Abx if e/o perforation, pain control

Disposition
- Admit to ICU if symptomatic

CELLULAR ASPHYXIATES

Etiology
- By-product of nitroprusside, acrylonitrile (nail polish, plastics, some tattoo ink), cyanogenic glycosides (apricot pits, cassava), cyanide gas (house fires)
- Mechanism: Binds to cytochrome oxidase, blocks aerobic utilization of O_2, leading to cellular asphyxia

History
- Difficulty breathing, confusion, HA, n/v, AMS, syncope, sz, cardiovascular collapse
- Sxs develop immediately after inhalational exposure, delayed sxs after exposure to nitroprusside, cyanide salts, acrylonitrile, cyanogenic glycosides

Physical Exam
- O_2 saturation often nl; dyspnea/tachypnea, confusion, tachycardia; agonal respirations & cardiovascular collapse a/w severe poisoning
- "Bitter almond" smell (unreliable), bright red venous blood due to high venous O_2 content

Evaluation
- **Labs:** BMP, ↑↑ lactate, ABG (metabolic acidosis), VBG (assess venous/arterial O_2 gradient), cyanide level, carboxyhemoglobin (if smoke inhalation)

Treatment
- Supportive: Maintain airway, O_2 therapy, IV fluids
- Activated charcoal (presenting <2 h)
- Cyanide antidote:
  - Cyanocobalamin adult: 5 g (child: 70 mg/kg) IV over 15 min
  - Cyanide kit (amyl nitrite, sodium nitrite, sodium thiosulfate) – causes methemoglobinemia

Disposition
- Admit: All pts; consider ICU for pts w/ szs, coma, acidosis, hypotension

---

CARBON MONOXIDE POISONING AND METHEMOGLOBINEMIA

Etiology
Carbon Monoxide
- Smoke inhalation, methylene chloride exposure
- Mechanism: Reduces O_2 carrying capacity, shifts O_2 dissociation curve to L

Methemoglobinemia
- Nitrites, dapsone, sulfa drugs, lidocaine/benzocaine, antimalarials, water contamination
- Mechanism: Disequilibrium of methemoglobin to hemoglobin; overwhelmed methemoglobin reductase

History
Carbon Monoxide
- Mild: Mild HA, DOE; mod: HA, N/V, dizziness, poor concentration; severe: CP, syncope, coma, LOC & persistent AMS

Methemoglobinemia
- SOB, HA, light-headedness, fatigue, nausea, tachycardia, CP, syncope

Physical Exam
Carbon Monoxide
- Lethargy, szs, tachycardia, tachypnea, rales, confusion, red skin, or cyanosis

Methemoglobinemia
- "Chocolate" cyanosis, tachycardia; coma, sz, D a/w severe exposure

Evaluation
- ABG & Pulse ox: May be falsely reassuring

Labs
- CO
  - CO oximeter, CO level (mild: 10–20%, mod: 20–40%, severe: >40%), urine hCG; mod/severe: ABG (metabolic acidosis), BMP, CBC, cardiac enzymes, UA, CPK, lactate, consider cyanide level
  - ECG: Arrhythmias, signs of MI
- Methemoglobinemia
  - CO oximeter, methemoglobin level; severe exposure: ABG, hemolysis labs (LDH, peripheral smear, haptoglobin, reticulocyte count), type & crossmatch
  - Bedside test: Drop of blood on white filter paper will turn chocolate brown (compared to regular venous blood)

Treatment
Carbon Monoxide
- O_2: 100% NRB until sxs improved
- Hyperbaric O_2: Sz, respiratory failure, LOC, CO level >25% (if pregnant, >15%), infants, severe acidosis, neuro deficits, CV dysfxn, exposure >24 h, age >36 yr

Methemoglobinemia (symptomatic exposures, level >20%)
- Methylene blue (reducing agent): 1–2 mg/kg of 1% solution IV qh × 2 doses
- Exchange transfusion/hyperbaric O_2: Severe sxs not responsive to methylene blue or if methylene blue is contraindicated (eg, G6PD deficiency)

Disposition
- Admit if CO level >25%, methemoglobin level >20%, dapsone tox, LOC, pts w/ underlying cardiac/neurologic/respiratory dz

Pearls
- Do NOT use methylene blue in pts w/ G6PD deficiency (hemolytic anemia)
- Large amounts of methylene blue may paradoxically elevate methemoglobin levels

---

HYPOGLYCEMICS

History
- Oral ingestion of sulfonylureas, meglitinides (eg, repaglinide), or SC/IV insulin (oral insulin is not toxic)

- Agitation, coma, convulsions, confusion, blurry vision, n/v, rapid heartbeat, sweating, tingling of tongue & lips, tremor, dizziness, poor feeding; children may show sxs w/i 5 min of ingestion
- RF: Extremes of age, polypharmacy, renal or hepatic dz, suicide attempt

Physical Exam
- AMS, generalized weakness, diaphoresis, tachycardia, tachypnea, transient neurologic deficit, pallor, sz, cyanosis, coma, hypothermia

Evaluation
- **Labs:** FSG q1h, BMP, urine hCG; tox screen (if intentional overdose or ingestion unknown), C-peptide (present w/ endogenous insulin secretion)

Treatment
- Supportive: ABCs, activated charcoal if recent ingestion
- Dextrose:
  - Oral: Glucose paste, juice
  - IV: 0.5–1 g/kg IV $D_{50}W$ (adults), $D_{25}W$ (children), $D_{10}W$ (neonates) × 1 dose; persistent hypoglycemia: 0.5 g/kg/h $D_{10}W$ (titrate to glucose >100)
- Glucagon: 1 mg/dose IV/IM/SC (if <20 kg, 0.5 mg/dose)
- Octreotide for sulfonylurea or meglitinide overdose

Disposition
- Home: Pts w/ unintentional isolated insulin overdose may be treated & released after effect of insulin wears off depending on rapid vs. long-acting
- Admit: Pts w/ sulfonylurea overdose must be monitored for at least 8 h

OTHER INGESTIONS

Etiology, Hx, & Sxs of Other Ingestions		
Overdose	**Etiology**	**Sxs of Acute Toxicity**
Insecticides	**Organophosphate** nerve gas (Sarin, Tabun)	SLUDGE: Salivation, lacrimation, urinary incontinence, defecation, GI distress, emesis Other: Muscle weakness/paralysis, diaphoresis, bronchospasm, miosis, bronchorrhea, tachycardia, HTN, sz, respiratory depression, garlic-like odor; AVOID succinylcholine
	Carbamates (used to treat myasthenia gravis)	Similar to organophosphates but shorter acting & may not have neuro sxs
	Chlorinated Hydrocarbons (DDT, chlordane, lindane)	Tremors, paresthesias, szs, AMS, muscle twitching, hyperthermia, arrhythmias, rhabdomyolysis, chemical pneumonitis
Iron	Any iron supplement, tox >20 mg/kg	<12 h: GI (emesis/diarrhea/abd pain; Severe: Bloody emesis/diarrhea, large fluid losses) 6–24 h: Latent phase w/o sxs 24–72 h: Hepatorenal failure 2–6 wk: Chronic GI strictures
Phenytoin/ fosphenytoin		Lethargy, dysarthria, ataxia, dizziness, confusion, horizontal nystagmus, N/V
Hydrocarbons/ volatiles	Baby oil, mineral oil, furniture polish, paint thinner, petroleum jelly, solvents, gasoline, lamp oil kerosene, lighter fluid	Hydrocarbon odor, glue sniffer's rash, chemical pneumonitis, aspiration, confusion, depression, dysrhythmias, N/V, liver failure, burns, cerebellar dysfxn
Herbicides	Paraquat, diquat, Roundup (glyphosate), Glufosinate, Atrazine, Mecoprop, Acetochlor, Dicamba, Pentachlorophenols, Chlorophenoxy, Nitrophenolic, Metolachlor	Dermatologic irritant, mediastinitis, peritonitis, N/V/D, liver failure, CV shock, coma, sz, muscle weakness, renal failure/tubular necrosis/ myoglobinuria, rhabdomyolysis, pulmonary edema, pulmonary fibrosis (paraquat), ICH (diquat)

Overdose	Etiology	Sxs of Acute Toxicity
Heavy metals	Arsenic, bismuth, cadmium, chromium, cobalt, copper, lead, manganese, mercury, nickel, selenium, silver, thallium, zinc	Varies based on poisoning; in general N/V, GI distress, renal failure/ATN, pneumonitis, encephalopathy, abd pain; zinc smells like fish
Rodenticides	Red squill, strychnine, yellow phosphorous, warfarin type/brodifacoum	Red squill: Cardiac glycoside-like sxs Strychnine: Sz-like appearance w/ extensor posturing, rhabdomyolysis Yellow phosphorous: Garlic odor, oral burns, vomiting, phosphorescent smelling feces, GIB, electrolyte abnl, sz, arrhythmias, renal/hepatic failure Warfarin type/brodifacoum: Long-acting anticoagulation, bleeding risk
Household products	Acids (toilet bowel cleaners), bases (bleach, ammonia), detergents, all-purpose cleaners (glass cleaner, pine oil, turpentine), chlorine, cosmetics	Bases/acids: GI irritation Bases: Pneumonitis, pneumomediastinum Perfume/mouthwash: Depends on alcohol level Pine oil/turpentine: Hemorrhagic pulmonary edema Detergents: GI irritants/corrosives, pulmonary edema Glass cleaner: Ocular, o/w well tolerated

Eval & Tx of Other Ingestions		
Overdose	Labs/Imaging	Tx
Organophosphates	BMP, ECG, plasma cholinesterase level, lactate, CK, LFTs, CXR	Decontamination; atropine (2–5 mg) IV q5min (endpoint = dried secretions); 2-PAM 1–2 g IV over 30–60 min, 500–1000 mg/h (will not work on skeletal muscle); BZD (prn szs/agitation)
Carbamates	Same as organophosphates	Supportive, decontamination, atropine (dose same as organophosphates)
Chlorinated hydrocarbons	Electrolytes (metabolic acidosis, ATN), ECG (arrhythmias), CK (rhabdomyolysis)	Supportive, decontamination, activated charcoal, cholestyramine (do not use in bowel obstruction), BZD (prn sz/agitation), βB
Iron	Fe level q4h; check BMP, LFTs, lactate, CBC, coags if symptomatic; KUB may show radiopaque tablets	Decontamination & whole bowel irrigation; supportive/IVFs; deferoxamine 15 mg/kg/h (max 1 g/h) over 6 h (for severe sxs, may induce hypotension)
Phenytoin/ fosphenytoin	Check phenytoin or fosphenytoin level; calculate free phenytoin level, albumin level, ECG, BMP	Supportive, activated charcoal, treat hypotension w/ fluids/ pressors
Hydrocarbons & other Volatiles	BMP (renal tubular acidosis, hypokalemia), ECG, LFTs (elevated); CXR (infiltrate, bronchovascular markings)	Remove all exposed clothing; supportive care – if intubated, PEEP beneficial

Overdose	Labs/Imaging	Tx
Herbicides	BMP (tubular necrosis, hypernatremia), lipase, CK, urine myoglobin, ECG (dysrhythmias), LFTs, CXR	Irrigate all areas of exposure (skin, eyes, gastric lavage), IVFs, electrolyte replacement, BZD (sz, agitation); activated charcoal Paraquat/Diquat/Glufosinate: Hemoperfusion Chlorophenoxy: Alkaline diuresis via 1–2 amps bicarb + KCl (urine output: 4–6 cc/kg/h) Pentachlorophenols/ nitrophenolic: Aggressive cooling, treat hyperkalemia/ rhabdomyolysis
Heavy metals	Send off individual levels, BMP (electrolyte abnl, renal failure), CBC (HCT), CXR (pneumonitis)	Supportive; may require intubation BAL: Copper, arsenic, lead, mercury NAC: Chromium, cobalt D-Penicillamine: Copper EDTA: Cobalt, lead MDAC: Thallium Prussian Blue: Thallium Selenium: Silver Succimer: Lead, copper, arsenic
Rodenticides	CXR, BMP, LFTs, EKG, CXR, CK, Urine hCG, PT/PTT, may check individual levels	Decontaminate, activated charcoal, whole bowel irrigation, supportive, renal failure may require dialysis, exchange transfusion for severe hemolysis
Household material	BMP (hypernatremia w/ bleach), CXR (aspiration PNA)	Supportive: IVFs, intubation if necessary; copious irrigation of skin, eye Ingestion: Water, milk to reduce irritation; Pine oil/turpentine: GI decontamination, endoscopy

AIRWAY MANAGEMENT

Approach
- Assess need for intubation

Indications for Intubation
Inability to oxygenate
Inability to ventilate
Impending clinical course

- Anticipated need for airway management in pts at risk for deterioration
- Assess difficulty of intubation early
- In pts w/ acute respiratory failure, BVM ventilation or noninvasive positive pressure ventilation (NiPPV) can be a bridge, but not a substitute, to intubation
- **Choose appropriate intubation algorithm**

Airway Algorithms	
Clinical Presentation	**Algorithm**
Standard	RSI
Anticipated difficult airway	Awake, sedated airway
Failed airway: Can't intubate	BVM + oral airway, EGD
Failed airway: Can't intubate, can't ventilate	Cricothyrotomy
Crash airway (near D)	BVM, intubation by any means

- **Choose appropriate intubation tool**
  - VL: 1st choice, if available; higher 1st pass success rate vs. DL
  - DL: Most commonly used (Mac or Miller blade)
  - Awake sedated airway (when difficult laryngoscopy is anticipated): Inhalation ± topical application of local anesthetic, parenteral sedation, evaluate airway, intubate via VL or fiber optic, paralyze/sedate when airway established → requires cooperative pt, noncrash airway

Pearls
- Have rescue devices at the ready: EGD, cricothyrotomy kit
  Consider glycopyrrolate 0.2 mg IV to w/ ketamine to minimize secretions
- Good BVM technique saves lives

RAPID SEQUENCE INTUBATION

The "7 Ps"
Preparation, **P**reoxygenation, **P**retreatment, **P**ositioning, **P**aralysis w/ induction, **P**lacement w/ proof, **P**ostintubation management

- Preparation
  - Monitor O_2 sat, BP, rhythm, ≥1 IV
  - BVM, **suction**, ET CO_2 detector, oral airway, Bougie
  - Intubation equipment (eg, laryngoscope): Blade, backup blade, check video monitor/light
  - ETT: 7.5–8 (male), 7–7.5 (female); check cuff, load stylet/10-cc syringe; pediatrics tube size: = 4 + (age in y/4) → or use Broselow tape
  - RSI medications/doses
  - Assess for difficult BVM, difficult intubation, & difficult cricothyrotomy → prepare appropriately

Assessing Difficult BVM → MOANS	
Measure	**Comment**
M – mask seal	Beard, lower facial trauma
O – obesity, obstruction	Includes angioedema, Ludwig angina, trauma, etc.
A – age	Age >55 yr
N – no teeth	Difficulty obtaining seal
S – stiff	Stiff lungs (asthma/COPD, PNA, ARDS, etc.)

Assessing Difficult Airway → LEMON	
Measure	**Comment**
L – look externally	Overall gestalt of difficulty
E – evaluate 3-3-2	Can fit 3 fingers into open mouth, 3 fingers b/w tip of chin & chin/neck jxn, 2 fingers b/w chin/neck jxn & thyroid notch
M – Mallampati class	From I (soft palate, uvula, pillars seen) to IV (only hard palate seen)
O – obesity/obstruction	Look for muffled voice, difficulty handling secretions, stridor, sense of dyspnea
N – neck mobility	Eg, C-spine immobilization, ankylosing spondylitis, RA

Assessing Difficult Cricothyrotomy → SHORT	
Measure	**Comment**
S – surgery	Eg, Halo device, recent thyroid surgery
H – hematoma	Anything distorting neck anatomy (includes infection, abscess)
O – obesity	Also consider short neck, SC emphysema
R – radiation	Distorts anatomy
T – tumor	Distorts anatomy, ↑ bleeding

- Preoxygenation: BVM (provides ~100% FiO_2) × 3 min or 8 vital capacity breaths
- Consider passive/apneic oxygenation: Place NC on high flow throughout intubation, prolongs time to desaturation
- Pretreatment: Give 3 min prior to intubation—lidocaine 1.5 mg/kg IV (↓ ICP, in pts w/ ↑ ICP, ↓ bronchospasm in pts w/ reactive airway dz); fentanyl 3 μg/kg IV (↓ ICP in pts w/ ↑ ICP, ↓ HTN response in pts w/ cardiac ischemia, aortic dissection, head bleed)
- Paralysis w/ induction: Always induce prior to paralysis
- Induction: Etomidate (0.3 mg/kg IV), midazolam (0.3 mg/kg IV), ketamine (1–3 mg/kg IV), thiopental (3 mg/kg IV)
- Paralysis: Succinylcholine (1.5 mg/kg IV, if no CI), rocuronium (1–1.2 mg/kg IV)
  - Succinylcholine CIs: Large burns, paralysis, crush injury (w/ in 3 d–6 mo), abd sepsis (>3 d), elevated ICP or intraocular pressure, hx of MH, neurologic d/o (muscular dystrophy, MS, Amyotrophic Lateral Sclerosis)
  - Rocuronium has no CIs but longer half-life often leads to delayed sedation
- Positioning: ± Cricoid pressure (prevents gastric regurgitation but may worsen DL view) before/during intubation until tube placement confirmed
- Placement w/ proof: Insert ETT via direct visualization of vocal cords, inflate cuff
- Confirm placement: ET CO_2 detector, auscultate lungs (assess for R-side intubation)
- Secure ETT, release cricoid pressure
- Postintubation management: Oral gastric tube, CXR, sedation (benzos, propofol) ± paralytics (vecuronium 0.1 mg/kg IV), analgesia (fentanyl), initiate mechanical ventilation

CRICOTHYROTOMY

Purpose
- Failed airway (can't intubate/can't oxygenate or ventilate); severe facial trauma, trismus, upper airway obstruction

Equipment
- Scalpel (11 blade), Trousseau dilator, tracheal hook, Bougie, tracheostomy tube (6.0–6.5 ET tube if none immediately available)

Positioning
- Pt supine, hyperextend neck if no CI

Procedure
- Sterile technique if time allows; see *RSI for preparation & postintubation management*
- **Open Technique:**
  - Hold larynx w/ nondominant hand
  - Make **vertical incision** w/ dominant hand from thyroid cartilage to cricoid membrane (2–3 cm), through skin & soft tissue
  - Palpate cricothyroid membrane through incision using nondominant index finger, **not** visualization

- Make **horizontal incision** <1 cm through cricothyroid membrane
- Place finger into stoma, then replace w/ tracheal hook-pointed caudad, then rotate cephalad. Alternatively, place Bougie (instead of tracheal hook) deep into stoma then slide ETT over Bougie & into place.
- Place Trousseau dilator in stoma w/ handle **perpendicular** to neck & dilate **vertically**
- Rotate dilator **parallel** to neck, then place tracheostomy tube w/ obturator in place, thumb over the obturator or ET tube
- Remove obturator (if tracheostomy tube), inflate cuff, suture in place

Complications
- Bleeding, misplaced tube, vocal cord damage
- Contraindicated in children <10 y/o, consider needle cricothyrotomy in peds

Pearl
- The hardest part of performing cricothyrotomy is deciding to do it → therefore, always consider this procedure in your airway algorithm

PRIMARY SURVEY

Definition
- Initial survey of the trauma pt for rapid identification of life-threatening injuries

Approach
- Eval in ABCDE order: Airway, breathing/ventilation, circulation, disability, exposure/environmental control

1° Survey	
Airway maintenance w/c-spine immobilization	Talking → airway patent → frequent reassessment Unable to talk → eval for FB/facial fractures/tracheal/laryngeal injury/other obstruction → if obstruction not reversible w/ chin lift jaw/thrust or GCS <8 → intubation w/c-spine immobilization Severe facial/neck trauma to be prepared for surgical airway (see Chapter 17 for further details of airway management)
Breathing/ventilation	Eval chest wall excursion/bilateral breath sounds/chest wall (flail chest, crepitance, open chest wound, tracheal injury) → identify/repair injuries that impair ventilation; tension ptx (needle decompression/finger or tube thoracostomy), flail chest w/ pulm contusion, massive hemothorax (tube thoracostomy → >1500 cc blood out or >200 cc/h or unstable HD → OR), open ptx
Circulation	Hypotension/altered MS/confusion/mottled skin/thready pulse/diminished pulse = hemorrhage/hypovolemia until proven o/w → place multiple large-bore IVs/control external hemorrhage → resuscitate w/ 2 L NS → persistent hypotension; transfuse PRBC (males O⁺, females O−), consider massive transfusion protocol (1 PRBC:1 FFP:1 PLTs) if persistent transfusion requirements, consider permissive hypotension (SBP 70–100 mmHg) & restrictive use of fluids FAST exam to evaluate for intra-abd hemorrhage → + FAST + persistent hypotension = OR
Disability	Rapid neurologic assessment; AVPU (**A**lert, responds to **V**erbal stimuli, responds to **P**ainful stimuli, **U**nresponsive), GCS
Exposure/environmental	Remove clothes, avoid hypothermia (massive transfusions/environmental exposures) can lead to coagulopathies (warmed blankets/IVF)

Glasgow Coma Scale
Eye opening
4—Open eyes spontaneously
3—Open eyes to command
2—Open eyes to pain
1—No eye opening
BEST motor response
6—Obeys commands
5—Localizes pain
4—Withdraws to pain
3—Decorticate posturing (abnl flexion)
2—Decerebrate posturing (abnl extension)
1—None (flaccid)
Verbal response
5—Oriented, fluent speech
4—Confused conversation
3—Inappropriate words
2—Incomprehensible words
1—No speech

Best possible score, 15; worst possible score, 3.

HEAD TRAUMA

Background
* Leading cause of traumatic D in pts <25
* 80% mild (GCS 14–15), 10% mod (GCS 9–13), 10% severe (GCS <9) injuries
* CPP = MAP – ICP, poor outcome if CPP <70 mmHg, CPP constant when MAP b/w 50 & 160
* 1° brain injury: Mechanical, irreversible damage caused by mechanical cell damage
* 2° brain injury: Alteration in cerebral blood flow → cerebral ischemia, membrane disruption, cerebral edema, free radical generation

Approach
* Careful hx: Associated sxs (photophobia, vomiting, visual Δ, ocular pain), focal neurologic sxs
* Assess for head or neck trauma, medications, substance abuse
* Check fingerstick blood sugar to r/o hypoglycemia as cause for AMS
* Warning signs for neuroimaging: severe HA, vomiting, worsening over days, aggravated by exertion or Valsalva, neck stiffness, AMS, abnl neuro exam, peri- or retro-orbital pain

Skull Fractures
History
* Direct blow to the head, pt c/o pain

Findings
* Skull depression
* Basilar skull fx: Periorbital ecchymosis (raccoon eyes), retroauricular hematoma (Battle sign), otorrhea & rhinorrhea (CSF leak), 7th nerve palsy, hemotympanum

Evaluation
* Noncontrast head CT. CBC, Chem, coags, type & screen, tox screen; plain films not indicated
* CTA to eval for vascular injury if basilar skull fx present

Treatment & Disposition
* Airway management; management guided by underlying brain injury
* Linear skull fx: If no other IC injury may be observed 4–6 h & D/C
* Depressed skull fx: Admit to NSGY, surgical elevation if depressed skull fx > thickness of skull, update tetanus, give ppx abx & consider anticonvulsants
* Basilar skull fx: Admit to NSGY

Pearl
* GCS more indicative of underlying brain injury or hemorrhage

Scalp Laceration
History
* Direct blow to the head, direct bleeding from scalp

Findings
* Often blood has clotted upon ED arrival; has potential for large blood loss
* Blood loss may not be evident in ED, eval for blood loss in field

Evaluation
* Noncontrast head CT if indicated. CBC, Chem, coags, type & screen, tox screen if significant blood loss
* Thoroughly evaluate & explore skull for depressions & large lacerations

Treatment
* Hemostasis & irrigation: Wounds often contaminated despite rich blood supply, direct venous drainage into the venous sinuses can cause significant CNS infections
* Staples can be used if galea not involved
* Interrupted or vertical mattress sutures w/ 3-0 nylon or Prolene
* Galea must be repaired w/ absorbable sutures if lacerated; continued bleeding → subgaleal hematoma that often becomes infected

Disposition
* If no other injuries, can d/c. Otherwise admission & observation.

Pearl
* Abx not indicated for properly managed head wound unless gross contamination

Head Injury Classifications			
	Mild	**Moderate**	**Severe**
GCS	14–15	9–13	<9
Hx	Transient LOC, amnestic to event	LOC, amnestic to event	Pt unable to provide hx
Sxs	Mild HA, nausea	Confused or somnolent, often unable to follow commands	Obtunded, cannot follow simple commands
Head CT	Only if indicated (head CT rules); usually neg	All pts	All pts
Eval	Evaluate C-spine, no other testing needed	CBC, glucose, Chem, tox, coags, UA, hCG	CBC, glucose, Chem, tox, coags, UA, hCG
Tx	Observation w/ neuro checks, d/c w/ careful return instructions	24-h admission even if head CT neg, repeat CT if ↓ GCS, AMS	Intubation, NSGY eval, IVF, tight BP control (SBP >90), treat ↑ ICP (mannitol, hypertonic NS, sz tx)

Canadian Head CT Imaging Rule; Must Have Initial GCS 13–15
Indications for CT Scan
GCS <15 at 2 h postinjury
Suspected open or depressed skull fx
Age >64
Retrograde amnesia to event at >30 min
Any sign of basilar skull fx
2 or more episodes of vomiting
Dangerous mechanism

Postconcussive Syndrome
History
• Closed head injury, ± LOC (brief); HA, memory problems, dizziness, etc. may last 6 wk

Findings
• nl neurologic exam, wide spectrum of mild neuro complaints

Evaluation
• Noncontrast CT shows no bleed but clinically insignificant SAH may have occurred

Treatment
• Symptomatic HA control

Disposition
• D/c w/ careful head injury instructions
• Progressive return to full activity only after complete resolution of concussive sxs

Pearls
• Thought to be secondary to stretching of white matter fibers at time of injury
• 2nd head injury more dangerous than 1st

Intracerebral/Intraparenchymal Hemorrhage
History
• Depends on size & location of bleed

Findings
• Pts commonly c/o HA, N/V

Evaluation
• Noncontrast head CT; CBC, Chem, coags, type & screen

Treatment
• Airway management
• Emergent neurosurgical eval although most pts are managed nonoperatively; ICP monitor if significant bleed present
• Mannitol for ↑ ICP, anticonvulsant medication to all pts
• Reverse coagulopathy emergently w/ appropriate agent (Vit K vs. FFP vs. PCC vs. factor conc) depending on underlying cause of coagulopathy

Disposition
- Follow

Pearl
- Frontal lobe hematoma may cause disinhibition & personality Δ

Subarachnoid Hemorrhage (SAH)
History
- Pt c/o "worst HA of life"; acute onset & rapid progression, meningismus, vomiting, photophobia; can often pinpoint exact moment of onset
- Spontaneous (ruptured cerebral aneurysm [~75%], AVM [~10%]) or traumatic

Findings
- HA, N/V, sz, syncope, acute distress
- Acute AMS is indicative of large bleed, usually requires emergent intervention

Evaluation
- Noncontrast CT scan of head, ancillary studies (CBC, BMP, coags, T&S)
- Head CT 95–99% sens for acute SAH (w/i 6–24 h); perform LP if CT neg
- If concern for ruptured cerebral aneurysm, should also obtain CT angiogram
- Large # RBC in CSF, may not be present in large numbers after 12 h or may not be present at all after 2 wk
- Xanthochromia highly suggestive of bleed b/w 12 h & 2 wk (yellow discoloration due to RBC breakdown)
- Check fingerstick blood sugar to R/O hypoglycemia as cause for AMS

Treatment
- Airway management if comatose or not protecting airway, neurosurgical consultation
- ICP & BP monitoring if bleed is significant; a-line, elevate head of bed to 30°
- SPB b/w 90 & 140 mmHg, HR b/w 50 & 90 bpm, nicardipine or labetalol prn
- Mannitol for significant bleed w/ increased ICP
- Nimodipine to decrease vasospasm 60 mg PO q4h × 21 d
- Sz prophylaxis (phenytoin, Keppra)

Disposition
- To neurologic ICU

Pearls
- Outcome directly related to amount of intracranial blood
- 30–50% have "sentinel HA" days to weeks prior to SAH

Clinical Findings of SAH	
Findings	**Frequency**
HA	95–100%
Meningismus	Frequent
Transient LOC/syncope	50%
Retinal subhyaloid hemorrhage	6–30%

Hunt–Hess Scale for SAH		
Grade		**Percent Survival (%)**
I.	Asymptomatic or mild HA	70
II.	Mod-to-severe HA, nuchal rigidity, no neuro deficits or other CN palsy	60
III.	Confusion, drowsiness, mild focal signs	50
IV.	Stupor or hemiparesis	40
V.	Coma, moribund appearance, posturing	10

Subdural Hematoma (SDH)
History
- Often caused by acceleration/deceleration tearing injury of bridging veins
- Can be acute (<48 h), subacute (2 d–3 wk) or chronic (>3 wk)

Findings
- Varied. Range from HA w/ nausea to comatose & flaccid

Evaluation
- Noncontrast head CT shows crescent-shaped mass. Check CBC, Chem, Coags, type & screen

Treatment
- Airway management, emergent neurosurgical eval
- If e/o ↑ ICP or midline shift, mannitol & anticonvulsant
- Reverse coagulopathy emergently w/ appropriate agent (Vit K, PCC, FFP, factor conc.)

Disposition
- Follow

Pearls
- More common than epidural hematoma
- Comatose & flaccid pts w/ SDH have an extremely poor prognosis, should discuss w/ family

Epidural Hematoma
History
- Brief LOC followed by "lucid interval," then rapidly progressive deterioration
- Head injury usually in area of temporal bone, causes damage to middle meningeal artery

Findings
- Ipsilateral pupil deviation, occasionally contralateral hemiparesis, N/V, sz, hyperreflexia, + Babinski

Evaluation
- Noncontrast CT often shows lenticular biconcave mass, possible fx of temporal bone
- CBC, Chem, coag panel, type & screen

Treatment
- Airway management, emergent neurosurgical consultation
- Mannitol & anticonvulsant
- Reverse coagulopathy emergently w/ appropriate agent (Vit K, PCC, FFP, factor conc.)

Disposition
- Follow

Pearl
- Bleeding b/w the dura mater & skull

Indications for Sz Prophylaxis
Depressed skull fractures
Paralyzed & intubated, severe head injury
Sz at the time of injury or during ED presentation
Penetrating brain injury
GCS ≤8
Acute SDH, EDH, or ICH
Hx of szs prior to injury

Diffuse Axonal Injury (DAI)
History
- Result of tremendous shearing forces seen in high-speed MVCs

Findings
- Pts often present in coma; document best neuro response: May have prognostic value

Evaluation
- Noncontrast CT often nl, must r/o bleed
- CBC, Chem, coag panel, type & screen, tox; look for other etiology for coma
- MRI (nonemergent) will show Δ & can guide prognosis

Treatment
- Airway management
- Emergent neurosurgical consultation for ICP monitor to avoid 2° injury from edema
- Mannitol & anticonvulsants

Disposition
- Follow

Pearl
- Prognosis determined by clinical course & difficult to predict

MAXILLOFACIAL INJURY

Definition
- Injuries to the soft tissue or bones of the face (50% caused by MVCs)

Approach
Inspection
- Deformities, enophthalmos (orbital blowout fracture), jaw malocclusion, dentition step-offs, nasal septal/auricular hematomas, rhinorrhea (CSF leak), trigeminal/facial nerve deficits, abnl EOM, diplopia, gross visual acuity

Palpation
- Facial prominences for tenderness/bony defects/crepitance/false motion, FB

Radiology
- Panoramic x-ray for mandibular/dental fractures, maxillofacial CT scan for most injuries, CTA in injuries at high risk for vascular trauma

Soft Tissue Injury
Definition
- Injury to the soft tissue of the face

History
- MVC/bites/assault

Evaluation
- CT only if bony injury/FB suspected

Treatment
- Irrigate/eval for FB/1° closure w/ in 24 h, abx (cefazolin, Ampicillin/Sulbactam, amoxicillin/clavulanate) for contaminated wounds (eg, bites), plastic surgery repair for nerve damage/extensive repair

Disposition
- Home

Septal/Auricular Hematomas
Definition
- Hematoma of nasal septum/ear

History
- Direct trauma to the nose (a/w nasal bone fractures)/ear (classically in wrestlers)

Physical Findings
- Swelling/purple discoloration

Treatment
- Septal: Apply topical anesthetic, incise/evacuate w/ elliptical incision, pack bilateral nares, abx (amoxicillin/clavulanate) (failure to drain → cartilage necrosis → saddle nose deformity)
- Auricular: Anesthetize area (lidocaine 1%) or auricular block, needle aspiration (chronic hematomas) or incise along skin folds, evacuate, apply compression dressing (failure to drain/compress → cauliflower ear/infection)

Disposition
- Home, f/u in 24 h

Nasal Fractures
Definition
- Fractures of the nasal bone

History
- Direct trauma to the nose

Physical Findings
- Swelling/deformity note: Patency of nares & appearance of septum

Evaluation
- CT only if significant deformity/persistent epistaxis/rhinorrhea

Disposition
- Isolated nasal fractures → Most home w/ plastic/ENT f/u in 5–7 d for reduction, consider reduction in ED if displaced, (pediatric pts → 3 d, ↑ risk for growth dysplasia)

Pearl
- Septal hematoma requires immediate I&D to prevent necrosis

Zygomatic Fracture

Definition
- Fractures of the zygomatic arch or fracture at the zygomaticotemporal suture/ zygomaticofrontal suture/infraorbital foramen (tripod fracture)

History
- Direct trauma to face

Physical Findings
- Shallow depression over temporal region, trismus, edema, diplopia/vertical dystopia/ infraorbital nerve anesthesia (tripod fracture)

Evaluation
- Maxillofacial CT

Treatment
- ENT/OMFS/Plastics consult

Disposition
- Home, ENT/OMFS/plastics f/u for delayed ORIF, sinus precautions

Mandibular Fractures

Definition
- Fracture of the mandible (>50% multiple fracture sites)

History
- Direct trauma to mandible (assaults usually = body/angle fractures, MVC usually = symphysis/condylar fractures)

Physical Findings
- Malocclusion, trismus, associated dental & lingual injury

Evaluation
- Panorex (isolated mandibular fractures): Can miss condylar fracture, maxillofacial CT (preferred): Condylar fractures/additional facial trauma

Treatment
- OMFS or plastic surgery consult: Temporary immobilization (wiring of jaw) or delayed ORIF, abx (PCN, clindamycin) if gingival bleeding

Disposition
- Home

Pearls
- Pts D/C w/ temporary wiring must be D/C w/ wire cutters
- Tongue blade test has high sens for mandibular fx

Maxillary Fractures

Definition
- Fracture of the maxilla, rare in isolation, a/w significant mechanism, greatest risk of airway compromise, traditionally classified by Le Fort system

History
- Significant mechanism trauma to the face (high-speed MVC)

Physical Findings
- Midface swelling/mobility, malocclusion of mandible, CSF rhinorrhea

Evaluation
- Maxillofacial CT
- CTA in Le Fort II & III should be strongly considered

Treatment
- Airway management (eval for difficult airway, Le Fort II/III highest risk), hemorrhage control (nasal packing/nasal Foley/elevation of head), abx (ceftriaxone) for CSF communication, ENT/OMFS consult

Disposition
- Admit

Le Fort Classification	
Le Fort I	Involves only maxilla at level of nasal fossa; Free-floating jaw
Le Fort II	Involves maxilla, nasal bones, & medial aspects of the orbits & is described as pyramidal Dysfxn
Le Fort III	Involves the maxilla, zygoma, nasal bones, & ethmoids. Extends through the maxillary sinuses & infraorbital rims bilaterally across the bridge of the nose. Is described as craniofacial Dysfxn

EYE INJURY

Definition
- Injury to eye caused by trauma

Approach
- Assess visual acuity (use lid retractors if needed) & extraocular muscles (EOM), remove contact lenses

Orbital Fracture
Definition
- Fracture to the wall of the orbit (floor/medial wall most common)

History
- Blunt trauma to eye by object larger than the orbital rim

Physical Findings
- Periorbital swelling/crepitance, tenderness/irregularities to bony orbit, vertical diplopia/limited range of motion (ROM) w/ upward gaze (inferior rectus/inferior oblique entrapment), diplopia/limited ROM w/ lateral gaze (medius rectus entrapment), hypoesthesia of lower lid/cheek (infraorbital nerve entrapment), enophthalmos, ptosis

Evaluation
- Orbital CT (opacification of maxillary sinus = orbital floor fracture)

Treatment
- Abx (cover sinus flora), ophthalmology consult (rarely require surgery unless diplopia/entrapment) if any EOM entrapment or visual acuity Δ, "sinus precautions" (no nose blowing/sneezing, no sucking on straws/smoking)

Disposition
- Home

Pearls
- Orbital floor fractures are rare but a/w CNS trauma/infection
- Pts are at ↑ risk zygomatic tripod fractures/Le Fort II & III fractures

Globe Rupture
Definition
- Full-thickness defect in the cornea/sclera

History
- Blunt (most common at muscle insertion sites/corneoscleral junction) or penetrating (more common) trauma, decreased vision, pain

Physical Findings
- ↓ visual acuity, teardrop-shaped pupil, hyphema, + Seidel test (bright stream of aqueous humor after fluorescein) for corneal perforations, intraocular content extrusion, flattening of anterior chamber, oculocardiac reflex can cause bradycardia

Evaluation
- Orbital/head CT (for FB/intracranial injury), US—but must be careful to not apply pressure

Treatment
- Ophthalmology consult (for surgical repair), tetanus, abx (fluoroquinolones, vanc/gent), avoid pressure on eye/topical agents/Valsalva (antiemetics), protective shield

Disposition
- Admit

Chemical Burns

Definition
- Burns to sclera/conjunctiva/cornea/lid caused by alkali (oven cleaner, dish soap, detergents, cement, bleach) or acid (less severe)

History
- Chemical exposure, severe pain, FB sensation, photophobia

Physical Findings
- ↓ visual acuity, conjunctival injection, corneal edema, lens opacification, limbal blanching

Evaluation
- pH testing of effluent in fornixes

Treatment
- Topical anesthetics, irrigation (>2 L NS), use Morgan lens/manual retraction to keep eye open, check pH every 30 min until pH 7.3–7.7 & 10 min later, ↑ IOP treat like glaucoma, cycloplegics (cyclopentolate, tropicamide) if ciliary spasm, antibiotic ointment, ophthalmology consult for corneal haziness/perforation/conjunctival blanching

Disposition
- Admit for increased IOP/intractable pain, minor burns: f/u in 24 h

Pearls
- Hydrofluoric acid exposure: Administer 1% calcium gluconate drops during irrigation
- If no pH paper available can use urine dipstick, for nl pH compare to unaffected eye

Retrobulbar Hematoma

Definition
- Bleeding in the space surrounding the globe

History
- Blunt trauma, recent eye surgery, pain, vomiting, ↓ visual acuity

Physical Findings
- Afferent papillary defect, restricted EOM, ↑ IOP, proptosis, periorbital ecchymosis, subconjunctival hemorrhage

Evaluation
- Orbital CT

Treatment
- Immediate ophthalmology consult, treat ↑ IOP (timolol, acetazolamide), decompress w/ lateral canthotomy

Disposition
- Admit

Retinal Detachment

Definition
- Detachment of the retina

History
- Floaters/flashing lights, "mosca volante"—solitary large floater, ↑ IOP, visual loss (macula involvement)

Physical Findings
- Visual field deficit (curtain being pulled down), dilated retinal exam: Retinal tears/ detachment

Evaluation
- β-scan u/s w/ undulating, hyperechoic membrane

Treatment
- NPO, bed rest, restrict EOM, immediate ophthalmology consult for surgical repair

Disposition
- Admit

Hyphema

Definition
- Accumulation of blood in the anterior chamber caused by rupture iris root vessel (trauma) or sickle cell/DM/anticoagulation

History
- Blunt or penetrating trauma to the globe, dull eye pain, photophobia

Physical Findings
- Microhyphemas: Visualized w/ slit lamp, larger hyphemas: Visualized w/ tangential pen light, total hyphema (high association w/ globe rupture): ↑ IOP

Evaluation
- INR if on Coumadin
- If any FH of hemoglobinopathy pt should be screened

Treatment
- Immediate ophthalmology consult for >10%/↑ IOP, treat ↑ IOP (timolol, acetazolamide), metal eye shield, cycloplegics (cyclopentolate, tropicamide) if ciliary spasm
- HOB >45% (upright allows blood to settle in anterior chamber/avoid retinal staining)
- Topical anesthesia if no globe rupture, PO/IV analgesia
- Topical steroids may help prevent rebleeding & synechiae

Disposition
- Admit for >50%, ↑ IOP, coagulopathy or sick cell
- Urgent ophthalmology f/u

Pearls
- Sickle cell: Avoid acetazolamide/pilocarpine/hyperosmotic, ↑ risk of rapid ↑ IOP → optic nerve injury
- Avoid ASA/NSAIDs 2/2 ↑ rebleed risk
- 10% rebleed (usually more severe) in 2–5 d

Vitreous Hemorrhage
Definition
- Blood in the vitreous humor

History
- Blunt trauma, floaters, blurry vision, vision loss, sickle cell/DM

Physical Findings
- Loss of light reflex, poorly visualized fundus

Evaluation
- β-scan u/s: For associated retinal detachment
- Consider noncontrast CTH if a/w trauma

Treatment
- Immediate ophthalmology consult, HOB >45%, bed rest

Disposition
- Admit if retinal tear/unknown cause

Pearl
- Avoid ASA/NSAIDs b/c ↑ risk rebleed

Subconjunctival Hemorrhage
Definition
- Hemorrhage b/w the conjunctiva & sclera caused by trauma, Valsalva (coughing/straining/vomiting), HTN, coagulopathy

History
- Painless red eye

Physical Findings
- Blood b/w the conjunctiva & sclera

Treatment
- BP control, avoid Valsalva, avoid ASA/NSAIDs, artificial tears for comfort

Disposition
- Home, ophthalmology f/u in 1 wk

Pearls
- Resolution in 2 wk
- Blood chemosis (large/circumferential) ↑ risk globe rupture

NECK TRAUMA

Definition
- Injuries soft tissue & structures of the neck

Approach
- Evaluate 3 main categories: vascular, pharyngoesophageal, laryngotracheal (do not place NGT if esophageal/laryngeal injury suspected)

Inspection
- Violation of platysma (↑ incidence of underlying structure injury, may indicate need for surgical exploration) (*Trauma 1979;19:391*), pulsatile/expanding hematomas

Penetrating Trauma Zones
- Anterior triangle: Bordered by anterior SCM, midline, mandible. Posterior: Posterior to SCM, anterior to trapezius, superior to clavicle, most significant structures are anterior
- Zone I: Below cricoid cartilage (highest mortality), Zone II: B/w cricoid & angle of mandible, Zone III: Above angle of mandible

Recommended Imaging for Penetrating Neck Injury	
Injury	**Imaging**
Vascular	Unstable → OR for exploration/angiography
	Zone I & III → CTA/angiography (high incidence of vascular injury)
	Zone II → CTA or exploration in OR
Pharyngoesophageal	CTA, Gastrografin/barium swallow study, endoscopy
Laryngotracheal	Unstable → bronchoscopy in OR
	Stable → CT scan (sens for detecting glottic/cartilaginous injury)

Penetrating Neck Trauma
Definition
- Injury to the neck from GSW, stabbings, projectile objects (shrapnel/glass)

Physical Findings
- Laryngotracheal injuries may have stridor, respiratory distress, hemoptysis, SQ air, dysphonia
- Esophageal injuries may have dysphagia, hematemesis, SQ air
- Vascular injuries may have neuro deficits, expanding/pulsatile hematoma/bleeding, bruit/thrill, hypotension

Evaluation
- CXR/(ptx/htx), lateral neck x-ray in trauma bay, CT, CTA
- Trauma labs: CBC, BMP, type & cross, PTT/PT, ABG

Treatment
- Airway management (may be difficult airway), surgical consultation if platysma violation, abx (if ↑ risk contamination from aerodigestive perforation)
- Treat as trauma resuscitation (ABCs, transfusion, etc.)

Disposition
- Admit if surgical intervention/observation needed

Pearl
- Arrest due to penetrating neck trauma is indication for ED thoracotomy

Strangulation
Definition
- Neck trauma due to strangulation (3500 D/y)

History
- Strangulation, voice Δ, attempt to obtain "height of drop" from EMS

Physical Findings
- Dysphonia/dyspnea (indicators serious injury), petechial hemorrhages (Tardieu spots), ligature/finger marks, neuro deficits/coma

Treatment
- Airway management (may be difficult airway), surgical consultation (if needed), consider CTA, abx (if ↑ risk contamination from aerodigestive perforation)

Disposition
- Admit if needed

Pearls
- ↑ incidence of ARDS & long-term neuropsychiatric sequelae (selective vulnerability of hippocampus to anoxic injury)
- Self-inflicted hanging rarely a/w C-spine injury, see Hangman fracture (Chapter 18)

CERVICAL SPINE TRAUMA

Definition
- Injury to the bony/ligamentous structure of the cervical spine (C2 24%, C6 20%, C7 19%)

Approach
- Maintain C-spine immobilization until cleared clinically w/o imaging (see table) or radiographically

Palpation
- Midline cervical tenderness, step-offs, neurologic deficits

Radiology
- Plain c-spine x-rays: 52% sens (limited use); C-spine CT: 98% sens → persistent midline tenderness/obtunded → Flex/ex films: 94% sens for ligamentous injury if adequate ROM (30° flexion/extension), MRI: 98% sens for ligamentous injury (*J Trauma* 58(5):902; 53(3):426)

Cervical Spine Clearance	
NEXUS Low-risk Criteria	**Canadian Cervical Spine Rule**
No posterior midline tenderness	Age ≥ 16
No focal neurologic deficits	GCS 15
nl alertness	nl VS (RR 10–14, SBP > 90 mmHg)
No intoxication	Injury w/i 48 h
No painful distracting injury (long bone fracture, visceral injury, large laceration, degloving, burns, injury causing functional impairment)	Blunt trauma
	No paralysis/paresthesia
	No known vertebral dz
	Not evaluated previously for same injury
	Not pregnant
	Not high high (<65 y/o, dangerous mechanism: MVC rollover/ejection/>62 mph, fall from ≥3 ft, bicycle accident)
	Presence of ≥1 low risk finding (simple rear-end MVC, sitting position in ED, ambulatory after trauma, delayed onset neck pain, no midline tenderness)
	Able to rotate neck 45% L & R
99.6% sens, 12.9% spec for significant C-spine injury	99.4% sens, 45.1 spec for significant C-spine injury

(*NEJM* 2000;342:94; 2003;349:2510)

C1 Burst Fracture (Jefferson Fracture)
Definition
- Unstable burst fracture of atlas (C1) causing widening of lateral masses (33% a/w C2 fracture)

History
- Axial load

Physical Findings
- C1 tenderness, neurologic deficit rare (wide canal at C1)

Evaluation
- CT/CTA, MRI for ligamentous injury

Treatment
- C-spine immobilization, spine consult for operative management

Disposition
- Admit

C2 Hangman Fracture
Definition
- Unstable fracture of bilateral C2 pedicles (↑ risk of C2 anterior subluxation/C2–C3 disk rupture → high mortality)

History
- Hyperextension
- Named due to judicial hangings in which knot is in front of pt & "height of drop" is at least as long as victim

Physical Findings
• C2 tenderness, high-impact trauma, neurologic deficits

Evaluation
• CT/CTA, MRI for ligamentous injury

Treatment
• C-spine immobilization, spine consult for operative management

Disposition
• Admit

Odontoid Fracture (C2 Dens)
Definition
• Fracture through the dens w/ variable stability (see table)

History
• Flexion injury

Physical Findings
• C2 tenderness

Evaluation
• CT scan, MRI for ligamentous injury

Treatment
• C-spine immobilization, spine consult

Disposition
• Likely admit

Dens Fracture Classification	
Classification	**Findings**
Type I	Avulsion fracture through upper part of odontoid process Stable & does not require surgical intervention
Type II	Fracture at the junction of the odontoid process w/ the vertebral body Potentially unstable fracture Nondisplaced: Halo often used to treat Displaced/angulated: Surgery often performed
Type III	Fracture at base of odontoid that extends down into body of atlas Immobilize w/ halo, does not usually require surgical intervention

Tear Drop Fracture
Definition
• Unstable avulsion of cervical vertebral body at insertion of anterior ligament in extension injury (C2 common) or posterior in flexion injury (C5–C6)

History
• Flexion (MVC, diving in pool) or extension (elderly fall on chin)

Physical Findings
• C-spine tenderness, anterior cord syndrome (flexion), central cord syndrome (extension)

Evaluation
• CT/CTA, MRI for ligamentous injury

Treatment
• C-spine immobilization, spine consult

Disposition
• Admit

Clay Shoveler Fracture
Definition
• Stable avulsion fracture of spinous process (most common in low C-spine, >C6)

History
• Forceful flexion (as when clay sticks to a shovel when trying to throw it)

Physical Findings
• C-spine tenderness, no neurologic deficits

Evaluation
• CT scan

Treatment
- C-spine immobilization, spine consult

Disposition
- D/c

Subluxation/Ligamentous Injury
Definition
- Unstable rupture of ligaments w/o bony injury, anterior slipping of vertebrae one over the other

History
- Flexion

Physical Findings
- C-spine tenderness, no neurologic deficits

Evaluation
- CT/CTA scan, MRI

Treatment
- C-spine immobilization, spine consult

Disposition
- May require admission

THORACIC/LUMBAR/SACRAL SPINE TRAUMA

Definition
- Injury to the bony/ligamentous structure TLS spine

Approach
- Maintain logroll precautions
- Palpation: Spinal tenderness, step-offs, neurologic deficits

Anterior Wedge/Compression Fracture
Definition
- Stable compression fracture of the vertebral body (wedge → only anterosuperior vertebral body endplate). May be unstable if >50% height loss of vertebral body

History
- Flexion

Physical Findings
- Focal tenderness, no neurologic deficits

Evaluation
- CT scan

Treatment
- Spine consult

Disposition
- D/c if pain controlled

Burst Fracture
Definition
- Stable compression fracture of anterior & posterior vertebral body (may be complicated by retropulsed bony fragments → cord injury)

History
- Axial load/vertical compression

Physical Findings
- Focal tenderness, ± neurologic deficit

Evaluation
- CT scan

Treatment
- Spine consult, bracing/orthosis

Disposition
- Likely admit

Chance Fracture

Definition
- Often stable fracture through the vertebra, can also include body/pedicles/laminae

History
- Back pain after head-on MVC when wearing only a lap belt from flexion injury

Physical Findings
- Focal tenderness, rare neurologic deficit

Evaluation
- CT scan

Treatment
- Spine consult, orthosis

Disposition
- Admit

Sacral Fracture

Definition
- Fractures of the sacrum (may be a/w pelvic fractures in above S4)

History
- Buttock/perirectal/posterior thigh pain after direct trauma to sacrum (fall or force from behind)

Physical Findings
- Focal tenderness, neurologic deficits (above S4), careful eval for cauda equina

Evaluation
- CT scan

Treatment
- Spine consult

Disposition
- D/c if isolated & stable

Anterior Cord Syndrome

Definition
- Injury to the anterior cord from blunt or ischemic injury

History
- Flexion/axial load (major trauma), minor trauma (arthritis/spinal stenosis/OA/spinal cord pathology)

Physical Findings
- Bilateral loss of motor/pain/temperature sensation, dorsal column intact (proprioception/vibratory sense) (See *Sensory & Motor deficit tables*)

Evaluation
- MRI

Treatment
- Spine consult

Disposition
- Admit

Central Cord Syndrome

Definition
- Trauma to central cord → injury of corticospinal motor tracts of UE > tracts of LE (buckling of ligamentum flavum)

History
- Hyperextension of neck, hx of elderly, arthritis, OA, spinal stenosis

Physical Findings
- Loss of motor fxn in UE >LE, variable sensory loss (See *Sensory & Motor deficit tables*), loss of pain & temperature if nontraumatic

Evaluation
- MRI

Treatment
- Spine consult

Disposition
• Admit

Brown–Sequard Syndrome (Lateral Cord Syndrome)
Definition
• Hemicord transection from penetrating trauma

History
• Penetrating trauma

Physical Findings
• Ipsilateral motor/proprioception/vibration loss, contralateral pain/temperature sensation loss, deficits occur 2 levels below lesion

Evaluation
• MRI

Treatment
• Spine consult

Disposition
• Admit

Deficit by Level of Spinal Injury			
Sensory-deficit Landmarks		**Motor-deficit Landmarks**	
C2	Occiput	C5	Elbow flexion
C4	Clavicular region	C7	Elbow extension
C6	Thumb	C8	Finger flexion
C8	Little finger	T1	Finger abduction
T4	Nipple line	L2	Hip flexion
T10	Umbilicus	L3	Knee extension
L1	Inguinal region	L4	Ankle dorsiflexion
L3	Knee	S1	Ankle plantar flexion
S1	Heel		
S5	Perineal area		

Spinal Shock
Definition
• Loss of vascular tone caused by cord trauma lasting 24–48 h, rarely can last several weeks

History
• Spinal cord trauma

Physical Findings
• Hypotension, bradycardia, flaccid paralysis, hyporeflexia

Treatment
• Phenylephrine (Neosynephrine peripheral alpha agonist) for BP support

Disposition
• Admit

Pearls
• There is NO evidence to support the administration of steroids in spinal trauma
• SCIWORA (spinal cord injury w/o radiologic abnl): In pediatric pts, if focal tenderness/neurologic deficits → treat as cord injury regardless of imaging

THORACIC TRAUMA

Definition
• Injuries to the thorax & its structures caused by penetrating or blunt trauma (25% all trauma Ds; immediate: heart/great vessel injury, early: Airway obstruction/tamponade/tension PTX, Late: PNA/PE)

Approach
• Evaluate anatomical categories although many injuries do not occur in isolation: Cardiac/vascular, pulmonary, skeletal, esophageal, diaphragmatic

Inspection
- External trauma: Open wounds (do not probe wounds: Clot dislodgement → hemorrhage), exit/entrance wounds, flail segments (may require external fixation or PPV), seat belt marks, impaled objects (stabilization → removal in OR)

Palpation
- Crepitance (PTX), unequal pulses (vascular trauma, mediastinal hematoma), wounds below nipple line/tip of scapula ↑ risk abd trauma (25% have both intra-abd + thoracic trauma) (*J Trauma* 1998;45:87)

Radiology
- See table

Thoracotomy
- Blunt Traumatic Arrest
  - CPR >10 min, do not perform
  - CPR <10 min or profound refractory shock
- Penetrating Trauma Arrest
  - CPR >15 min, do not perform
  - CPR <15 min or profound refractory shock or CPR <5 min penetrating neck or extremity trauma
- Do not transport pt only if pulseless & no electrical cardiac activity in field
- Survival rate in pt w/ arrest from blunt trauma 1.6%, survival rate for arrest from penetrating trauma w/ some signs of life is 31.1% (*J Trauma Acute Care Surg* 2012;73(6):1359)

Thoracic Trauma Treatment Guidelines	
Thoracic Trauma	**General Guidelines**
Blunt trauma	If e/o thoracic trauma exists: CXR, chest CT
Penetrating trauma— traverses mediastinum	Agonal: Thoracotomy Unstable: Place bilateral chest tubes Stable: CXR, chest CTA, esophagoscopy, bronchoscopy
Penetrating trauma—does not traverse mediastinum	CXR &/or chest CT for intrathoracic or extrathoracic injury

Traumatic Aortic Rupture
Definition
- Traumatic rupture of the aorta (descending aorta → fixed to thorax) caused by deceleration injury (fall from height, high-speed MVC, T-boned MVC)

History
- Retrosternal/intrascapular pain (80% die immediately)

Physical Findings
- Exam has poor sens for detecting injury, must have high index of suspicion w/ high mechanism
- Hypotension, asymmetric pulses/BP

Evaluation
- CXR (>8 cm widening of mediastinum, esophageal/trachea deviation, loss of aortic knob/aortopulmonary window, L apical cap, fractures of 1st rib/2nd rib/sternum, widening of paravertebral strip), CTA, TEE

Treatment
- BP control (labetalol/esmolol/nitroprusside): Allow permissive hypotension (SBP 70–90), surgical consult

Disposition
- Admit

Pearl
- 90% who survive have contained hematoma near ligamentum arteriosum
- nl CXR does not rule or aortic injury

Pneumothorax
Definition
- Air in the plural space (simple: w/o shift/communicating w/ outside air, tension: Injury acts as one-way valve/increased intrapleural pressures, open: wall deficit/collapse on inspiration/expansion on expiration/ineffective ventilation)

History
- Blunt (simple) or penetrating (tension/open) trauma

Physical Findings
- Decreased BS, hyperresonance, tension: Tracheal deviation/neck vein distension/hypotension, open: Chest wound w/ "sucking"

Evaluation
- US, CXR (treat tension PTX prior to imaging), chest CT

Treatment
- 100% O_2
- Tension: Needle decompression (large-bore needle/IV catheter → 2nd intercostal space, midclavicular line), chest tube to 4th–5th intercostal space mid/anterior axillary line
- Open: Sterile occlusive dressing to taped down on 3 sides → allows efflux/not influx of air, chest tube
- Simple: <10% → serial CXR, mod/large → chest tube directed anteriorly/serial CXR
- Occult: No tx other than O_2
- PPx abx indicated in tube thoracostomy in setting of trauma (*World J Surg* 2006;30:1843)

Disposition
- Admit

Pearl
- Chest tube must be placed if mechanical ventilation required

Hemothorax
Definition
- Blood in the plural space, most common from lung lacerations

History
- Blunt/penetrating trauma

Physical Findings
- Pain, decreased BS, dullness to percussion

Evaluation
- CXR: Costophrenic angle blunting (upright)/diffuse haziness (supine), US, chest CT

Treatment
- Large-bore chest tube directed inferiorly, surgical consult → OR if >1.5 L bloody output initially (>20 mL/kg)/>200 cc/h (>3 mL/kg/h) or if unstable (↑ likelihood of injury to intercostal/internal mammary/hilar vessels)
- PPx abx indicated in tube thoracostomy in setting of trauma

Pearl
- ~300 cc needed to see hemothorax on CXR

Disposition
- Admit

Flail Chest
Definition
- Fracture >3 or more ribs in 2 or more places → discontinuous segment of chest wall → paradoxical movement w/ respiration (5% of thoracic trauma)

History
- Blunt trauma, SOB

Physical Findings
- Respiratory distress, tenderness, crepitus, paradoxical movement of chest wall

Evaluation
- CXR

Treatment
- External stabilization (pillow), CPAP (1st line if poor oxygenation/ventilation in awake/cooperative pt → lower mortality/PNA rates vs. intubation) (*EMJ* 22(5):325), ± chest tube placement, pain control (rib block catheter/epidural is best), intubate only if necessary (obtunded, airway obstruction, respiratory distress)

Disposition
- Admit

Pearl
- 35–50% mortality → related to underlying injuries & cx (pulmonary contusions, PNA)

Pulmonary Contusion

Definition
• Injury to lung parenchyma → hemorrhage/edema → V/Q mismatch

History
• Blunt trauma, SOB

Physical Findings
• Respiratory distress, tenderness, tachypnea, tachycardia, hemoptysis, hypoxia ↑ 1–2 d/ resolve 7 d

Evaluation
• CXR: May be nl initially, bilateral alveolar infiltrates

Treatment
• Restrict IVF goal euvolemia, intubate if needed

Disposition
• Admit

Cardiac Tamponade

Definition
• Hemopericardium → constriction of the heart → decreased CO, most commonly due to penetrating injury (rarely blunt trauma)

History
• Penetrating trauma

Physical Findings
• Beck triad (hypotension/JVD/muffled heart sounds), tachycardia, pulsus paradoxus

Evaluation
• Bedside/formal US: Pericardial effusion/diastolic collapse of RA/RV, ECG: Low voltage/ electrical alternans, CXR: Usually unremarkable

Treatment
• Aggressive IVF (preload dependent)
• Hypotension + pericardial effusion → OR/pericardiocentesis (blood usually clotted, if fresh may be in RV)
• Arrest → thoracotomy

Disposition
• Admit

Pearl
• JVD is rare in trauma pts given hypovolemia

Cardiac Contusion

Definition
• Contusion of the myocardium/coronary vessels/valves/septum

History
• Blunt trauma

Physical Findings
• Tachycardia, hypotension

Evaluation
ECG: New BBB, dysrhythmias (rare after 1st 24 h), ST Δ /conduction abnl/RV Dysfxn, ± cardiac enzymes (poor sens, levels not predictive of outcome)

Treatment
• IV fluid resuscitation (RV damage → preload dependence), see table

Disposition
• Admit to Tele

Pearl
• New ECG Δ consider 1° cardiac event → trauma

Cardiac Contusion	
Asymptomatic, no ECG Δ, no dysrhythmias	Can be D/C home
ECG Δ or dysrhythmia in HD stable pt	24 h of cardiac monitoring
ECG Δ or dysrhythmia in HD unstable pt	Echo ± cardiology consult
Life-threatening dysrhythmias	ACLS guidelines

Esophageal Injury

Definition
- Injury to the esophagus most commonly from penetrating trauma (possible w/ significant epigastric blunt trauma)

History
- Penetrating trauma

Physical Findings
- Respiratory distress, neck/chest crepitus, hematemesis
- Often will have severe other injuries in blunt trauma

Evaluation
- CXR: Mediastinal/deep cervical air, neck films: Esophageal + laryngeal injury → air column in the esophagus, flexible esophagoscopy + esophagram (90% sens), CT

Treatment
- Surgical consult for operative management, broad-spectrum abx

Disposition
- Admit

Tracheobronchial Tear

Definition
- Tear to trachea/bronchus, most commonly due to penetrating trauma

History
- Penetrating trauma or severe deceleration injury, often die at scene

Physical Findings
- Crepitance, large persistent air leak or recurrent ptx after chest tube placement (if cervical injury may not have air leak)

Evaluation
- CXR: PTX/pneumomediastinum/"fallen lung sign," chest CT, bronchoscopy (gold standard, may miss injuries >2 cm above carina)

Treatment
- Fiberoptic intubation (in major bronchial lesions → consider double lumen ETT), chest tube placement (may require >1 chest tube)

Disposition
- Admit

Pearl
- May p/w difficulty passing ETT/difficulty w/ ventilation after ETT intubation

ABDOMINAL TRAUMA

Definition
- Trauma to the abdomen & its structures

Approach
Evaluate 4 Main Areas
- Anterior abdomen: nipple line → inguinal ligaments/pubic symphysis → anterior axillary line, Flank: B/w anterior & posterior axillary lines from 6th rib → iliac crest, Back: Inf scapular tips → iliac crest, gluteal region: Iliac crest → gluteal fold

Inspection
- Entrance/exit wounds (check b/w buttock/thigh/axilla/neck), seat belt sign (↑ risk mesenteric tear/avulsion, bowel perforation, aorta/iliac thrombosis, chance fracture of L1/L2), do not remove objects, cover eviscerated organs in saline soaked gauze

Palpation
- Peritoneal signs (operative management), rectal exam (high-riding prostate/blood/tone)

Labs
- CBC (Hct may be nl initially in setting of hemorrhage), ABG, lactate, LFTs, lipase, UA

Radiology
- FAST (90–100% sens for hemoperitoneum, not spec), CXR (abd free air), pelvic x-ray (loss of psoas shadow → retroperitoneal injury, location of bullets), CT (definitive test, low sens for early pancreatic/diaphragmatic/bowel injury)

Diagnostic Peritoneal Lavage (DPL)
• Rarely used given FAST/CT scans, positive study → >10 cc gross blood or enteric contents, blunt trauma >100000 RBCs, penetrating trauma >5000–10000 RBC

Liver Laceration
Definition
• Laceration to liver (most commonly injured organ)

History
• Blunt or penetrating trauma

Physical Findings
• ± RUQ tenderness

Evaluation
• LFTs, HCT, FAST, CT scan: Grading of laceration (I–VI)

Treatment
• Surgical consultation for operative vs. conservative management (HD stable, serial exams/HCT)

Disposition
• Admit ICU vs. floor

Approach to Abd Trauma			
Abd Trauma	Examples	Most Common Injuries	General Guidelines
Blunt trauma	Motor vehicle crash, falls, assaults	Spleen, liver, intestine, kidney	Unstable + distention → OR Unstable → FAST Stable → CT (IV contrast only), FAST, or serial abd exams
Penetrating trauma—anterior abdomen	GSW, SW	Small bowel, colon, liver, & vascular structures (GSW); liver, small bowel, diaphragm	GSW to anterior abdomen → OR Unstable w/ non-GSW trauma → OR Stable w/ non-GSW trauma → local wound exploration, CT
Penetrating trauma—flank & back	GSW, SW		Unstable → OR. Stable GSW → triple contrast (IV, PO, PR) Stable non-GSWs → local wound exploration, CT, serial exams

Notes:
(1) 1° objective is to identify need for surgical exploration.
(2) Peritoneal irritation often seen w/ hollow viscus injury, but not w/ hemoperitoneum.
(3) If fascia penetration is found, f/u w/ DPL, CT, or ex lap. If not pt can be D/C after wound care.
(4) Intra-abd organ injury occurs in 20% of non-GSW flank injuries & 5–10% of non-GSW back injuries.

Splenic Laceration
Definition
• Laceration to spleen (most commonly injured organ in blunt trauma)

History
• Blunt or penetrating trauma, L shoulder pain (Kehr sign)/chest/flank/upper quadrant pain

Physical Findings
• LUQ pain

Evaluation
• FAST, CT scan: Grading of laceration (I–V)

Treatment
• Surgical consultation for operative vs. conservative management (HD stable, serial exams/HCT), IR for embolization

Disposition
• Admit ICU vs. floor

Splenic Laceration Grading	
Grade	
Grade I	Subcapsular hematoma <10% surface area, capsular tear <1 cm depth
Grade II	Subcapsular hematoma 10–50%, intraparenchymal hematoma <5 cm diameter, parenchymal laceration 1–3 cm not involving vessels
Grade III	Subcapsular hematoma >50% or expanding, ruptured subcapsular/ intraparenchymal hematoma, intraparenchymal hematoma >5 cm, splenic laceration >3 cm/involving trabecular vessels
Grade IV	Laceration of segmental or hilar vessels → devascularization of >25%
Grade V	Shattered spleen, hilar vascular injury → complete devascularization

Small Bowel Injury

Definition
• Injury to small bowel (GSW > SW > blunt trauma)

History
• Blunt or penetrating trauma, classically handlebar injury

Physical Findings
• Seat belt sign (MVC), peritoneal signs (may be delayed)

Evaluation
• Unstable → FAST/DPL, Stable → CT scan (low sens, fluid collection/bowel-wall thickening/ stranding/free air) CXR (rarely shows free air), Lumbar XR (Chance fracture)

Treatment
• Surgical consultation for operative management (perforation or devascularization), abx (ampicillin/ciprofloxacin/metronidazole)

Disposition
• Admit

Colorectal Injury

Definition
• Injury to colon or rectum (transverse colon most common)

History
• Penetrating trauma (GSW)

Physical Findings
• Hypoactive bowels, peritoneal signs, gross rectal blood

Evaluation
• Triple contrast CT scan (Gastrografin, barium is irritating), KUB (air lining psoas), f/u sigmoidoscopy

Treatment
• Surgical consultation for operative management (perforation or devascularization), abx (ampicillin/ciprofloxacin/metronidazole)

Disposition
• Admit

Duodenal Injury

Definition
• Injury to duodenum (80% a/w other injury)

History
• Penetrating trauma, N/V (obstructing hematoma)

Physical Findings
• Epigastric tenderness, heme positive stool, bloody NGT aspirate

Evaluation
• Upright CXR (free air), CT scan (duodenal wall hematoma), Upper GI ("coiled spring" area)

Treatment
• Surgical consultation for operative management (perforation or devascularization), abx (ampicillin/ciprofloxacin/metronidazole), NGT placement

Disposition
• Admit

Pearls
- 2nd portion most commonly injured (contains bile/pancreatic duct openings)
- Mortality 40% if dx delayed 24 h

Gastric Injury
Definition
- Injury to stomach, uncommon

History
- Penetrating trauma

Physical Findings
- Epigastric tenderness, heme positive stool, bloody NGT aspirate

Evaluation
- Upright CXR (free air)

Treatment
- Surgical consultation for operative management, abx (ampicillin/ciprofloxacin/metronidazole)

Disposition
- Admit

Pancreatic Injury
Definition
- Injury to pancreas (75% penetrating trauma)

History
- Penetrating trauma, direct epigastric trauma (steering wheel, bicycle handles)

Physical Findings
- Minimal epigastric tenderness (retroperitoneal structure)

Evaluation
- CT scan (low sens early), lipase (may be nl), ERCP for ductal injury

Treatment
- Surgical consultation

Disposition
- Admit

Pearl
- A/w other injuries 90% of the time

Vascular Trauma
Definition
- Injury to abd vasculature (10% of SW, 25% of GSW)

History
- Penetrating trauma

Physical Findings
- Distension, expanding hematoma, Grey–Turner sign (flank ecchymosis)/Cullen sign (periumbilical ecchymosis) → retroperitoneal hemorrhage

Evaluation
- FAST, CT scan (if stable), wound exploration

Treatment
- Surgical consultation, unstable → OR

Disposition
- Admit

Pearl
- Avoid LE venous access

Diaphragmatic Tear
Definition
- Tear to diaphragm from blunt trauma, ↑ lateral impact (large, L-sided 2–3× more likely than R, posterolaterally located) or penetrating trauma (small but enlarge w/ time)

History
- Penetrating/blunt trauma, delayed presentation; pain, ± obstruction

Physical Findings
- BS over chest

Evaluation
- CXR (50% sens): Hemothorax/PTX (penetrating), abnl diaphragmatic shadow (blunt), US, CT scan, careful NGT placement (may be seen in hemithorax)

Treatment
- Respiratory distress → NGT placement for decompression, surgery consult for operative repair. CXR may be misinterpreted as hemothorax, avoid chest tube placement

Disposition
- Admit

Pearl
- Intrapericardial diaphragmatic rupture/bowel herniation → tamponade

GENITOURINARY TRAUMA

Definition
- Trauma to the structures of the genitourinary tract, uncommon to be life-threat unless significant renal/vascular injury

Approach
Inspection
- Blood at meatus (urethra trauma), blood in vagina, perineal lacerations (do not probe → hemorrhage), scrotal ecchymosis/lacerations, flank bruising

Palpation
- Rectal exam (high-riding prostate/boggy → membranous urethral injury, blood → rectal laceration), testicular disruption

Labs
- UA (microscopic hematuria → no eval, gross blood → serious GU trauma)

Radiology
- RUG: Males w/ blood at meatus before Foley placement (to prevent full urethral tear/false passage), inject 50 cc contrast into urethra → pelvic x-ray for extravasation
- Cystogram: Instill 400–500 cc contrast into bladder via Foley → AP film or CT scan → repeat image after contrast is washed out (posterior bladder tears)
- IV pyelogram: Rarely indicated
- CT scan (IV contrast): Complete eval of kidneys

Renal Laceration
Definition
- Laceration to kidney (major: Extend to medulla/collecting system, minor: No involvement of collecting system/medulla, no extraversion of urine, pedicle: injury to renal vasculature)

History
- Penetrating trauma

Physical Findings
- Flank wound, gross hematuria, ± hypotension

Evaluation
- CBC, UA, other trauma labs as needed, CT scan: Eval extent of injury

Treatment
- Surgery consult, minor lacerations may be nonoperative

Disposition
- Admit

Renal Contusion
Definition
- Contusion to kidney

History
- Blunt trauma

Physical Findings
- Flank ecchymosis

Evaluation
• UA (if neg → no further testing), CT scan

Treatment
• Surgery consult, subcapsular hematoma → 24 h observation/serial HCT/serial UA/bed rest, microscopic hematuria → avoid strenuous exercise/repeat UA in 2 d + until clear

Disposition
• Admit: Major/subcapsular hematoma
• Home: Microscopic hematuria

Renal Pedicle/Vascular Injury
Definition
• Injury to renal pedicle or vasculature

History
• High-velocity deceleration, penetrating trauma

Physical Findings
• Flank ecchymosis, hypotension

Evaluation
• UA, CBC, Coags, BMP, CT scan: Nonenhancing kidney/± perirenal hematoma

Treatment
• Surgery consult for operative management → repair (20% salvage rate in pedicle lacerations) vs. nephrectomy

Disposition
• Admit

Renal Pelvis Rupture
Definition
• Rupture of the renal pelvis

History
• High-velocity deceleration, penetrating trauma

Physical Findings
• Flank ecchymosis, hypotension

Evaluation
• UA, CBC, Coags, BMP, CT scan: Extravasation of urine in perirenal space

Treatment
• Urology consult for operative repair

Disposition
• Admit

Pearl
• ↑ risk of infection in delayed repair

Ureteral Injuries
Definition
• Injury to ureter (very rare), majority are iatrogenic from gyn/uro procedures

History
• Hyperextension, penetrating trauma, forced flexion of L-spine → rupture below UPJ, delayed necrosis from microvascular injury after GSW (rare)

Evaluation
• UA, HCT, CT scan: Extravasation of urine, IVP (limited sens)

Treatment
• Urology consult for operative ureterouretostomy

Disposition
• Admit

Intraperitoneal Bladder Rupture
Definition
• Laceration at dome of bladder w/ intraperitoneal communication

History
• MVC, blunt trauma (burst injury)

Physical Findings
- Lower abd tenderness, ↓ UOP, hematuria

Evaluation
- UA, HCT, CT cystogram/cystogram: Extravasation of urine

Treatment
- Urology consult for urgent operative repair

Disposition
- Admit

Extraperitoneal Bladder Rupture
Definition
- Rupture of the bladder w/ extraperitoneal spillage

History
- MVC, blunt trauma

Physical Findings
- Lower abd tenderness, ↓ UOP, hematuria

Evaluation
- UA, HCT, CT cystogram/cystogram w/ washout: Extravasation of urine

Treatment
- Urology consult (usually nonoperative unless extends to bladder neck), Foley 10–14 d

Disposition
- Admit

Male Urethral Injuries
Definition
- Injury to posterior (prostatomembranous) urethra (a/w pelvic fractures, esp bilateral or both ipsilateral pubic rami fx & posterior disruption injuries) & anterior (bulbous/penile) urethra (a/w direct trauma to penis/penile fracture/saddle injuries/falls/GSW)

History
- Blunt or penetrating trauma

Physical Findings
- Blood at meatus, gross hematuria, inability to void

Evaluation
- UA, HCT, RUG (prior to Foley)

Treatment
- Suprapubic bladder decompression if needed, urology consult for 1° repair/fluoroscopic catheter placement/suprapubic cystotomy

Disposition
- Admit

Female Urethral Injuries
Definition
- Injury to female urethra associated most commonly w/ pelvic fractures (rarely saddle injuries, falls, GSW, instrumentation)

History
- Blunt or penetrating trauma, much less common than in males

Physical Findings
- Vaginal bleeding, inability to place Foley, labial edema

Evaluation
- RUG not useful, passage of Foley precludes complete tear

Treatment
- Suprapubic bladder decompression if needed, urology consult for surgical repair

Disposition
- Admit

Testicular Contusion/Rupture
Definition
- Blunt trauma to the testicle leading to contusion or rupture (disruption of tunica albuginea)

History
- Blunt trauma, pain, swelling

Physical Findings
- Ecchymosis, edema, tenderness, inability to palpate testicle due to dislocation

Evaluation
- Testicular US (mod sens/spec for rupture)

Treatment
- Urology consult for surgical repair/clot evacuation (early intervention → ↓ morbidity)

Disposition
- Admit

Penile Fracture
Definition
- Blunt injury to the erect penis when penis is forcefully bent leading to rupture of the tunica albuginea/rupture of corpora cavernosa

History
- "Cracking sound" usually during sexual activity → severe pain

Physical Findings
- Swelling, discoloration (vascular engorgement), ecchymosis, blood at meatus (10–20% a/w urethral injury)

Evaluation
- RUG for urethral injury (concomitant injury in 15–20%)

Treatment
- Urology consult for surgical urethral repair/clot evacuation

Disposition
- Admit

Penile Amputation/Laceration
Definition
- Complete or partial amputation/laceration of the penis

History
- Penetrating trauma, zipper injury

Evaluation
- RUG or testicular US if associated injuries suspected

Treatment
- Amputation: Urology consult (best results in reimplanted in 18 h)
- Simple laceration: Repair w/ absorbable suture
- Zipper injury: Remove zipper w/ mineral oil/wire cutters at zipper median bar to break apart

Disposition
- D/C unless reimplantation required

Female Genital Injuries
Definition
- Injury to ovary, uterus, fallopian tube, vagina (difficult to Dx usually found when evaluating for other injury), a/w pelvic fractures

History
- Blunt or penetrating trauma, vaginal bleeding

Physical Findings
- Blood in vaginal vault, lower abd tenderness

Evaluation
- CT scan, pelvic US (in gravid pt, ↑ risk)

Treatment
- Open vaginal lacerations open → abx (ampicillin, gentamicin, Flagyl) GYN consult
- Simple vaginal lacerations: Repair w/ absorbable suture

Disposition
- Admit if needed

HIP/PELVIC TRAUMA

Definition
- Trauma to hip or pelvis

Approach
Pelvis Anatomy
- Sacrum, coccyx, & R/L innominate bones (ileum, ischium, pubis) fuse at acetabulum

Inspection
- Perineal edema/lacerations/ecchymosis, deformities (length discrepancy, internal/external rotation)

Palpation
- Rectal exam (blood, high-riding prostate, tone), pulses, pelvic stability (limit manipulation if unstable → clot dislodgement), neurologic exam (strength, sensation, DTRs), in females pelvic exam

Radiology
- AP pelvis (can miss sacral fractures/SI joint disruptions → inlet/outlet views), CT scan (superior for acetabular fractures/associated injuries), hip x-ray

Pelvic Fractures
Definition
- Fractures of the pelvis usually caused by significant mechanism (↑ association w/ other injuries)

History
- Blunt trauma, lateral/AP compression, vertical shear (fall)

Physical Findings
- External contusion/abrasion/ecchymosis, caution w/ manual compression/distraction of pelvis (may dislodge clot → hemorrhage), evaluate for open pelvic fx as these have 40–50% mortality, hypotension (42–50% mortality), blood at meatus, perineal trauma, neurologic abnl (cauda equina syndrome, plexopathies, radiculopathies)

Evaluation
- FAST, AP pelvis, CT scan, evaluate carefully for intra-abd trauma as >15% w/ pelvic fx will have intra-abd injury

Treatment
- Unstable: Temporizing measures (wrapped sheet/external binders/external clamps), immediate orthopedic & trauma surgery consult (reduction/external fixation & pelvic packing), IR for hemorrhage control
- Stable: Orthopedic consult

Disposition
- Admit

Pearls
- Type A (inferior pubic rami/avulsion) & type B2 (bucket handle) → most common
- Type B3 (open book) & C (70% have major associated injuries) → most life-threatening

Pelvic Fracture Classification (Tile Classification System)	
Type	
Type A: Stable pelvic ring fracture	A1: Avulsion of innominate bone → sudden muscle contraction, Iliac wing (Duverney) fracture → direct lateral to medical trauma
	A2: Stable or minimally displaced fracture of pelvic ring (ramus/ischium) → elderly fall
	A3: Transverse fracture of sacrum/coccyx → fall in sitting position
Type B: Partially stable pelvic ring injuries (rotationally unstable/vertically stable)	B1: Unilateral open book (disruption symphysis pubis + SI joint hinge rotation) → AP compression
	B2: Bucket handle fractures → lateral compression
	B3: Bilateral open book fracture → severe AP compression
Type C: Unstable pelvic ring fractures	Distracting vertical sacral fractures/other vertical shear fractures → vertical shear injuries

Vascular Pelvic Injuries

Definition
- Injury to vascular structures of pelvis a/w pelvic fractures (most commonly AP trauma or vertical shear)

History
- Blunt trauma, lateral/AP compression, vertical shear (fall)

Physical Findings
- Unstable pelvis, hypotension resistant to resuscitation

Evaluation
- FAST, AP pelvis, CT scan (if stable), pelvic angiography, consider DPA if FAST neg but HD unstable

Treatment
- Stabilization of pelvis, orthopedic & trauma surgery consult (external fixation & pelvic packing to control hemorrhage), IR embolization for continued hypotension (less effective for venous bleed → high collateralization)

Disposition
- Admit

Acetabular Fractures

Definition
- Fractures to the acetabulum (MVC → knee striking dashboard or lateral intrusion), fall in elderly

History
- Blunt trauma, pain w/ movement of hip

Physical Findings
- Pain w/ movement of hip/compression of sole of foot or greater trochanter

Evaluation
- AP pelvis, lateral hip films (± Judet views), CT scan (if plain films unrevealing)
- 3 types (although some fit in multiple categories
- Wall: Anterior, posterior, posterior wall/column, transverse/posterior wall
- Column: Anterior, posterior, both, posterior wall/column, anterior/transverse
- Transverse: Transverse, T, transverse/posterior wall, anterior column/transverse

Treatment
- Orthopedic consult for operative management

Disposition
- Admit

Hip Fractures

Definition
- Fractures of the hip (femoral head/neck/trochanter)

History
- Elderly → fall from standing, young → significant mechanism trauma (MVC)

Physical Findings
- External rotation, shortening of leg

Evaluation
- AP pelvis, lateral hip films, CT (if unable to bear weight + neg plain films)

Treatment
- Orthopedic consult for operative management (femoral neck fractures → ↑ risk avascular necrosis of femoral head, surgical repair in <6 h)

Disposition
- Admit

Pearl
- Hip fracture in elderly → 25% 1-y mortality

Hip Fractures	
Type	
Intracapsular	Femoral head: Rare in isolation, a/w posterior dislocations Femoral neck: ↑ risk avascular necrosis of femoral head, most common in elderly women
Extracapsular	Intertrochanteric: Markedly externally rotated/shortened, elderly fall Subtrochanteric: ↑ risk bleeding into thigh, elderly fall/MVC

Hip Dislocations

Definition
- Dislocation of femoral head from acetabulum (90% posterior)

History
- Elderly fall w/ hx of hip total hip replacement, MVC (knee hitting dashboard, a/w other injuries), athlete running & lands w/ hip flexed/internally rotated & adducted

Physical Findings
- Flexed/adducted/internally rotated hip (posterior)

Evaluation
- AP pelvis, lateral hip films

Treatment
- Orthopedic consult if fracture or prosthetic hip, reduction under conscious sedation (in <6 h, ↑ risk avascular necrosis of femoral head)

Disposition
- Admit if needed

EXTREMITY INJURY

Definition
- Injuries to the extremities (vascular/bony/soft tissue/nerve)

Approach
History
- Last tetanus (booster if >5 y), hand dominance, time of injury, mechanism (crush/penetrating), neurologic deficit (loss of sensation/motor), environmental exposures (burn/cold), preinjury functional status

Inspection
- Color (discoloration/ecchymosis/perfusion), soft tissue defects (control hemorrhage during 1° survey), deformities (angulations/shortening), swelling

Palpation
- Pulses, all joints/bones (tenderness), FB, crepitance, strength, sensation, DTRs, range all joints, joint effusions

Radiology
- Plain films guided by PE

Consults
- Orthopedic &/or vascular for open fractures/amputations/vascular injuries/compartment syndrome, hand surgery for significant hand injuries

Extremity Vascular Injury
Definition
- Injury to the vasculature of the extremities

History
- Blunt trauma (fracture/dislocation → tearing of vessels) or penetrating trauma

Physical Findings
- Obvious vascular compromise → pulseless/pallor/pain/paresthesia/cold, indicators of vascular injury → swelling/pain/↓ cap refill/mottled skin/↓ pulses

Evaluation
- Plain films (blunt trauma), CTA, or angiography (if stable), Ankle/Brachial index or Ankle/Ankle index: Abnl if <0.9

Treatment
- Vascular surgery consult for immediate surgical repair (↓ salvage rate if >6 h)

Disposition
- Admit if needed

Extremity Orthopedic Injuries
Definition
- Bony fractures or joint dislocations of the extremities

History
- Blunt trauma or penetrating

Physical Findings
- Deformities, pain, swelling, crepitance, neurologic deficits, diminished pulses

Evaluation
- Plain films, image joint above & below for significant fracture, CT in certain injuries (tibial plateau)

Treatment
- Open fractures: Immediate orthopedic consult for operative washout/fixation (<6 h), abx (cefazolin 1–2 g)
- Closed UE fractures + intact neuro exam: Splint, outpt f/u (see table)
- Closed LE fractures + intact neuro exam: Splint, outpt f/u if able to use crutches (see table)
- Dislocations: ED reduction, pt f/u

Disposition
- Admit if needed

Principles of Immobilization & Referral		
Fracture Sites	**Splint/Immobilization Technique**	**Referral Guidelines**
Femoral fractures	Temporary traction splints	Emergent ED consult
Knee injuries (w/ no e/o dislocation & no neurovascular compromise)	Knee immobilizer/long leg cast w/ leg flexed 10°	Orthopedic f/u w/i 1 wk
Tibia fractures (not tibial plateau)	Lower leg posterior splint	Orthopedic f/u in 1–2 d
Ankle fractures	Lower leg posterior U-splint	If fracture fragments well aligned, orthopedic f/u in 1 wk. If angulation or distraction, needs next-day f/u
Hand fractures	Thumb & index finger—radial gutter splint Middle, ring, & little fingers—ulnar gutter splint	If fracture fragments well aligned & fracture is closed, f/u w/ hand surgeon w/i 1 wk
Wrist fractures	Wrist splint/immobilizer unless scaphoid fracture then thumb spica cast	Orthopedic f/u in 7–10 d unless scaphoid displacement—then f/u in 1–2 d
Distal radius/ulna fractures	Short arm cast	Orthopedic f/u in 1–2 d unless closed reduction results in good anatomic alignment—then f/u in 7–10 d
Humerus fractures	Sling, coaptation splint rarely used	Orthopedic f/u in 7–10 d, sooner if articular surface or tuberosity
Shoulder dislocations	Sling, early ROM to prevent frozen shoulder	Orthopedic f/u in 7–10 d

Pearls
- 5th MCP fractures or "Boxer fractures" have a high rate of infection secondary to breaks in skin from opponent's tooth. Always r/o FB w/ plain radiographs & f/u in 1–2 d in ED or in hand clinic
- Scaphoid tenderness w/o radiologic e/o fracture requires splinting & orthopedic f/u & repeated x-rays w/i 7 d

ED, emergency department; MCP, metacarpal

Extremity Soft Tissue Injury
Definition
Injury to the soft tissue of the extremities

History
Blunt trauma or penetrating (polytrauma, industrial accidents)

Physical Findings
Soft tissue defects, FBs

Evaluation
- Plain films for FB/underlying fractures, US, CPK (if extensive injury)

Treatment
- Irrigate, explore for FB (↑ risk wound infection → poor cosmetic outcome), plastic surgery consult (extensive injuries), hand consult for palmar injuries as exploration w/ potential for iatrogenic injury, abx (grossly contaminated wounds)

Disposition
- Admit if extensive, e/o rhabdomyolysis/compartment syndrome

Extremity Nerve Injury
Definition
- Injury to the nerves of the extremities (a/w fractures/dislocations/lacerations/ vascular ischemia/compartment syndrome)

History
- Blunt trauma or penetrating

Physical Findings
- See table

Evaluation
- Plain films for fracture/dislocation

Treatment
- Reduce fracture/dislocation (↓ pressure on nerve), fasciotomy (compartment syndrome), orthopedic/plastic surgery consult

Disposition
- Admit if needed

Extremity Nerve Injuries			
Nerve	Motor	Sensation	Injury
Ulnar	Index finger abduction	Tip of little finger	Elbow injury
Median (distal)	Thenar opposition	Tip of index finger	Wrist dislocation
Median (anterior interosseous)	Index tip flexion		Supracondylar fx of humerus in children
Musculocutaneous	Elbow flexion	Lateral forearm	Anterior shoulder dislocation
Radial	Thumb, finger MCP extension	1st dorsal web space	Distal humeral shaft, anterior shoulder dislocation
Axillary	Deltoid	Lateral shoulder	Proximal humerus fx, anterior shoulder dislocation
Femoral	Knee extension	Anterior knee	Pubic rami fx
Obturator	Hip adduction	Medial thigh	Obturator ring fx
Posterior tibial	Toe dorsiflexion	Sole of foot	Knee dislocation
Superficial peroneal	Ankle eversion	Lateral dorsum of foot	Fibular neck fx, knee dislocation
Deep peroneal	Ankle/toe dorsiflexion	Dorsal 1st to 2nd web space of foot	Fibular neck fx, compartment syndrome
Sciatic	Plantar & dorsiflexion	Foot	Posterior hip dislocation
Superior gluteal	Hip abduction		Acetabular fx
Inferior gluteal	Gluteus maximus hip extension		Acetabular fx

Compartment Syndrome
Definition
- A condition in which perfusion pressures < tissue pressures in closed space (fascial compartments) → ↓ circulation/tissue fxn (↑ risk injuries: Tibial/forearm fractures, crush injuries, burns, immobilized injuries in tight dressing/cast)

History
* Blunt trauma or penetrating, pain > than expected/worse w/ passive muscle stretching

Physical Findings
* Tenderness, tense swelling, classically: Pain, pallor, paresthesias, paralysis, pulselessness (late finding). Pain w/ passive stretching is early sign but not always reliable

Evaluation
* Compartment pressures (measure w/ Stryker or 18 G IV + arterial line transducer) >30 mmHg or <20–30 mmHg difference b/w DBP & compartment pressure (if hypotensive necrosis occurs at ↓ pressures), CK

Treatment
* Remove restrictive dressings/casts, elevate extremity, correct BP, surgery consult for fasciotomy (do not delay fasciotomy for surgical availability)

Disposition
* Admit

Crush Syndrome/Rhabdomyolysis
Definition
* Crush injury → release in cellular contents of muscle cells → CK levels >5000 U/L

History
* Crush injury

Physical Findings
* May have minimal external injury, dark brown/orange urine

Evaluation
* CK levels >5000 U/L, ↑ Cr (15–47% a/w ARF), ↑ potassium, UA (+ myoglobin), observe closely for reperfusion syndrome, esp if in field

Treatment
* IV fluids for UOP >1 mL/g/h, traditionally alkalization of urine (sodium bicarbonate, 1 amp/1 L NS → urine pH >7 → prevents tubular precipitation of myoglobin) → no difference than NS in prevention of renal failure, treat hyperkalemia (*J Trauma* 2004;56:1191)

Disposition
* Admit

Partial/Complete Amputation
Definition
* Amputation of extremity

History
* Blunt or penetrating trauma (polytrauma, industrial accident)

Physical Findings
* Document motor/neurologic/vascular fxn in remaining limb

Evaluation
* Plain films of stump + amputated fragment, ± angiography (if not going directly to OR)

Treatment
* Limit mobility, hemostasis w/ direct pressure, immediate surgery consult for replantation, abx (cefazolin 1–2 g IV), pack stump w/ sterile NS soaked gauze, wrap amputated part in cold NS soaked gauze/place on ice (do not place in direct contact w/ ice or NS)

Disposition
* Admit

Pearl
* Replantation depends on age, vocation, injury severity

WOUND MANAGEMENT

Approach
History
Time of event (>12 h → irrigate/heal by secondary intention or delayed 1° closure, face/significant soft tissue defect → 1° closure in <24 h), location (suture selection/time until removal), mechanism (↑ risk FB/contamination), tetanus (booster if >5 y)

Inspection
- FB, wound approximation

Palpation
- Pulses, strength, sensation distal to injury

Laceration
Definition
- Cut or tear to skin & soft tissues

History
- Penetrating or blunt trauma

Physical Findings
- Skin defect, ↓ pulses/sensation/motor (neurovascular injury)

Evaluation
- Plain films only if FB/fracture suspected

Treatment
- Hemostasis: Direct pressure, lidocaine w/ epinephrine if needed (avoid in digits, nose, ears, penis), hemostatic agents (eg, thrombin, Surgicel), proximal tourniquet
- Analgesia: Use regional blocks when possible (↓ wound distortion/amount of analgesic needed)

Commonly Used Local Anesthetics						
Agent	Trade Name	Class	Concentrations (%)	Maximum Safe Dose	Onset	Duration
Lidocaine w/ epinephrine	Xylocaine	Amide	0.5–2	4.5 mg/kg 7 mg/kg	~5 min	1–2 h 2–4 h
Bupivacaine w/ epinephrine	Marcaine	Amide	0.125–0.25	2 mg/kg 3 mg/kg	~5 min	4–8 h 8–16 h
Procaine w/ epinephrine	Novocaine	Ester	0.5–1	7 mg/kg 9 mg/kg	~5 min	15–45 min 30–90 min

- Irrigation: >500 cc NS (no benefit over tap water) (Ann Emerg Med 1999;34:356), 8 psi of pressure (18 g IV catheter or Zerowet splash shield in 30–60 cc syringe), caution on delicate tissues (eye lids)
- Exploration (through a full ROM): FB, tendons (including in position of injury), fascial planes
- Repair:

Suture Choice		
Body Part	Suture Size	Remove Sutures on Day
Scalp	Staples or 4-0	7
Face	5-0, 6-0	4–5
Chest	3-0, 4-0	7–10
Back	3-0, 4-0	10–14
Forearm	4-0, 5-0	10–14
Finger/hand	5-0	7–10
LE	4-0, 5-0	10–12

- Abx: Not routinely required (must be given for certain bites)

Disposition
- Home

Pearls
- Scarring: Take up to 1 y to fully develop, apply sunscreen/keep covered even on cloudy days, apply Vit E
- Hand flexor tendon lacerations: Emergent 1° repair by hand surgeon, splint (wrist 30° flexion, MP joint 70° flexion, DIP/PIP 10° flexion)
- Hand extensor tendon lacerations: Zone IV & VI repair 1° in ED, splint, hand surgery f/u

Foreign Body

Definition
- Retained FB in wound (most common hand/foot) → ↑ risk delayed infection/granuloma/formation/local compression of structures/embolization/allergic rxns (reactive FBs: Wood, organic matter, clothing, skin fragments)

History
- Know FB, ↑ risk wounds: Stepping on glass/punching windows/MVC w/ glass exposure/fall on gravel/pain at IVD site/persistent wound infections/failure to heal (41% wounds caused by glass)

Physical Findings
- Visible/palpable FB

Evaluation
- Explore wound (adequate anesthesia/hemostasis/probe w/ instrument), plain films for radiopaque FBs (glass, metal, bone, teeth, graphite, gravel), US (use 100 cc bag of NS or other transducing material for superficial FB location)

Treatment
- Not all FB require removal (deep, small, inert, asymptomatic, away from vital structures), removal (significant pain, functional impairment, reactive, contamination, near vital structures, cosmetic concerns): May require wound extension, irrigation, fine tip forceps

Disposition
- D/C

Fingertip Wounds

Definition
- Amputations/laceration/crush to fingertip (skin/volar pulp/distal phalanx/nail/nail bed)

History
- Cutting/crushing injury

Physical Findings
- Amputation, nail bed lacerations, subungual hematoma

Evaluation
- Finger plain film (FB, fracture)

Treatment
- Amputation: Distal to DIP joint → wound care/secondary intention (may need to trim back bone/should always be covered by soft tissue)/abx, significant bone/soft tissue loss → emergent hand surgery consult
- Subungual hematoma: Large → nail trephination, small → no intervention
- Nail bed laceration: 1° repair → remove nail, repair w/ 6-0 absorbable suture, replace nail into nail fold (suture or secure w/ tape) to splint nail bed/maintain nail fold (nail growth → 70–160 d)

Disposition
- D/C

ABUSE

Approach

History
- Delays in seeking care, hx inconsistent w/ injury, multiple past injuries, injuries in various stages of healing

Team Approach
- Social work, child protective services, trained sexual assault nurses, pt advocate

Documentation
- Record factual events/injuries, avoid judgments, informed consent for forensic collection/release of information, mandatory reporting for child/elder abuse

Child Abuse
History
- Story inconsistent w/ injuries/child's developmental age, inconsistent stories by caretakers

Physical Findings
- Child neglect: Flattening/alopecia of occiput (supine for long periods of time), decreased SC tissue/prominent ribs/loose skin over buttocks (FTT)
- Child abuse: Bruises/fracture varying stages, bruises in areas not prone to trauma (lower back, buttock, thighs, cheeks, ear pinna), geometric-shaped bruising (belts, cords), scald burns w/o splash marks or in "dip" pattern, multiple deep contact burns, unexplained extremity swelling (long bone spiral fracture, metaphyseal chip fractures, femur fractures in <3 y), posterior rib fractures, MS Δ (shaken baby), suspicious oral/facial trauma (torn frenulum, dental trauma present in 50% of abuse)
- Child sexual assault: Penile/vaginal d/c (STDs), UTI, genital/rectal trauma (inner thigh bruising, rectal tears, loss rectal tone), often no physical findings if delay in presentation

Evaluation
- Skeletal series (children <5), head CT (suspected intracranial injury), dilated eye exam (retinal detachment/hemorrhage → shaken baby), CBC, Coags, LFTs, tox screen, growth measurements, vaginal/rectal/oral swabs

Treatment
- Social work/child protective services, treat injuries as appropriate

Disposition
- D/C per child protective services

Pearls
- 2–3% children (physical abuse associated low SES)
- ↑ risk in children w/ mental/physical disabilities/chronic medical problems
- Consider Munchausen syndrome by proxy in cases w/ extensive/neg prior w/u
- Most important to suspect abuse & allow trained specialists to opine if abuse occurred

Sexual Assault
History
- Time, date, number/description of assailants, threats made, weapons used, type of assault, drugs used, LOC, post assault activity (Δ of clothing, urination, showering, tampon use), last time of voluntary intercourse

Physical Findings
- Document: Appearance of clothes, scratches, bruising, lacerations (can use toluidine dye to identify vaginal lacerations), d/c

Evaluation
- Imaging as needed, have pt advocate present, pregnancy test, ± STD testing, full rape kit if <72 h (modify as appropriate), vaginal/rectal secretions for acid phosphatase/glycoprotein p30, tox screen
- Many areas will have SANE services available & pt may need transfer for SANE exam must medically clear pt 1st

Treatment
- Pregnancy prophylaxis (levonorgestrel 0.75 q12h × 2 doses), STD prophylaxis (gonorrhea: Ceftriaxone 125 mg IM × 1, Chlamydia: Azithromycin 1 g PO × 1, Hep B: 1st of 2 vaccines, HIV), antiemetics

Disposition
- D/C w/ f/u counseling

Pearl
- 1/5 women is sexually assaulted in lifetime, only 7% reported

Intimate-partner Violence
History
- Story inconsistent w/ injuries, frequent ED visits, vague medical complaints, chronic pain (>abd pain), overbearing/controlling partner, injury during pregnancy

Physical Findings
- Injuries face/head/neck/areas covered by clothes (most common)

Evaluation
• Imaging as needed

Treatment
• Photographs as appropriate, determine safety of home/immediate risk (escalating violence, treats, firearms), devise safety plan (avoid sedative/arguments in small rooms/access to firearms, teach children to call 911), social work consult

Disposition
• D/C to shelter if unsafe home

Pearls
• ↑ risk during pregnancy/attempts to leave partner
• Universal screening for all pts should be done in the ED

Elder Abuse

History
• Delayed presentation, hx of med noncompliance/missed appointments, often lives w/ abuser, have dementia, are dependent on abuser for ADLs, RFs for abusive caretaker: Mental illness, substance abuse, hx of family violence/financial stress/stress of being caretaker

Physical Findings
• Poor hygiene, malnutrition, decubitus ulcers, "urine rash," unexplained injuries to face/head/torso/back/buttocks/limb contractures (restraints)/bilateral upper extremities (grabbing)

Evaluation
• Imaging as needed, CBC, BMP, CK (rhabdomyolysis)

Treatment
• Photographs as appropriate, arrange for support services to relieve stress on caretaker (VNA, meals-on-wheels), arrange for home safety eval

Disposition
• Admit if unsafe to go home

Pearls
• May be as high as 5–10% in elderly
• Decreased reporting for fear of institutionalization

ABBREVIATIONS

A/P	assessment and plan	BPH	Benign prostatic hyperplasia
a/w	Associated with	BPPV	Benign paroxysmal positional vertigo
AAA	Abdominal aortic aneurysm		
βB	Beta-blocker	BSUS	bedside ultrasound
ABC	Airway, berthing, circulation	BVM	Bag-valve mask
ABG	Arterial blood gas	BZD	Benzodiazepines
ABI	Ankle-brachial index	c/o	Complaint of
abnl	Abnormal	c/w	Compared with
abnlty	Abnormality	CABG	Coronary artery bypass graft
abx	Antibiotics	CAD	Coronary artery disease
AC	Acromioclavicular	CAP	Community-acquired pneumonia
ACE-I/	Angiotensin-converting		
ACEI	enzyme inhibitor	CBC	Complete blood count
ACS	Acute coronary syndrome	CBD	Common bile duct
ADH	Antidiuretic hormone	CCB	Calcium channel blocker
ADHD	Attention-deficit hyperactivity disorder	CCU	Coronary care unit
		CHF	Congestive heart failure
AED	Antiepileptic drug	CKD	Chronic kidney disease
AF	Atrial fibrillation	CI	Contraindication
AFL	Atrial flutter	CMP	Cardiomyopathy
AG	Aminoglycoside	CMV	Cytomegalovirus
AGE	Arterial gas embolism	CN	Cranial nerve
AI	Aortic insufficiency	CNS	Central nervous system
AIDS	Acquired immunodeficiency syndrome	CO	Carbon monoxide, cardiac output
AIVR	Accelerated idioventricular rhythm	CO_2	Carbon dioxide
		COPD	Chronic obstructive pulmonary disease
AKD	Acute kidney disease		
AKI	acute kidney injury	CP	Chest pain
ALI	Acute lung injury	CPAP	Continuous positive airway pressure
ALT	Alanine transaminase		
ALTE	Apparent life-threatening event	CPK	Creatine phosphokinase
		CPP	Cerebral perfusion pressure
AMS	Acute mountain sickness	CPR	Cardiopulmonary resuscitation
ANC	Absolute neutrophil count		
APAP	Acetaminophen	Cr	Creatinine
ARB	Angiotensin receptor blocker	CRAO	Central retinal artery occlusion
		CRP	C-reactive protein
ARDS	Acute respiratory distress syndrome	CRVO	Central retinal vein occlusion
		CSF	Cerebrospinal fluid
ARF	Acute renal failure	CT	Computed tomography
AS	Aortic stenosis	CTA	Computed tomography angiography
ASA	acetylsalicylic acid (aspirin)		
ASD	Atrial septal defect	CTH	Chronic tension headache
AST	Aspartate aminotransferase	cTn	Cardiac troponin
AT	Atrial tachycardia	CTV	Computed tomography venography
ATN	Acute tubular necrosis		
AVA	Aortic valve area	CTX	ceftriaxone
AVM	Arteriovenous malformation	CVA	Cerebral vascular accident
AVN	atrioventricular node	cx	Complications
AVNRT	AV node re-entrant tachycardia	CXR	Chest x-ray
		d	Day(s)
AVR	Aortic valve replacement	D/C	Discharge
AVRT	AV reciprocating tachycardia	DAI	Diffuse axonal injury
b/c	Because	DBP	Diastolic blood pressure
b/w	Between	DCS	Decompression sickness
BAL	Blood alcohol level	DDx	Differential diagnosis
BBB	Bundle branch block	DI	Diabetes insipidus
BiPAP	Bilevel positive airway pressure	DIC	Disseminated intravascular coagulation
BMP	Basic metabolic panel		
BMS	Bare metal stent	DIP	distal interphalangeal joint
BNP	brain natriuretic peptide	DKA	Diabetic ketoacidosis
BP	Blood pressure	DL	Direct laryngoscopy

DMS	Altered mental status
DOAC	direct oral anticoagulant
DOE	Dyspnea on exertion
DP	Dorsalis pedis
DPA	Diagnostic peritoneal aspiration
DPL	Diagnostic peritoneal lavage
DTR	Deep tendon reflex
DUB	Dysfunctional uterine bleeding
DVT	Deep vein thrombosis
Dx	Diagnosis
Dysfxn	Dysfunction
dz	Disease
e/o	Evidence of
EBV	Epstein–Barr virus
ED	Emergency Department
EDH	Epidural hemorrhage
EEG	electroencephalogram
EF	Ejection fraction
EGD	Extraglottic device
EKG	electrocardiogram
EMS	Emergency medical services
EOM	Extraocular muscles
EP	Electrophysiologist
ERCP	Endoscopic retrograde cholangiopancreatography
ESBL	extended spectrum beta-lactamase
esp	Especially
ESR	Erythrocyte sedimentation rate
EtOH	Ethanol
ETT	Endotracheal tube
eval	Evaluation
f/b	followed by
f/u	Follow-up
FAST	Focused assessment with sonography for trauma
FB	Foreign body
FFP	Fresh frozen plasma
FH	Family history
FHH	Familial hypocalciuric hypercalcemia
FSG	Fingerstick glucose
FTT	Failure to thrive
FUO	Fever of unknown origin
G6PD	Glucose-6-phosphate dehydrogenase
GC	Gonococcal
GCS	Glasgow coma scale
GERD	Gastroesophageal reflux
GI	Gastrointestinal
GIB	Gastrointestinal bleeding
GNR	gram-negative rods
GP	glycoprotein
GSW	Gunshot wound
GVHD	Graft versus host disease
h	Hour(s)
H&P	history and physical
HA	Headache
HACE	High altitude cerebral edema
HAPE	High altitude pulmonary edema
HCAP	Health-care associated pneumonia
Hct	Hematocrit
HD	Hemodialysis, hemodynamically
HEENT	head, eyes, ears, nose, and throat
HELLP	Hemolysis, Elevated Liver enzymes, and Low Platelets
HHS	Hyperosmolar hyperglycemic state
HI	Homicidal ideation
HIDA	Hydroxy iminodiacetic acid
HIT	Heparin-induced thrombocytopenia
HIV	human immunodeficiency virus
HK	Hypokinesis
HL	Hyperlipidemia
HLD	Hyperlipidemia
HOB	Head of bed
HR	Heart rate
HRUS	High-resolution ultrasound
HSCT	hematopoietic stem cell transplantation
HSP	Henoch–Schönlein purpura
HSV	Herpes simplex virus
HTN	Hypertension
HUS	Hemolytic uremic syndrome
hx	History
I&D	Incision and drainage
IABP	Intra-aortic balloon pump
IBD	Inflammatory bowel disease
ICH	Intracranial hemorrhage
ICP	Intracranial pressure
ICU	intensive care unit
IFA	Immunofluorescence antibody
ILD	Interstitial lung disease
inpt	inpatient
INR	International normalized ratio
IO	Intraosseous
IOP	Intraocular pressure
IPH	Intraparenchymal hemorrhage
IR	Interventional radiology
ITP	Immune thrombocytopenic purpura
IVDA	Intravenous drug abuse
IVDU	Intravenous drug use
IVIG	Intravenous immunoglobulin
IVP	Intravenous pyelogram
JVD	Jugular venous distension
JVP	Jugular venous pressure
KUB	Kidney ureter bladder
L	Left
LAD	Lymphadenopathy, Left-axis deviation
LAE	Left atrial enlargement
LAFB	Left anterior fascicular block
LBBB	Left bundle branch block
LBP	Lower back pain
LDH	Lactate dehydrogenase
LE	Lower extremity
LFT	Liver function test
LGIB	Lower gastrointestinal bleeding
LLL	Left lower lobe
LLQ	Left lower quadrant

LMN	Lower motor neuron
LMP	Last menstrual period
LOC	Loss of consciousness
LP	Lumbar puncture
LPFB	Left posterior fascicular block
LV	Left ventricle
LVAD	Left ventricular assist device
LVH	Left ventricular hypertrophy
MAHA	Microangiopathic hemolytic anemia
MAP	Mean arterial pressure
MAT	Multifocal atrial tachycardia
MCP	Metacarpophalangeal
MDR	Multiple drug resistance
MDRO	multi-drug resistant organism
MDS	myelodysplastic syndrome
MH	Malignant hyperthermia
MI	Myocardial infarction
min	Minute(s)
MM	Mucous membrane
mo	Month(s)
mod	Moderate
MR	Mitral regurgitation
MRA	Magnetic resonance angiography
MRCP	mental retardation/cerebral palsy
MRI	Magnetic resonance imaging
MRSA	Methicillin-resistant *Staphylococcus aureus*
MRV	Magnetic resonance venography
MS	Mitral stenosis
MSK	musculoskeletal
MV	Mitral valve
MVC	Motor vehicle collision
MVP	Mitral valve prolapsed
N/V	Nausea/vomiting
NAPQI	N-acetyl-p-benzoquinone imine
NCHCT	non-contrast head computed tomography
NEC	Necrotizing enterocolitis
neg	Negative
NGT	nasogastric tube
NHL	non-Hodgkin's lymphoma
NIF	Negative inspiratory force
NIPPV	non-invasive positive-pressure ventilation
NIV	Noninvasive ventilation
nl	Normal
NMS	Neuroleptic malignant syndrome
NPJT	Nonparoxysmal junctional tachycardia
NPO	Nil per OS
NPV	Negative predictive value
NRB	Nonrebreather
NSAID	Nonsteroidal anti-inflammatory drug
NSTEMI	Non-ST-elevation MI
NSTV	Nonsustained ventricular tachycardia
NTG	Nitroglycerin
o/w	Otherwise

O_2	Oxygen
OA	Osteoarthritis
OCP	Oral contraceptive pill
OE	Otitis externa
OM	Otitis media
OMFS	Oral and maxillofacial surgery
OR	Operating room
ORIF	Open reduction and internal fixation
OSA	Obstructive sleep apnea
OTC	Over-the-counter
otw	otherwise
outpt(s)	Outpatient(s)
p/w	Presents with
PAN	Polyarteritis nodosa
PCI	Percutaneous coronary intervention
PCKD	Polycystic kidney disease
PCN	Penicillin
PCOS	Polycystic ovary syndrome
PCP	Pneumocystis jirovecii pneumonia, primary care physician
PCR	Polymerase chain reaction
PDA	Patent ductus arteriosus
PE	Pulmonary embolism
PEEP	Positive end-expiratory pressure
PEFR	Peak expiratory flow rate
PGE_1	Prostaglandin E_1
PHT	Pulmonary hypertension
PID	Pelvic inflammatory disease
PIP	Proximal interphalangeal joint
pl	Pleural
PLT	Platelet
PM	Pacemaker
PMH	Past medical history
PMR	Polymyaliga rheumatica
PMV	Percutaneous mitral valvuloplasty
PNA	Pneumonia
PND	Paroxysmal nocturnal dyspnea
PostTP	Posttest probability
PPM	Permanent pacemaker
PPV	Positive predictive value, positive pressure ventilation
PQRST	Palliation, quality, radiation, severity, timing
PRBC	Packed red blood cell
PreTP	Pretest probability
PRWP	Poor R-wave progression
PS	Pulmonary stenosis
PT	Prothrombin time, Posterior tibialis
pt(s)	Patient(s)
PTX	Pneumothorax
PUD	Peptic ulcer disease
PVD	Peripheral vascular disease
Qw	Q wave
R	Right
r/o	Rule out
RAD	Right axis deviation
RAE	Right atrial enlargement
RBBB	Right bundle branch block
RF	Risk factor

RLQ	Right lower quadrant
RMSF	Rocky Mountain spotted fever
ROM	Range of motion
ROS	Review of systems
ROSC	Return of spontaneous circulation
RPR	rapid plasma reagin
RR	Respiratory rate
RSI	Rapid sequence intubation
RSV	Respiratory syncytial virus
RTA	Renal tubular acidosis
RUG	Retrograde urethrogram
RUQ	Right upper quadrant
RV	Right ventricle
RVH	Right ventricular hypertrophy
RVOT	Right ventricular outflow tract
rxn	Reaction
SAH	Subarachnoid hemorrhage
SBE	Subacute bacterial endocarditis
SBO	Small bowel obstruction
SBP	Systolic blood pressure
SCD	Sickle cell disease
SCFE	Slipped capital femoral epiphysis
SCM	Sternocleidomastoid
SDH	Subdural hemorrhage
sec	Second(s)
sens	Sensitive, Sensitivity
SFV	Superficial femoral vein
SI	Suicidal ideation
SIRS	Systemic inflammatory response syndrome
SJS	Stevens–Johnson syndrome
SLE	systemic lupus erythematosus
SMA	Superior mesenteric artery
SOB	Shortness of breath
spec	Specific, Specificity
SS	Serotonin syndrome
SSRI	Selective serotonin reuptake inhibitor
SSSS	Staphylococcal scalded skin
ST	Sinus tachycardia
ST-T	ST-segment-T wave
STD	Sexually transmitted disease
STEMI	ST-segment elevation MI
SVC	superior vena cava
SVT	Supraventricular tachycardia
sxs	Symptoms
sz	Seizure
T+S	type and screen
TAH	total abdominal hysterectomy
TB	Tuberculosis
TBI	Traumatic brain injury
TBW	Total body weight
TCA	Tricyclic antidepressants

TCP	Thrombocytopenia
TEE	Transesophageal echocardiogram
Tele	Telemetry
TEN	Toxic epidermal necrolysis
TIA	Transient ischemic attack
TM	Tympanic membrane
TMJ	Temporomandibular joint
TOA	Tubo-ovarian abscess
tox	toxicity
TRACO	transfusion-associated circulatory overload
TRALI	transfusion-associated lung injury
TSH	thyroid stimulating hormone
TSS	Toxic shock syndrome
TTE	Transthoracic echocardiogram
TTP	Thrombotic thrombocytopenic purpura
TWI	T-wave inversion
tx	Treatment
TXA	tranexamic acid
u/s	Ultrasound
UA	Urine analysis, Unstable angina
UAG	Urinary anion gap
Ucx	Urine culture
UGIB	Upper gastrointestinal bleeding
UH	unfractionated heparin
UMN	Upper motor neuron
UOP	Urinary output
UPJ	Urinary pelvic junction
URI	Upper respiratory infection
UTI	Urinary tract infection
V/D	Vomiting/diarrhea
VBG	Venous blood gas
VCUG	voiding cystourethrogram
VL	Video laryngoscopy
VN	Visiting Nurse (Association)
VRE	vancomycin-resistant enterococcus
VS	Vital signs
VSD	Ventricular septal defect
VT	Tidal volume
vWD	von Willebrand disease
vWF	von Willebrand factor
VZV	Varicella zoster virus
w/	With
w/i	Within
w/o	Without
w/u	Workup
WBC	white blood cell
WCT	Wide-complex tachycardia
wk	Week(s)
WPW	Wolff–Parkinson–White Syndrome
XRT	Radiation therapy
y/o	Year old
yr	Year(s)
Δ	Change

PEDIATRIC ADVANCED LIFE SUPPORT (PALS)

		Drugs Dosages Used in PALS		
Medication	**Route**	**nl Dose**	**Incremental Dose**	**Maximum**
Adenosine	Rapid IV push	0.1 mg/kg (up to 6 mg)	0.2 mg/kg	12 mg
Amiodarone	Rapid IV/IO	5 mg/kg		15 mg/kg/d
Atropine	IV/IO/ET	0.02 mg/kg	0.04 mg/kg	0.5 mg single dose
Calcium chloride	IV/IO	20 mg/kg		
Dobutamine	IV/IO	2–20 μg/kg/min		Titrate to effect
Epinephrine PEA, bradycardia	IV/IO: 0.01 mg/kg (1:10000) ET: 0.1 mg/kg (1:1000)		q3–5min during CPR	0.1 mL/kg
Glucose	IV/IO	0.5–1 g/kg		2–4 mL/kg 25%
Lidocaine	IV/IO/ET	1 mg/kg		
Mg sulfate	IV/IO	25–50 μg/kg		2 g
Naloxone		If <5 yr or <20 mg: 0.1 mg/kg If >5 yr or >20 kg: 2 mg		Titrate to effect

	Cardioversion in PALS	
Reason	**nl Dose**	**Incremental Dose**
Tachycardia	0.5–1 J/kg	2 J/kg if ineffective
VF/pulseless VT	2–4 J/kg	4 J/kg if ineffective w/i 30–60 sec after med

MECHANICAL VENTILATION

(NEJM 2001;344:1986)

Approach
- Choose invasive ventilation vs. NIV → choose type of NIV or invasive mode → adjust settings
- In the ED, NIV is used to avoid intubation, esp in acute COPD/RAD or CHF/pulm edema

	Indications for Ventilation	
Type of Ventilation		**Indications**
Noninvasive	CPAP	Hypoxemia (ie, CHF exacerbation)
	BiPAP	Hypoventilation (ie, COPD)
Invasive		Apnea, impending respiratory failure, airway protection, failed NIV

Noninvasive Ventilation	
CPAP	**BiPAP**
Opens atelectatic alveoli, can improve respiratory mechanics & hemodynamics	CPAP + pressure support → directly reduces work of breathing
In ACPE → ↓ intubation, mortality	In COPD, PNA → ↓ intubation, mortality
Relative CIs: Aspiration risk, vomiting, UGIB/epistaxis, agitation or lethargy precluding compliance, hemodynamic instability	

	Invasive Ventilation	
Invasive Ventilation Modes	**Description**	**Comments**
Assist control	All breaths fully assisted by vent	Most useful in apneic pts (eg, chemically paralyzed)

Invasive Ventilation Modes	Description	Comments
Synchronized intermittent mandatory ventilation	Set # of supported breaths, synchronized to pt's effort; all other pt-initiated breaths determined by pt	Useful for weaning pts from ventilator
Volume targeted	Set TV for assisted breaths	Standard setting
Pressure targeted	Set inspiratory pressure for assisted breaths	Useful for pts at risk for barotrauma

Other Ventilator Settings	
Standard initial settings	Assist control ventilation, TV 4–8 mL/kg, RR 12–14, FiO₂ 100%, PEEP 5 cm H₂O, Wean FiO₂ as quickly as tolerated
Other modes	See above
PEEP	Positive pressure present during exhalation → maintains patent alveoli → ↓ shunting & ↑ oxygenation (cardiac effects dictate CO & oxygenation); 5 cm H₂O = "physiologic" PEEP Preload: Decreased via ↑ intrathoracic pressure → ↓ venous return Afterload: Decreased via ↓ transmural cardiac pressure
Auto-PEEP	Presence of flow at end expiration due to "breath stacking": ↓ time for exhalation → incomplete expiration → lungs "trap" air → leading to potential compromise of respiratory mechanics & hemodynamics (↓ preload)
Inspiratory flow rate	↑ Flow rate → ↓ inspiratory time → ↑ expiratory time (ie, ↓ I:E ratio) → improves ventilation & minimizes auto-PEEP in obstructive dz (asthma, COPD)
Pplat	Plateau pressure, measured at end expiration; determined by respiratory system compliance ↑ Pplat w/ obesity, pulmonary edema, ARDS → auto-PEEP, asynchronous breathing
PIP	Peak pressure measured during inspiration affected by airway resistance plus lung/chest wall compliance If ↑ PIP & nl Pplat → cause = airway resistance (bronchospasm, secretions, etc.)

Making Changes to the Ventilator	
Improve oxygenation	↑ PEEP, ↑ FiO₂
Improve ventilation	↑ TV, ↑ RR
Reduce auto-PEEP	↓ RR, ↑ expiratory time, ↑ insp flow rate
Permissive hypercapnia	Low TV (4–6 mL/kg) to reduce baro/volutrauma in ALI/ARDS

ANALGESIA & CONSCIOUS SEDATION

Opioids				
Medication	nl Dose	Incremental Dose	Onset of Action	Duration
Morphine	0.1 mg/kg	½ nl dose	5–10 min	3–4 h
Hydromorphone	0.5–2 mg	½ nl dose	3–5 min	2–4 h
Fentanyl	0.5–1 µg/kg (25–100 µg)	25 µg	1–2 min	10 min–1 h

Benzodiazepines				
Medication	nl Dose	Incremental Dose	Onset of Action	Duration
Diazepam	5–10 mg	2.5 mg	1–5 min	30 min–2 h
Midazolam	1–5 mg	0.5–1 mg	1–2 min	15–60 min

Conscious Sedation Medications				
Medication	**nl Dose**	**Incremental Dose**	**Onset of Action**	**Duration**
Ketamine*	1–2 mg/kg IV or 2–4 mg/kg IM	1 mg/kg	1–2 min	10–30 min
Chloral hydrate**	50–75 mg/kg prn	25–75 mg/kg	20–30 min	2–6 h
Propofol	1–3 mg/kg	0.5–5 mg/kg	<1 min	8–10 min
Etomidate	0.2–0.5 mg/kg	0.05 mg/kg	<1 min	5–8 min
Nitrous oxide	30–50%	Constant	1–2 min	5 min

*Consider administration w/ glycopyrrolate (0.01 mg/kg) or atropine (0.01 mg/kg) as an antisialogogue
**Pediatric only, rarely used

Reversal Agents				
Medication	**nl Dose**	**Incremental Dose**	**Onset of Action**	**Duration**
Naloxone (opioids)	0.4–2 mg	0.04 mg	1–2 min	30 min–1 h
Flumazenil (benzo)	1 mg	0.2 mg	1–2 min	30 min–1.5 h

ICU MEDICATIONS

ICU Medications		
Drug	**Class**	**Dose**
Pressors, Inotropes		
Phenylephrine	α_1	50–200 µg/min
Norepinephrine	$\alpha_1 > \beta_1$	0.05–0.5 µg/kg/min, max ~5 µg/kg/min
Vasopressin	V_1	0.04 U/min
Dopamine	D	0.5–2 µg/kg/min
	β, D	2–10 µg/kg/min
	α, β, D	>10 µg/kg/min, max 50 µg/kg/min
Dobutamine	$\beta_1 > \beta_2$	2–20 µg/kg/min
Epinephrine	$\alpha_1, \alpha_2, \beta_1, \beta_2$	0.05–0.5 µg/kg/min, max ~5 µg/kg/min
Vasodilators		
Nitroglycerin	NO	5–1000 µg/min
Nitroprusside	NO	0.1–10 µg/kg/min
Enalaprilat	ACEI	0.625–2.5 mg over 5 min then 0.625–5 mg q6h
Hydralazine	Vasodilator	5–20 mg q20–30min
Labetalol	$\alpha_1, \beta_1, \beta_2$ blockers	20 mg over 2 min then 20–80 mg q10min or 10–120 mg/h
Nicardipine	NO	2.5–15 mg/h
Antiarrhythmics		
Amiodarone	Class III	150 mg over 10 min, then 1 mg/min × 6 h, then 0.5 mg/min × 18 h
Lidocaine	Class IB (Na channel)	1–1.5 mg/kg (100 mg) then 1–4 mg/min
Procainamide	Class IA (Na channel)	17 mg/kg (1 g) over 60 min, then 1–4 mg/min
Ibutilide	Class III (K channel)	1 mg over 10 min, may repeat × 1
Propranolol	βB	0.5–1 mg q5min then 1–10 mg/h
Esmolol	β_1 blocker > β_2 blocker	500 µg/kg (20–40 mg) over 1 min, then 25–300 µg/kg/min (2–20 mg/min)
Verapamil	CCB	2.5–5 mg over 1–2 min repeat 5–10 mg in 15–30 min prn, 5–20 mg/h
Diltiazem	CCB	0.25 mg/kg (20 mg) over 2 min, reload 0.35 mg/kg (25 mg) × 1 prn, then 5–15 mg/h

Antiarrhythmics (Continued)		
Drug	**Class**	**Dose**
Adenosine	Purinergic	6 mg rapid push, if no response 12 mg rapid push, repeat × 1 prn
Sedation		
Morphine	Opioid	1–unlimited mg/h
Etomidate	Anesthetic	0.2–0.5 mg (100–300 mg)
Propofol	Anesthetic	1–3 mg/kg (50–200 mg) then 0.3–5 mg/kg/h (20–400 mg/h)
Diazepam	Benzo	1–5 mg q1–2h then q6 prn
Midazolam	Benzo	0.5–2 mg q5min prn or 5–4 mg then 1–10 mg/h
Ketamine	Anesthetic	1–2 mg/kg (60–150 mg)
Haloperidol	Antipsychotic	2–5 mg q20–30min
Paralysis		
Succinylcholine	Depolarizing	0.6–1.1 mg/kg (70–100 mg)
Pancuronium	nACh	0.08 mg/kg (2–4 mg) q30–90min
Rocuronium	nACH	0.6 mg/kg (60–100 mg)
Vecuronium	nACH	0.08 mg/kg (5–10 mg) over 1–3 min, then 0.5–0.1 mg/kg/h (2–8 mg/h)
Cisatracurium	nACH	5–10 µg/kg/min
Miscellaneous		
Insulin		0.1 U/kg/h
Glucagon		5–10 mg then 1–5 mg/h
Octreotide	Somatostatin analog	50 µg then 50 µg/h
Phenytoin	Antiepileptic	20 mg/kg (1–1.5 g) over 20–30 min
Fosphenytoin	Antiepileptic	20 mg/kg (1–1.5 g) over 10 min
Phenobarbital	Barbiturate	20 mg/kg (1–1.5 g) over 20 min
Thiopental	Barbiturate	3–5 mg/kg (200–400 mg) over 2 min
Mannitol	Osmotic	1.5–2 g/kg over 30–60 min, repeat q6–12h to keep oSm 310–320
Naloxone	Opioid antagonist	0.4–2 mg q2–3min to total 10 mg
Flumazenil	Benzo antagonist	0.2 mg over 30 sec then 0.3 mg over 30 sec, may repeat 0.5 mg over 30 sec to max 3 mg
Fentanyl	Opioid	50–100 µg then 50–unlimited µg/h

EQUATIONS

Metabolic

Anion Gap: $Na - (Cl + Bicarb)$

Delta/Delta = (actual anion gap − normal gap)/(normal HCO_3 − actual HCO_3)

Total body water (TBW) = weight (kg) × 0.6 (use 0.5 if female/elderly, 0.6 for infants)

Corrected Na = measured Na + [2.4 × (measured glucose −100)]

Calculated osmoles = (2 × Na) + (glucose/18) + (BUN/2.8) + (EtOH/4.6)

Osmolal gap = measured osmoles − calculated osmoles (nl)

Estimated Cr clearance $= \dfrac{[140 - \text{age (y)}] \times \text{wt (kg)}}{\text{Serum Cr (mg/dL)} \times 72} \times (0.85 \text{ in women})$

Pediatric fluid maintenance (4-2-1 Rule):

(4 cc/kg for 1st 10 kg) + (2 cc/kg for 2nd 10 kg) + (1 cc/kg for remainder kg)

Hyponatremia:

$$\Delta[Na]/\text{liter infusate} = \frac{[Na]_{infusate} \times [Na]_{serum}}{TBW + 1}$$

Rate of infusion (mL/h) $= \dfrac{1000 \times [TBW \times (\text{desired Na} - \text{serum Na})]}{[Na \text{ (mmol/L)}]_{infusate} \times \text{time (h)}}$

Hypernatremia:

Free water deficit = total body water $\times$ [(140/serum Na) $- 1$]

$$\Delta[\text{Na}]/\text{liter infusate} = \frac{([\text{Na}]_{\text{infusate}} + [\text{K}]_{\text{infusate}}) - [\text{Na}]_{\text{serum}}}{\text{TBW} + 1}$$

$$\textbf{Total infusion (L)} = \frac{\text{Desired [Na (mEq/L)]} - \text{Serum [Na (mEq/L)]}}{\Delta[\text{Na}]/\text{liter infusate}}$$

Rate of infusion (mL/h) = total infusion (mL)/24 h

CARDIOPULMONARY

A-a gradient = $PAO_2 - PaO_2$ (nl $\approx 4 + (\text{age}/4)$)
Stroke volume = cardiac output/heart rate

$$\textbf{Mean arterial pressure} = \frac{[\text{SBP} + (\text{DBP} \times 2)]}{3} \text{ (nl 70–100 mmHg)}$$

PROCEDURES

Common ED Procedures *(italicized procedures are discussed below)*	
Type	**Procedures**
Respiratory	Airway management (Ch. 17), mechanical ventilation (see above), *thoracentesis, tube thoracostomy*
Cardiac	Cardiac pacing, *pericardiocentesis*, ED thoracotomy
Vascular	*Arterial puncture/catheterization*, peripheral IV, *central venous catheterization & CVP monitoring*, venous cutdown, *IO placement*
Anesthesia	Conscious sedation, nerve blocks
Skin & soft tissue	Wound closure, FB removal, *I&D*
GI	*Nasogastric intubation*, balloon tamponade of esophageal varices, *paracentesis*, anorectal procedures
Orthopedic	Fracture/dislocation reductions, splinting, arthrocentesis, compartment pressure measurement
GU	Bladder catheterization (urethral, suprapubic)
OB	Emergency delivery
Neuro	*LP*, Dix–Hallpike/Epley maneuver
Ophtho	Eye irrigation, FB removal, lateral canthotomy
ENT	Peritonsillar abscess drainage, ear canal & nasal FB removal, drainage of auricular hematoma
Dental	Dental nerve blocks, abscess drainage, mandibular reduction

ARTERIAL PUNCTURE AND CATHETERIZATION

Purpose
- Puncture to obtain ABG; catheterization for continuous real-time BP monitoring or need for repeat arterial blood sampling

Equipment
- Puncture: Local anesthetic, 3-mL syringe, 22-gauge needle (or insulin syringe)
- Catheterization: Arm board, tape, angiocath (size depends on artery cannulated), guide-wire, pressure tubing, pressure transducer, suture, needle driver, sterile dressing

Positioning
- Ideally placed in the radial, femoral, or DP artery; brachial & axillary are also useable but they are terminal (no collateral supply) so worse prognosis if thrombosis occurs. Document Allen's test before & after catheterization of radial artery.

Procedure
- Sterilize area, use sterile gloves, but generally drape & gown are not required
- Puncture: Palpate artery w/ nondominant hand, insert needle distal to palpated artery at a 30° angle to skin, advance until flash in syringe or angiocath, remove 1–2 mL blood, remove air bubbles, & send immediately to lab *on ice*. US w/ sterile cover may help.

- Catheterization: Immobilize wrist in slight dorsiflexion using tape/arm board, insert needle as above until flash is observed, then advance another 2–3 mm, remove needle & leave catheter, pull back slowly until arterial blood flow is observed, pass guidewire into artery, advance catheter to hub along the guidewire, remove wire, check flow, attach to pressure tubing, suture in place, apply sterile dressing

Complications
- Hematoma, AV fistula, pseudoaneurysm, bleeding, PAIN. *Rarely:* Catheter infection, thrombosis or stenosis of artery, hand/limb ischemia

---

CENTRAL VENOUS CATHETERIZATION

Purpose
- Rapid volume resuscitation, emergency venous access, administration of spec medicines (ie, pressors, high concentration electrolytes), central venous pressure monitoring
- Sometimes used when peripheral access is not obtainable, but 1st consider external jugular, basilic, or cephalic vein catheterization, or IO access

Choice of Site
- Each site has advantages & disadvantages. Overall, no compelling evidence that one site is uniformly superior to others, or definite difference in infection risk. CDC recommends weighing risk/benefits for each pt, but avoiding femoral when possible ("*Guidelines for the Prevention of Intravascular Catheter-related Infections*", 2011, CDC: www.cdc.gov).

Comparison of Types of Central Venous Catheterization			
Site	**Pros**	**Cons**	**Comments**
Internal jugular	Bleeding easily controlled Low mechanical cx rate when used w/ U/S	Can be more time consuming w/ U/S Intermediate risk of infection	U/S guidance is now the standard of care for IJ
Infraclavicular subclavian	Fast, considered ↓ infection rate	↑ Risk of PTX ↓ Bleeding control	± U/S guided
Supraclavicular subclavian	Practical for cardiac arrest	↑ Risk of PTX ↓ Bleeding control	± U/S guided
Femoral	Fast, practical during arrest	Thought to have ↑ risk of infection	± U/S guided

Equipment
- Chlorhexidine, cap, mask, sterile drape/gloves/gown, catheter device kit (includes 1% lidocaine w/ 10-mL syringe & 25-gauge needle, catheterization needle/syringe, guidewire, scalpel, dilator, catheter, needle driver, scissors, suture, sterile dressing)

Positioning
- Supine pt, Trendelenburg position for IJ; can do subclavians upright (eg, in CHF)
- Internal jugular: Bedside U/S guidance recommended if available
  - Locate the IJ vein (compressible) & carotid artery (pulsatile, noncompressible) using a sterile U/S probe w/i the triangle created by the clavicle & the sternal & clavicular heads of the sternocleidomastoid muscle
  - Advance the needle toward the IJ vein & away from the carotid artery w/ needle at 30° angle to skin while observing the needle penetrate the vein on U/S towards ipsilateral nipple
  - Confirm venous cannulation via U/S once the wire is in place
- Infraclavicular: Insert needle 2 cm inferior & 2 cm lateral to the angle of the clavicle (located along the middle third), point toward spot just superior to the suprasternal notch & advance just posterior to the clavicle
- Supraclavicular: Insert needle at the junction of the middle & medial thirds of the clavicle, just posterior to the clavicle, point toward the contralateral nipple
- Femoral: Palpate femoral artery, then advance needle at 45° angle to skin toward the head just medial to the palpable artery

Procedure
- Rate of CVL-associated infection ↓ w/ use of observer & checklist (*NEJM* 2006;355:2725)
- Sterile technique. Attach catheterization needle to syringe, advance while aspirating.
- Remove syringe once vein is entered & check for free return of nonpulsatile blood
- Place the curved end of the guidewire into the needle & advance, check that the wire passes easily, & advance to estimated location of SVC

- Remove the needle while keeping the wire in position
- Make a 1-cm incision through the dermis where the wire meets the skin
- Advance the dilator over the wire several centimeters, then remove the dilator
- Advance catheter over wire, advance to the estimated location of the SVC, remove wire
- Suture in place, cover w/ sterile dressing, obtain CXR to r/o PTX (for all but femoral lines)

Complications
- Arterial puncture (if needle/wire puncture & compressible, apply prolonged pressure). If a major artery was *dilated*, leave in place & consult IR & vascular surgery.
- PTX: Always r/o w/ XR. Always stat XR if SOB during line placement.
- Bloodstream infection, air embolus, nerve injury (phrenic, brachial plexus, femoral)

Pearls
- A triple-lumen CVC has a slower infusion rate than most PIVs, consider percutaneous introducer if large-volume resuscitation needed

---

INCISION AND DRAINAGE

Purpose
- Definitive tx of a soft-tissue abscess

Equipment
- Consider bedside U/S prior to procedure to confirm fluid collection. Hemostat, scissors, forceps, scalpel, packing gauze, 1–2% lidocaine w/ 10-mL syringe & 25-gauge needle.

Procedure
- Anesthetize skin over the most fluctuant area. Make a single, linear incision w/ scalpel over the entire length of the abscess cavity
- Dissect wound using a hemostat & probe into all corners of the cavity to break up loculations & evaluate for an FB, then irrigate wound
- Place enough packing gauze to prevent wound closure but do not pack tightly

---

INTRAOSSEOUS CATHETERIZATION

Purpose
- Rapid temporary vascular access. Increasing use in adults & nonemergent cases.

Equipment
- IO needle w/ stylet & syringe, EZ-IO drill if available, gauze

Positioning
- Anteromedial aspect of the proximal tibia, 1–3 cm distal to the tibial tuberosity
- Secondary options include distal femur or proximal humerus

Procedure
- Sterile technique. Advance IO needle/stylet perpendicular to the bone w/ firm pressure & a twisting motion until the cortex is penetrated, remove stylet, attach syringe & aspirate to correct positioning of the needle. Secure in place w/ gauze pads.

Complications
- Infection, bleeding, fracture, retained FB, pain

LUMBAR PUNCTURE

Purpose
- Dx of meningitis (in the absence of elevated ICP), SAH, idiopathic intracranial HTN, other infectious, inflammatory, neoplastic processes

Equipment
- Careful neurologic exam beforehand (avoid in any pt w/ focal neurologic findings), sterile technique, 20–22-gauge spinal or Whitacre needle, LP tray (w/ collecting tubes, lidocaine 1%, manometer/stopcock, 25-gauge needle, 10-cc syringe, sterile drapes)
- Consider U/S in obese pts to identify nonpalpable landmarks
- Consider CTH prior to procedure if concern for mass effect/elevated ICP

Positioning
- Lateral decubitus w/ shoulders/hips perpendicular to the bed (preferable & necessary to measure opening pressure) or sitting up on the edge of the bed
- Have the pt maximally flex neck, hips, & knees, & arch back, into a fetal position
- L4 spinous process is found at the intersection of a line b/w the spine & the iliac crests; enter through the interspace above or below this location

Procedure
- Anesthetize locally w/ lidocaine 1% using 25-gauge needle, then advance needle while aspirating → inject lidocaine into the interspinous ligament
- Advance spinal needle toward the umbilicus w/ bevel pointed toward the pt's side (left or right) until a "pop" or sudden decrease in resistance is felt → remove the stylet
- Once clear fluid is obtained, attach the manometer & record opening pressure
- If fluid is not found, replace the stylet, pull back the needle to the level of SQ tissue, confirm that you are in midline, & reangle your needle slightly
- Obtain at least 1 cc in each collecting tube (more if extensive studies are necessary)
- Replace stylet, remove needle, place sterile dressing over wound
- Tests: Send for cell count (tubes #1, 4), protein/glucose (#2 or #3), gram stain & culture (#2 or #3)

Complications
- HA (5–40%), localized infection, epidural hematoma (rare), herniation (in cases of elevated ICP)

NASOGASTRIC INTUBATION

Purpose
- Aspiration of stomach contents in pts at risk for recurrent vomiting (eg, GI obstruction), stomach decompression during trauma or after intubation

Equipment
- 16- or 18-gauge NG tube, lubricant, 60-cc syringe, cup of water w/ straw, towel, tape, stethoscope, topical anesthetic jelly, nasal vasoconstrictor

Positioning
- Sitting up, chin down

Procedure
- Place towel over chest, estimate distance to stomach (from xiphoid to earlobe to stomach)
- Lubricate tube, spray patent nare w/ vasoconstrictor, apply anesthetic jelly, wait a few minutes
- Advance tube posteriorly along the floor of the nose until it enters the oropharynx, then have pt continuously sip water through straw while the tube is advanced into esophagus; once in the esophagus, quickly advance the tube to the desired distance
- Confirm placement by insufflating the NG tube w/ air using 60-cc syringe & listening over stomach for gush of air, & aspiration of GI contents. Obtain upright CXR if any concern.
- Secure tube using tape attached to the nose & wrapped around the tube from each side; tape should also be used to attach a 2nd segment of the NG tube to the gown

Complications
- Vomiting during placement, tracheal intubation, small risk of intracranial penetration (contraindicated in facial fractures), bleeding, esophageal rupture (hx of esophageal stricture/alkali injury), pain

---

PARACENTESIS

Purpose
- Diagnostic: Removal of peritoneal fluid in a pt w/ ascites to (a) diagnose the cause of new ascites; (b) assess for spontaneous bacterial peritonitis
- Therapeutic: Relieve sxs in pts w/ tense ascites (eg, hypoxia from mass effect)

Equipment
- Use bedside U/S prior to procedure to confirm ascites & identify large pocket
- Sterile technique
- 25-gauge needle, 1% lidocaine. For diagnostic tap, only need 20–22-gauge needle & large syringe to aspirate fluid. For therapeutic tap, use paracentesis kit w/ 18-gauge needle, catheter sheath, & vacuum-sealed collection bottles.

Positioning
- Supine; identify entry site: Usually 4–5 cm cephalad & medial to anterior superior iliac spine, lateral to the rectus muscle sheath, being careful to avoid any visible veins

Procedure
- Check for severe coagulopathy prior to procedure
- Perform w/ real-time bedside U/S if possible
- Anesthetize locally w/ lidocaine 1% using 25-gauge needle
- Z-tract: Pull the skin 2 cm caudad before advancing the larger-bore needle, then place the needle perpendicular to the skin, advance needle slowly while occasionally aspirating, until ascitic fluid is aspirated, then release skin
- It may be necessary to make a 0.5 cm stab incision at the dermis to allow passage of the needle/catheter
- After aspirating fluid, advance catheter 1–2 cm & remove needle → connect catheter to stopcock, & collect fluid into sterile containers
- Fluid: Send for cell count, albumin, culture. Consider total protein, glucose, LDH, amylase, gram stain

Complications
- Hypotension (can have severe fluid shifts in large-volume tap), ascitic fluid leakage, abdominal wall hematoma, infection, hemoperitoneum, viscera perforation

---

PERICARDIOCENTESIS

Purpose
- Emergent tx of pericardial effusion/tamponade in a pt w/ cardiac arrest (often PEA) or periarrest; hemorrhagic tamponade is best treated w/ thoracotomy

Equipment
- 16- or 18-gauge spinal needle attached to a 30- or 60-cc syringe

Positioning
- Supine pt, angle needle 30°–45° to the skin, insert b/w xiphoid process & left costal margin, aim needle toward left shoulder (parasternal technique: 90° angle above 5th/6th rib L sternal border)

Procedure
- Sterile technique. Bedside U/S guidance recommended if available. Advance needle slowly while aspirating until fluid is removed (presence of blood suggests ventricular puncture)

Complications
- "Dry tap," PTX, myocardial laceration, coronary vessel laceration, hemopericardium, ventricular penetration, visceral injury

---

THORACENTESIS

Purpose
- Diagnostic eval (new/unclear etiology) or therapeutic tx of pl effusion

Equipment
- 20- or 22-gauge needle w/ catheter or thoracentesis kit

Positioning
- Pt sitting upright, needle angled 90° to skin, insert in intercostal space above rib (no lower than 8th intercostal space) in midscapular line

Procedure
- Sterile technique. Bedside U/S guidance is recommended for locating height of effusion & distance of lung from the parietal pleura.
- Anesthetize locally w/ lidocaine 1% using 25-gauge needle, then advance needle while aspirating → inject lidocaine → advance while aspirating further, until pl fluid is aspirated
- Remove needle, make a small 0.5 cm incision at the insertion site, then insert 20- or 22-gauge needle w/ catheter → advance while aspirating
- After aspirating fluid, advance catheter & remove needle
- Connect catheter to stopcock, & collect fluid into sterile containers
- Goal: Diagnostic (50–100 mL), therapeutic (relief of dyspnea, up to 1500 mL)
- Fluid: Send for LDH, protein, glucose, cell count, amylase, cytology, gram stain, culture
- Obtain postprocedure CXR

Complications
- PTX, bleeding (caution if PLT <50000 or >1.5 × nl PT/PTT), cough, infection, hemothorax, diaphragmatic penetration

TUBE THORACOSTOMY

Purpose
- Drainage of air (PTX), blood (hemothorax), or fluid (pl effusion, empyema) in the pl space that threatens cardiac or pulmonary function

Equipment
- #10 scalpel, Kelly clamp, #0 or 1 suture, scissors chest tube (28F minimum, larger for hemothorax; may consider pigtail catheter for small PTX)

Positioning
- Supine pt, shoulder abducted (raised overhead), enter at midaxillary line @ 4th–5th intercostal space (nipple line), lateral to pectoralis major

Procedure
- Sterile technique
- Create wheal using lidocaine 1% w/ epinephrine (1:100000) & a 25- or 27-gauge needle, then advance needle while aspirating, & infiltrate broadly through muscle, periosteum & parietal pleura, staying above the rib; ±intercostal nerve block (at level, above, & below)
- Make 3–4 cm incision parallel & just over rib, through skin & fat overlying the rib
- Perform blunt dissection w/a Kelly or scissors down to the rib & just above it
- Apply firm pressure w/ the Kelly closed to pop through the parietal pleura
- Look/listen for rush of fluid or air. Leave Kelly in place & spread to open the pleura further.
- Insert finger into the chest wall (Kelly still in place) to verify that it is the pl space (feel lung, ensure no abdominal organs)
- Keep finger in place, remove Kelly, pass the tube over finger while gently spinning the tube
- Typically, direct tube superiorly & posteriorly (can go anteriorly if certain there is only air)
- Rotate the tube 360° to ↓ kinking & ensure all the tube holes are in the pl space
- Attach to water seal or suction. Never clamp a chest tube
- Confirm placement: Condensation w/ respiration, bubbles in water seal w/ coughing, CXR
- Suture in place, place petroleum gauze over wound, cover w/ dry gauze & tape in place

Complications
- Infection, intercostal vessel/nerve laceration, lung laceration, intra-abdominal entry, solid organ tube placement, subcutaneous placement